Challenging Concepts in Infectious Diseases
and Clinical Microbiology

Titles in the Challenging Concepts in series

Anaesthesia (Edited by Dr Phoebe Syme, Dr Robert Jackson, and Dr Timothy Cook)

Cardiovascular Medicine (Edited by Dr Aung Myat, Dr Shouvik Haldar, and Professor Simon Redwood)

Emergency Medicine (Edited by Dr Sam Thenabadu, Dr Fleur Cantle, and Dr Chris Lacy)

Infectious Diseases and Clinical Microbiology (Edited by Dr Amber Arnold and Professor George E. Griffin)

Interventional Radiology (Edited by Dr Irfan Ahmed, Dr Miltiadis Krokidis, and Dr Tarun Sabharwal)

Neurology (Edited by Dr Krishna Chinthapalli, Dr Nadia Magdalinou, and Professor Nicholas Wood)

Neurosurgery (Edited by Mr Robin Bhatia and Mr Ian Sabin)

Obstetrics and Gynaecology (Edited by Dr Natasha Hezelgrave, Dr Danielle Abbott, and Professor Andrew Shennan)

Oncology (Edited by Dr Madhumita Bhattacharyya, Dr Sarah Payne, and Professor Iain McNeish)

Oral and Maxillofacial Surgery (Edited by Mr Matthew Idle and Group Captain Andrew Monaghan)

Respiratory Medicine (Edited by Dr Lucy Schomberg, Dr Elizabeth Sage, and Dr Nick Hart)

Challenging Concepts in Infectious Diseases and Clinical Microbiology
Cases with
Expert Commentary

Edited by

Dr Amber Arnold

Specialty Registrar in Infectious Diseases and Medical Microbiology, St George's Healthcare NHS Trust, London

Professor George E. Griffin

Professor of Infectious Diseases and Medicine; Honorary Consultant Physician, Clinical Infection Unit, St George's Healthcare NHS Trust, London

Series editors

Dr Aung Myat BSc (Hons) MBBS MRCP

BHF Clinical Research Training Fellow, King's College London British Heart Foundation Centre of Research Excellence, Cardiovascular Division, St Thomas' Hospital, London, UK

Dr Shouvik Haldar MBBS MRCP

Electrophysiology Research Fellow & Cardiology SpR, Heart Rhythm Centre, NIHR Cardiovascular Biomedical Research Unit, Royal Brompton & Harefield NHS Foundation Trust, Imperial College London, London

Professor Simon Redwood MD FRCP

Professor of Interventional Cardiology and Honorary Consultant Cardiologist, King's College London British Heart Foundation Centre of Research Excellence, Cardiovascular Division and Guy's and St Thomas' NHS Foundation Trust, St Thomas' Hospital, London, UK

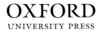

OXFORD
UNIVERSITY PRESS

UNIVERSITY PRESS

Great Clarendon Street, Oxford, OX2 6DP,
United Kingdom

Oxford University Press is a department of the University of Oxford.
It furthers the University's objective of excellence in research, scholarship,
and education by publishing worldwide. Oxford is a registered trade mark of
Oxford University Press in the UK and in certain other countries

Published in the United States of America by Oxford University Press
198 Madison Avenue, New York, NY 10016, United States of America

British Library Cataloguing in Publication Data
Data available

Library of Congress Control Number: 2014932764

ISBN 978-0-19-966575-4

Printed in Great Britain by
Ashford Colour Press Ltd, Gosport, Hampshire

To Noel, Alphege, Lynn, and Fabiola

PREFACE

Infectious diseases and microbiology continue to be part of a dynamic and continually evolving landscape. New infections emerge, older infections mutate, and the environment in which we live and harbour these infections constantly changes. In addition, new clinical trial data, laboratory studies, and discoveries at a cellular level all change the way we manage infections.

We as healthcare professionals must critically appraise the evidence base and apply it to everyday clinical practice so that we can give our patients the very best possible care that biomedical science will allow. Local, national, and international guidelines help, as does the expert consensus of opinion leaders and the advice of our colleagues and peers on the ground. We have tried in this publication to encapsulate this contemporary scheme of patient-focused care, with its foundation supported by guidelines and an evidence base.

We present 31 real-world clinical scenarios, each aiming to provide the reader with a holistic approach to dealing with a variety of challenging concepts in infectious diseases and microbiology. It has been our deliberate intention to include detailed reviews centred around individual cases which we may all encounter whether in the emergency department, the outpatient clinic, or on the ward. Indeed, we have tried to avoid presenting a compendium of the rare, weird, or wonderful. Each case has been written by a UK Specialty Trainee(s) and is punctuated by 'Learning points', 'Clinical tips', and 'Evidence base' summaries. These highlighted boxes are embedded alongside or within the main body of the case text and should help to aid memory and provoke thought.

We have then sought the peer review of an expert in the field for each of the clinical scenarios and have asked them to provide a narrative as the case proceeds in the form of 'Expert comments' boxes. These should provide the reader with a unique insight into how a specialist in the field would deal with the same clinical scenarios we all manage day in and day out.

We very much hope this text will appeal, first and foremost, to all specialty trainees in infection-based specialties as well as those in related specialties such as public health, genitourinary, emergency, acute, and general medicine. Allied to this the aim has been to make this book stimulating, transferable, and accessible to all those with an interest in infection-based medicine so in that respect general practitioners, other health professionals, core medical trainees, and medical students should all find this text relevant.

Amber Arnold
George E. Griffin

CONTENTS

EXPERTS

Chantal Bleeker-Rovers
Department of Internal Medicine
Radboud University Medical Centre in Nijmegen
The Netherlands

Mark Bower
Professor of Oncology
Chelsea and Westminster Hospital NHS Foundation Trust and
Imperial College London, UK

Tim Brooks
Head of Rare and Imported Pathogens Laboratory
PHE Microbiology Services Porton
Porton Down, UK

Mike Brown
Clinical Senior Lecturer and
Consultant Physician
London School of Hygiene and Tropical Medicine and
Hospital for Tropical Diseases at
University College London Hospital
London, UK

Andrew Carr
Professor of Medicine
University of New South Wales and
Head, HIV, Immunology and Infectious Diseases Unit and
Head, Clinical Research Program
Centre for Applied Medical Research
Sydney, Australia

Felix Chua
Consultant Respiratory and General Physician and
Honorary Senior Lecturer (SGUL)
St George's Healthcare NHS Trust
London, UK

Catherine Cosgrove
Consultant Physician Infectious Diseases and Acute Medicine
St George's Healthcare NHS Trust
London, UK

Tom Doherty
Consultant in Infectious Diseases and Tropical Medicine
University College London Hospital NHS Trust
London, UK

Hugo Donaldson
Consultant Medical Microbiologist
Imperial College Healthcare NHS Trust
London, UK

Daniel Forton
Consultant Hepatologist and Honorary Senior Lecturer
St George's Healthcare NHS Trust
London, UK

Patrick French
Consultant Physician in Genitourinary Medicine
The Mortimer Market Centre
London, UK

David E. Griffith
Professor of Medicine
Pulmonary and Critical Care Division Chief
The University of Texas Health Sciences Center
Texas, USA

Tom Harrison
Professor of Infectious Diseases and Medicine
and Joint Head of The Infection and Immunity Research Centre
St George's Healthcare NHS Trust
London, UK

Phillip Hay
Reader and Honorary Consultant
St George's Healthcare NHS Trust
London, UK

Carolyn Hemsley
Consultant in Infectious Diseases and Microbiology
Department of Infection
Guy's & St Thomas' NHS Foundation Trust
London, UK

Robert Hill
Unit Head
Antibiotic Resistance and Evaluation Unit
Public Health England Centre for Infections
London, UK

Matthew Laundy
Consultant Medical Microbiologist
St George's Healthcare NHS Trust
London, UK

Martin Llewelyn
Reader in Infectious Diseases and Therapeutics
Consultant in Infectious Diseases
Brighton and Sussex University Hospitals NHS Trust
Brighton, UK

Michael Loebinger
Respiratory Consultant
Royal Brompton Hospital
Honorary Senior Lecturer
Imperial College London
London, UK

Derek Macallan
Professor of Infectious Diseases and Medicine
St George's Healthcare NHS Trust
London, UK

David Moore
Reader Infectious Diseases and Tropical Medicine
London School of Hygiene and Tropical Medicine, UK

Elinor Moore
Consultant Physician in Infectious Diseases
Cambridge University Hospital NHS Foundation Trust
Cambridge, UK

William Newsholme
Consultant Physician
Department of Infection
St Thomas' Hospital
King's College Hospitals NHS Foundation Trust
London, UK

Sue O'Connell
Formerly Consultant Medical Microbiologist and
Head of the HPA's Lyme Borreliosis Unit
University Hospitals Southampton
NHS Foundation Trust
Southampton, UK

Chris Parry
Senior Clinical Consultant
Mahidol Oxford Tropical Medicine Research Unit
Angkor Hospital for Children
Siem Reap, Cambodia

Silke Schelenz
Clinical Senior Lecturer and
Consultant Microbiologist Norfolk and
Norwich University Hospitals Microbiology Department
Norwich, UK

Sorrush Soleimanian
Consultant Medical Microbiologist
North Middlesex University Hospital NHS Trust
London, UK

Claire P. Thomas
Consultant, Clinical Microbiology
Honorary Senior Lecturer, Infectious Diseases
Department of Infection
Imperial College Healthcare Trust
London, UK

Daniel Webster
Consultant and Senior Lecturer in Clinical Virology
Royal Free Hampstead NHS Trust
London, UK

CONTRIBUTORS

Daniel Bradshaw
Specialty Registrar in HIV and Genitourinary Medicine
Chelsea and Westminster Hospital NHS Foundation Trust
London, UK

Gayatri Chakrabarty
Specialty Registrar Gastroenterology
St George's Healthcare NHS Trust
London, UK

Naghum Dawood
Specialty Registrar in Infectious Diseases and Medical
Microbiology
Royal Free Hospital NHS Foundation Trust
London, UK

Rishi Dhillon
Consultant Microbiologist
University Hospital of Wales
Cardiff, UK

Tomas Doyle
Wellcome Trust Clinical Research Training Fellow
King's College London, UK

Ellen Dwyer
Specialty Registrar in HIV and Genitourinary Medicine
St George's Healthcare NHS Trust
London, UK

Nicholas Easom
Academic Clinical Fellow Infectious Diseases and
General Medicine
University College London Hospital
London, UK

Marcus Eder
Specialty Registrar in Infectious Diseases and Microbiology
Charing Cross Hospital
Imperial College Healthcare NHS Trust
London, UK

Kate El Bouzidi
Specialty Registrar in Infectious Diseases and Medical
Microbiology
St George's Healthcare NHS Trust
London, UK

Jayne Ellis
Academic Foundation Year 2 Doctor
St George's Healthcare NHS Trust
London, UK

Nicholas Feasey
Senior Clinical Lecturer
Liverpool School of Tropical Medicine
University of Liverpool, UK

Caoimhe Nic Fhogartaigh
Specialty Registrar in Infectious Diseases and Medical
Microbiology
Hospital for Tropical Diseases at
University College London Hospital
London, UK

James Hatcher
Specialty Registrar in Infectious Diseases and Medical
Microbiology
Hammersmith Hospital
Imperial College Healthcare NHS Trust
London, UK

Aseel Hegazi
Specialty Registrar in HIV and Genitourinary Medicine
St George's Healthcare NHS Trust
London, UK

Angela Houston
Specialty Registrar in Infectious Diseases and
Microbiology at St George's Hospital NHS Trust
London, UK

Julia Howard
Specialty Registrar in Medical Microbiology
Royal Free London NHS Foundation Trust
London, UK

Jasmin Islam
Specialist Registrar in Infectious Diseases and Medical
Microbiology
Brighton and Sussex University Hospitals NHS Trust
Brighton, UK

Jonathan Lambourne
Specialty Registrar in Infectious Diseases and
Microbiology
Rare and Imported Pathogens Laboratory
PHE Microbiology Services Porton
Porton Down, UK

Angela Loyse
Academic Clinical Lecturer
St George's Healthcare NHS Trust
London, UK

Mariyam Mirfenderesky
Specialty Registrar in Infectious Diseases and
Microbiology
St George's Healthcare NHS Trust
London, UK

Luke Moore
Specialty Registrar
Infectious Diseases and Medical Microbiology
Imperial College Healthcare NHS Trust
NIHR BRC Clinical Fellow
Division of Infectious Diseases and Immunity
Imperial College London, UK

Sally O'Connor
Specialty Registrar in Respiratory Medicine
St George's Healthcare NHS Trust
London, UK

James Price
Specialty Registrar in Infectious Diseases and Medical
Microbiology
Brighton and Sussex University Hospitals NHS Trust
Brighton, UK

Michael Rayment
Specialty Registrar in HIV and Genitourinary Medicine
Chelsea and Westminster Hospital NHS
Foundation Trust
London, UK

Catherine Roberts
Specialty Registrar Infectious Diseases and Microbiology
Department of Medicine
Imperial College London
London, UK

Georgina Russell
Specialty Registrar in Respiratory Medicine
St George's Healthcare NHS Trust
London, UK

Victoria Singh-Curry
Specialty Registrar in Neurology
Charing Cross Hospital
Imperial College NHS Foundation Trust
London, UK

Neill Storrar
Specialty Registrar Haematology
The Royal Infirmary of Edinburgh
Scotland, UK

Sathyavani Subbarao
Specialty Registrar in Infectious Diseases and Medicine
North Middlesex University Hospital NHS Trust
London, UK

Emily Wise
Specialty Registrar in Infectious Diseases
Royal Free London NHS Foundation Trust
London, UK

ABBREVIATIONS

3TC	lamivudine	BMT	bone marrow transplantation
5-FC	flucytosine	bPI	boosted protease inhibitor
^{18}F-FDG PET	^{18}F-fluorodeoxyglucose positron emission tomography	bpm	beats per minute
		BSAC	British Society for Antimicrobial Chemotherapy
AAD	antibiotic-associated diarrhoea		
ACDP	Advisory Committee on Dangerous Pathogens	BSMM	British Society for Medical Mycology
		CA	concomitant antibiotics
ACE	angiotensin converting enzyme	CA-MRSA	community-acquired MRSA
ACT	artemisinin combination therapy	CAP	cellulose acetate precipitation (test)
AFB	acid-fast bacillus	cART	combination antiretroviral therapy
AHR	adjusted hazard ratio	CC	clonal complex
AIDS	acquired immunodeficiency syndrome	cccDNA	covalently closed circular DNA
AII	airborne infection isolation room	CCHF	Crimean-Congo haemorrhagic fever
ALA	amoebic liver abscess	CDC	(United States) Centers for Disease Control
ALP	alkaline phosphatase		
ALT	alanine aminotransferase	CDI	*Clostridium difficile* infection
AmBd	amphotericin B deoxycholate	CDRN	*Clostridium difficile* Ribotyping Network
AML	acute myeloid leukaemia		
ANA	anti-nuclear antibody	CFU	colony forming units
ANCA	anti-neutrophil cytoplasmic antibody	CGD	chronic granulomatous disease
ARDS	adult respiratory distress syndrome	CHB	chronic hepatitis B
ART	antiretroviral therapy	CHOP	cyclophosphamide, doxorubicin, vincristine, and prednisolone
ASOT	anti-streptolysin O titre		
AST	aspartate transaminase; antimicrobial sensitivity testing	CI	confidence interval
		CIDP	chronic inflammatory demyelinating polyneuropathy
ATG	anti-thymocyte globulin		
ATN	acute tubular necrosis	CK	creatine kinase
ATS	American Thoracic Society	CLED	cystine-lysine-electrolyte deficient (agar)
ATV	atazanavir		
AUC	area under the curve	CLL	chronic lymphocytic leukaemia
BAL	broncho-alveolar lavage	CLSI	(United States) Clinical and Laboratory Standards Institute
Bb	*Borrelia burgdorferi*		
BCG	bacillus Calmette-Guérin	CM	cryptococcal meningitis
BCSH	British Committee for Standards in Haematology	CMV	cytomegalovirus
		CNS	central nervous system; coagulase-negative staphylococci
BCYE	buffered charcoal yeast extract		
BDG	beta-D-glucan	COPD	chronic obstructive pulmonary disease
BHL	bihilar (bilateral hilar) lymphadenopathy	CrAg	cryptococcal antigen
		CRMD	cardiac rhythm management devices
BI	bacterial infection	CRP	C-reactive protein
BIA	British Infection Association	CS	caesarean section
BJM	Bush-Jacoby-Medeiros group	CSF	cerebrospinal fluid
BLBLI	β-lactam β-lactamase inhibitors	CT	computed tomography

CVID	combined variable immunodeficiency
CVVH	continuous veno-venous haemofiltration
CXR	chest X-ray
D4T	stavudine
DAIR	debridement, antibiotics, and implant retention
D-AMB	amphotericin B dexoycholate
DAT	direct antiglobulin test
DCS	decreased ciprofloxacin susceptibility
DFA	direct fluorescent antibody
DIC	disseminated intravascular coagulation
DRAM	darunavir resistance-associated mutation
DRV	darunavir
DST	drug susceptibility testing
DTG	dolutegravir
EBUS	endobronchial ultrasound
EBV	Epstein–Barr virus
ECG	electrocardiogram
EEG	electroencephalogram
EFNS	European Federation of Neurological Societies
EFV	efavirenz
EGFR	estimated glomerular filtration rate
EIA	enzyme immunoassay
ELISA	enzyme-linked immunosorbent assay
EM	erythema migrans
EMA	European Medicines Agency
ENF	enfuvirtide
EORTC	European Organisation for Research and Treatment of Cancer
ESBL	extended spectrum β-lactamase
ESCAPPM	*Enterobacter, Serratia, Citrobacter freundii, Acinetobacter, Proteus vulgaris, Providencia*, and *Morganella morganii*
ESCMID	European Society of Clinical Microbiology and Infectious Diseases
ESR	erythrocyte sedimentation rate
ETV	etravirine
EUCAST	European Committee on Antimicrobial Susceptibility Testing
FC	fold change
FDA	(United States) Food and Drug Administration
FDG	fluorodeoxyglucose
FM	*falciparum* malaria
FMT	faecal microbiota transplantation
FNA	fine needle aspiration
FT	faecal transplant
FTC	emtricitabine
G6PD	glucose-6-phosphate dehydrogenase
GBR	genetic barrier to resistance
GCA	giant cell arteritis
GCS	Glasgow Coma Scale (score)
GDH	glutamate dehydrogenase
GI	gastrointestinal
GM	galactomannan
GMP	good manufacturing practice
GNB	Gram-negative bacillus
GUM	genitourinary medicine
GvHD	graft versus host disease
HAART	highly active antiretroviral therapy
HBcAb	hepatitis B core antibody
HBeAg	hepatitis B e-antigen
HBsAg	HBV surface antigen
HCT	haematopoietic cell transplant
HCV	hepatitis C virus
HDU	high dependency unit
HEPA	high-efficiency particulate air (filtration)
HHV	human herpes virus
Hib	*Haemophilus influenzae* type b
HIS	Hospital Infection Society
HIV	human immunodeficiency virus
HLA	human leucocyte antigen
HPA	Health Protection Agency
HR	hazard ratio
HRCT	high resolution computed tomography
HRP2	histidine-rich protein 2
HSIDU	high security infectious diseases unit
HSE	Health and Safety Executive
HSV	herpes simplex virus
HUS	haemolytic uraemic syndrome
hVISA	heterogenous vancomycin-intermediate *Staphylococcus aureus*
IA	invasive amoebiasis
IC50	concentration required to inhibit replication by 50%
ICP	intracranial pressure
ICT	immunochromatographic test
ID	infectious diseases
IDSA	Infectious Diseases Society of America
IE	infective endocarditis
IFAT	indirect fluorescent antibody test
IFD	invasive fungal disease
IgG	immunoglobulin G
IgM	immunoglobulin M

IGRA	interferon-gamma release assay		*Mtb*	*Mycobacterium tuberculosis*
IL-1,IL-2 etc.	interleukin 1, interleukin 2, etc.		MTCT	mother-to-child transmission
INH	isoniazid		MTD	*Mycobacterium tuberculosis* direct (test)
INI	integrase inhibitor		MVC	maraviroc
IRIS	immune reconstitution inflammatory syndrome		Na	nalidixic acid
			NAAT	nucleic acid amplification test
IVDU	intravenous drug user		NaR	nalidixic acid resistance
KS	Kaposi's sarcoma		NICE	National Institute for Health and Care Excellence
LANA	latency-associated nuclear antigen			
LB	Lyme borreliosis		NIH	(United States) National Institutes of Health
LFT	liver function tests			
LMIC	low and middle income countries		NNRTI	non-nucleoside reverse transcriptase inhibitor
LNB	Lyme neuroborreliosis			
LP	lumbar puncture		NPV	negative predictive value
LPV	lopinavir		NR	normal range; null responders
LS	leucocyte scintigraphy		NRTI	nucleoside reverse transcriptase inhibitor
LTT	lymphocyte transformation test			
LVOT	left ventricular outflow tract		NTM	non-tuberculous mycobacteria
mAb	monoclonal antibody		NTS	non-typhoidal salmonellae
MAC	*Mycobacterium avium* complex		NVT	non-vaccine type (pneumococcal disease)
MALDI	matrix-assisted laser desorption ionization		od	once daily
			OGD	oesophagogastroduodenoscopy
MARPA	multiple antibiotic resistance in *Pseudomonas aeruginosa*		OI	opportunistic infection
			OPAT	outpatient parenteral antibiotic therapy
MAT	microscopic agglutination test		OPG	orthopantomography
MBL	mannose-binding lectin; metallo-β-lactamase		OR	odds ratio
			PAS	periodic acid–Schiff; para-aminosalicylic acid
MCD	multicentric Castleman's disease			
MCV	mean cell volume; mean corpuscular volume		PBMC	peripheral blood mononuclear cells
			PCP	*Pneumocystis* pneumonia
MDR	multidrug resistant		PCR	polymerase chain reaction
MDS	myelodysplastic syndromes		PCV	pneumococcal conjugate vaccine
MDT	multidisciplinary team		PDC	potential diagnostic clue
MIC	minimum inhibitory concentration		pegIFN/RBV	pegylated interferon alpha and ribavirin
mKatG	*Mycobacterium tuberculosis* catalase-peroxidase		PEL	primary effusion lymphoma
			PEP	post-exposure prophylaxis
MLVA	multilocus variable number tandem repeat analysis		PET	positron emission tomography
			PFGE	pulsed-field gel electrophoresis
MRI	magnetic resonance imaging		PHE	Public Health England
MRL	Malaria Reference Laboratory		PI	protease inhibitor
MRSA	meticillin-resistant *Staphylococcus aureus*		PIC	preintegration complex
			PK	pharmacokinetics
MS	mass spectrometry		PLA	pyogenic liver abscess
MSCRAMM	microbial surface components recognizing adhesive matrix molecules		PLS	post-Lyme syndrome
			PMTCT	prevention of mother-to-child transmission
MSM	men who have sex with men			
MSSA	meticillin-sensitive *Staphylococcus aureus*		PNA	percutaneous needle aspiration
			PNSP	proportion not susceptible to penicillin
MSU	mid-stream urine		PPI	proton pump inhibitor

PPV	positive predictive value; pneumococcal polysaccharide vaccine	TB	tuberculosis
PR	partial responder	TBE	tickborne encephalitis
PSA	*Pseudomonas aeruginosa*	TBM	tuberculous meningitis
PTLD	post-transplant lymphoproliferative disease	TCC	transitional cell carcinoma
		TCR	T-cell receptor
PUO	pyrexia of unknown origin	TDF	tenofovir
PVL	Panton–Valentine Leukocidin	TDR	transmitted drug resistance
RAL	raltegravir	TIP	tipranivir
RAM	resistance-associated mutation	TNF	tumour necrosis factor
RAPD	random amplified polymorphic DNA analysis	TOE	transoesophageal echocardiography
		ToF	time of flight
R-CHOP	rituximab plus cyclophosphamide, doxorubicin, vincristine, and prednisolone	TPHA	*Treponema pallidum* haemagglutination assay
		TPN	total parenteral nutrition
RCT	randomized controlled trial	TPPA	*Treponema pallidum* particle agglutination assay
RDT	rapid diagnostic test	TST	tuberculin skin test
REA	restriction endonuclease analysis	TTE	transthoracic echocardiogram
RGM	rapidly growing mycobacteria	TTSS	type III secretion system
RIF	rifampicin	TURBT	transurethral resection of bladder tumour
RIPL	Rare and Imported Pathogens Laboratory		
ROS	reactive oxygen species	UD	undetectable
RPR	rapid plasma reagin	UTI	urinary tract infection
RT	reverse transcriptase	VATS	video-assisted thoracoscopic surgery
RT-PCR	reverse transcriptase PCR	VDRL	Venereal Disease Research Laboratory
SAB	*Staphylococcus aureus* bacteraemia	VFR	visiting friends or relatives
sACE	serum angiotensin converting enzyme	vIL-6	viral interleukin 6
SCID	severe combined immune deficiency	VISA	vancomycin-intermediate *Staphylococcus aureus*
SHEA	Society for Healthcare Epidemiology of America	VL	viral load
		VRE	vancomycin-resistant *Enterococcus*
SIADH	syndrome of inappropriate antidiuretic hormone secretion	VRSA	vancomycin-resistant *Staphylococcus aureus*
SOC	standard of care	VT	vaccine type (pneumococcal disease)
SOT	solid organ transplant	WCC	white cell count
ST	sequence type	WGS	whole genome sequencing
STI	sexually transmitted infection	XDR	extensively drug-resistant
SVR	sustained virological response	ZDV	zidovudine
TAM	thymidine analogue mutation		

REFERENCE INTERVALS

Haematology values

Haemoglobin	
men:	13–18 g/dL
women:	11.5–16 g/dL
Mean cell volume, MCV	76–96 fL
Platelets	$150–400 \times 10^9$/L
White cells (total)	$4–11 \times 10^9$/L
Neutrophils	40–75%
Lymphocytes	20–45%
Eosinophils	1–6%

Urea and electrolytes

Sodium	135–145 mmol/L
Potassium	3.5–5 mmol/L
Creatinine	70–150 μmol/L
Urea	2.5–6.7 mmol/L
Estimated glomerular filtration rate, EGFR	>90

Liver function tests

Bilirubin	3–17 μmol/L
Alanine aminotransferase, ALT	5–35 iu/L
Aspartate transaminase, AST	5–35 iu/L
Alkaline phosphatase, ALP	30–150 iu/L (*non-pregnant adults*)
Albumin	35–50 g/L
Protein (total)	60–80 g/L

Lipids and other biochemical values

Cholesterol	<5 mmol/L (*desired*)
Triglycerides	0.5–1.9 mmol/L
Amylase	0–180 Somogyi u/dL
C-reactive protein, CRP	<10 mg/L
Calcium (total)	2.12–2.65 mmol/L
Glucose, fasting	3.5–5.5 mmol/L

Pyrexia of unknown origin: the use of PET and PET-CT

1

Neill Storrar

Ⓔ **Expert commentary** Chantal Bleeker-Rovers

Case history

A 53-year-old white woman was referred to the cardiology team to rule out infective endocarditis when her general practitioner heard a new heart murmur. The patient had been to the GP several times over the last 3 months complaining of fatigue and 3 kg weight loss. She also complained of worsening sweats and hot flushes 6 months previously that were attributed to the menopause. The only other symptoms included long-standing low back pain which she did not think had significantly changed over the last year, and ongoing toothache for which she was awaiting tooth extraction. There were no other symptoms that might localize infection, and systemic enquiry was otherwise normal.

Her past medical history included persistent ventricular ectopic beats for which she had undergone an ablation procedure 12 months prior to admission. At that time she started antihypertensives. She suffered with mild depression and took fluoxetine. She had been prescribed hormone replacement therapy 3 months ago when she had first presented to her GP with sweats and hot flushes. She had not noticed any improvement in her symptoms.

She was an office worker and had smoked heavily for 20 years but had given up 10 years ago. She had not travelled outside the United Kingdom for several years, and never farther than Spain. She had a pet dog, and recalled a stray kitten scratching her a few months ago. She had had a trivial alcohol intake and no history of illicit drug use. There was no family history of note. She had no allergies.

On examination she appeared well, was apyrexial, and had no peripheral stigmata of endocarditis. Cardiovascular examination demonstrated a collapsing pulse and a loud early diastolic murmur at the left lower sternal edge consistent with significant aortic regurgitation. There was no palpable lymphadenopathy, no neurological abnormality, no abnormal abdominal mass, and the chest was clear. Dentition was indeed poor but there was no suggestion of an abscess on orthopantomography (OPG). Blood tests on arrival showed a neutrophilia and a markedly raised C-reactive protein (CRP) (Table 1.1).

The patient was admitted for investigations for infective endocarditis. On day 2 her temperature spiked at 38.6°C. However, over a 4-week admission she only had three further spikes over 38°C with her baseline temperature at the higher end of the normal range (37.5°C). She had multiple negative blood cultures. Transthoracic then transoesophageal echocardiography (TOE) showed severe aortic regurgitation and moderate LV impairment, but no vegetation or aortic root dilatation/abscess. Following maxillofacial review she had several teeth extracted but there was no evidence of root abscess and her symptoms and inflammatory markers were unchanged afterwards.

Table 1.1 Investigations on arrival at hospital

Test	Results
Hb (g/dL)	11.2
MCV (fL)	89.2
WCC (× 10^9 cell/L)	15.5
–Neutrophils	10.1
–Lymphocytes	4.2
Platelets (× 10^9/L)	548
Na (mM)	135
K (mM)	4.0
U (mM)	3.5
Cr (μM)	85
Bil (μM)	7
ALT (iu/L)	15
ALP (iu/L)	75
Albumin (g/L)	31
ESR mm/hr	114
CRP mg/L	233
Chest radiography	No abnormalities identified

Unable to fulfil the Duke criteria for infective endocarditis, the differential diagnosis was broadened to that of a pyrexia of unknown origin (PUO) and she underwent considerable investigations after consultation with the infectious diseases (ID), rheumatology, and haematology teams (Box 1.1).

Box 1.1 Negative or normal investigations

Microbiology

6 blood cultures (off antibiotics)
Serology for HIV, hepatitis B, C, cytomegalovirus (CMV), Epstein–Barr virus (EBV), atypical pneumonia, syphilis, *Borrelia*, and *Bartonella*
Anti-streptolysin O titre (ASOT)
T-SPOT interferon gamma release assay for tuberculosis (TB)
3 induced sputa for acid-fast bacilli (AFB) and mycobacterial culture

Others

Autoimmune serology: anti-nuculear antibody (ANA), anti-neutrophil cytoplasmic antibody (ANCA), liver autoantibodies, rheumatoid factor
C3 and C4
Immunoglobulins, serum protein electrophoresis, urinary Bence Jones protein
Thyroid function tests

⊕ **Clinical tip** Differential diagnosis

Aetiology of PUO differs according to region, time, and age. Infection has traditionally been seen as the largest aetiological group, accounting for 30–50% of cases, followed by malignant causes and connective tissue disease. However, this distribution is not always the case. Infection is more likely in older Western studies (e.g. 1950s compared to present-day), studies from tropical and low-income countries, and in younger patients [1]. There is also a suggestion in more recent studies from high-income countries that a higher proportion of patients remain undiagnosed [2]. These differences are likely due to the incidence of TB and ease of obtaining cross-sectional imaging, changing the population of the PUO. Many patients are no longer diagnosed as having PUO because, for example, a CT scan is performed early.

In older patients, as with our patient, the aetiology of PUO is much more likely to be due to multisystem and connective tissue diseases, with giant cell arteritis (GCA) being particularly common.

(continued)

Results of a study in Belgium on the aetiology of PUO in 47 patients over 65 years [3] are as follows:

- Infective 12 (25%)
- Malignant 6 (12%)
- Non-infectious inflammatory conditions 15 (31%) including vasculitis, e.g. temporal arteritis (most common), rheumatoid disease, polymyalgia rheumatica, and sarcoidosis
- Miscellaneous 8 (drug fever 3 [6%], other 5 [10%])
- Undiagnosed 6 (12%)

Due to the broad differential it is important to involve physicians from a range of specialties to help in the differential diagnosis, prioritizing of investigations, and interpretation of test results.

❝ Expert comment

Serological tests are not very useful if there are no clues for these infections. In this case, cat scratch disease should be included in the differential diagnosis because of the scratch from a kitten some time before the complaints started. Patients with cat scratch disease can present with PUO without other guiding symptoms, but this is more common in children than in adults. I would not have requested serology for hepatitis B and C, atypical pneumonia, CMV and EBV. In PUO without clues for specific infections, it has been shown that microbiological serological tests are never helpful in establishing a diagnosis. In addition, a *Borrelia* infection is usually not characterized by fever.

A CT scan of thorax-abdomen-pelvis found no evidence of infective collection, lymphadenopathy, or malignancy. An MR scan of the lumbar spine—to look for occult osteomyelitis in view of her back pain—demonstrated only degenerative changes.

Over the month-long admission her CRP continued to remain raised between 200 and 300 mg/L and she developed a mildly microcytic anaemia (Hb 98 g/L, MCV 75 fL). She did not experience any haematemesis or altered bowel motions. Both upper gastrointestinal (GI) endoscopy and virtual CT colonoscopy were reported as normal.

A technetium 99m white cell scan was attempted, but due to a technical problem in the labelling of cells this could not be performed. A bone marrow aspirate and trephine was negative for infection, malignancy, and infiltrative disease; slides were reported as showing only non-specific reactive changes.

✪ Learning point Nuclear medicine techniques in PUO—leucocyte scintigraphy (LS) and [67] gallium citrate

Leucocyte scintigraphy (LS)

A sample of the subject's white cells are incubated with indium-111 (^{111}In) or technetium-99 (^{99}Tc), then reinjected; their localization is followed radiographically. A prospective study compared 23 patients with PUO who underwent both LS and PET [4] (see Table 1.2).

Table 1.2 Comparison of FDG-PET and LS in 23 patients with PUO

	PET	LS
Sensitivity	86%	20%
Specificity	78%	100%
Positive predictive value	86%	100%
Negative predictive value (NPV)	78%	40%

Source: Data from *Journal of Infection*, Volume 65, Issue 1, N Seshadri et al, Superiority of 18F-FDG PET compared to 111In-labelled leucocyte scintigraphy in the evaluation of fever of unknown origin, pp. 71–79, Copyright © 2012 The British Infection Association. Published by Elsevier Ltd. All rights reserved.

(continued)

Negative LS strongly predicts absence of infection but does not rule out other conditions where leucocyte concentration is not a prominent feature such as malignancy—patient population should be considered. There can be technical problems where labelling fails (as in this case), white cell count (WCC) is very low, or venesection is difficult.

Gallium-67 (^{67}Ga) citrate

^{67}Ga citrate can be injected intravenously. It is thought to bind to transferrin, and extravasate at inflamed sites with increased vascular permeability. This allows identification of sites of infection and inflammation. There are few data to help assess its utility in PUO. In a prospective comparison of PET with ^{67}Ga citrate, 18 patients underwent both scans as part of a workup for PUO [5]. PET appeared to have better performance (see Table 1.3).

Table 1.3 Comparison of FDG-PET and ^{67}Ga citrate scanning in 18 patients with PUO

	PET	Gallium
Sensitivity	81%	67%
Specificity	86%	78%
Positive predictive value	90%	75%
NPV	75%	70%

Source: Data from J Meller et al, Fever of unknown origin: prospective comparison of [18F]FDG imaging with a double-head coincidence camera and gallium-67 citrate SPET, *European Journal of Nuclear Medicine and Molecular Imaging*, Volume 27, Issue 11, pp. 1617–1625, Copyright © Springer-Verlag 2000.

Other limitations of ^{67}Ga citrate scanning include long radioactive half-life (78 hours) and relatively high radiation dose, and the pattern of excretion (initially renal, then hepatobiliary) makes assessment of disease in these areas limited.

In further consultation, (^{18}F)-fluorodeoxyglucose positron emission tomography with computed tomography (^{18}FDG PET-CT) was performed. This was primarily intended to assess for vasculitis or lymphoma. The test was not readily available in the patient's hospital, but was obtained on referral to another hospital in the region.

This test showed markedly abnormal uptake of labelled glucose in the ascending and descending aorta, and subclavian and iliac arteries (Figure 1.1 and 1.2). These findings are typical of large vessel vasculitis and the patient was diagnosed based on imaging.

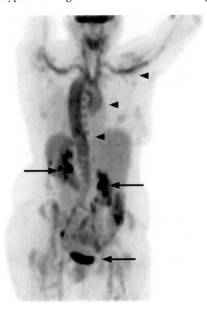

Figure 1.1 Positron emission tomograph (PET) images demonstrating the diagnosis of large vessel vasculitis. Increasing PET activity corresponds with darker appearance on the image. There is pathologically avid FDG uptake in the subclavian arteries, ascending aorta, aortic arch and descending aorta (arrow heads). Physiological concentration of FDG in the renal collecting system and bladder is shown (lined arrows) and PET activity elsewhere is normal (see Learning Point 'How does PET-CT work?')

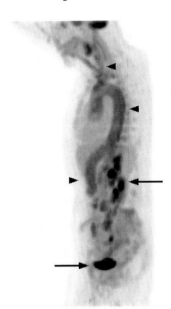

Figure 1.2 Positron emission tomograph (PET) images demonstrating the diagnosis of large vessel vasculitis. Increasing PET activity corresponds with darker appearance on the image. There is pathologically avid FDG uptake in the subclavian arteries, ascending aorta, aortic arch and descending aorta (arrow heads). Physiological concentration of FDG in the renal collecting system and bladder is shown (lined arrows) and PET activity elsewhere is normal (see Learning Point 'How does PET-CT work?').

✪ **Learning point** How does PET-CT work?

In positron emission tomography (PET) the patient is injected with a radio-labelled glucose solution—(^{18}F)-fluoro-2-deoxy-D-glucose (FDG)—which localizes to areas of high glucose uptake primarily mediated by GLUT-1 and GLUT-3 transporters. The half-life of FDG is 110 minutes. *In vivo* decay of ^{18}F results in positron emission which in turn causes emission of gamma rays detected by a gamma camera.

Areas of high glucose uptake/concentration appear as 'FDG-avid' regions. Due to the physiologically high signals in the brain, in kidneys and ureter where isotope is excreted, and variable uptake in the GI system and heart, this modality is less useful for identifying pathology in these areas. Pathological areas of high glucose metabolism such as bacterial infections (BIs), areas of inflammation (high uptake by leucocytes), and many malignancies will also demonstrate high FDG avidity. It is possible to improve the accurate localization of abnormal signal by overlaying PET images with conventional CT images: PET-CT.

Since the modality relies on abnormal localization of glucose, the majority of indications are for detection of focal disease, and are less useful for diffuse diseases (such as drug fever). The test also has a minimal resolution of 5 mm and so cannot easily identify medium or small vessel vasculitides, or cases of vasculitis limited to the temporal arteries.

ⓖ **Expert comment**

FDG-PET/CT is a very useful diagnostic test in patients with PUO because it shows increased uptake in infection, inflammation, and malignancy. The cause of PUO can be found in any of these disease categories. Although one of the advantages of FDG-PET/CT when compared to LS is its ability to detect vasculitis and lymphoma, the value of FDG-PET/CT is not limited to these specific diseases. Other advantages of FDG-PET/CT are the higher resolution, higher sensitivity in chronic low-grade infections, and high accuracy in the central skeleton. Disadvantages of ^{67}Ga-citrate scintigraphy and labelled LS when compared to FDG-PET/CT are handling of potentially infected blood products (labelled LS), higher radiation burden (^{111}In-labelled leucocyte and ^{67}Ga-citrate scintigraphy), instability of the labelling (^{99m}Tc-labelled LS), and the long time span between injection and diagnosis (^{67}Ga-citrate scintigraphy). Several studies directly comparing FDG-PET/CT with ^{67}Ga-citrate scintigraphy and LS in patients with PUO showed a higher accuracy of FDG-PET/CT.

⭐ **Learning point** Large vessel vasculitis

Vasculitides are usefully classified by the size of vessels affected. The large vessel forms include giant cell GCA and Takayasu's arteritis and are common diagnoses in PUO case series. Both conditions involve large, named arteries, and histology demonstrates granulomatous inflammation of arterial wall. While there are raised inflammatory markers (ESR, CRP), autoantibodies such as ANA and ANCA are not detected. There is clinical overlap, as in the case presented here, but Table 1.4 gives characteristic features.

Table 1.4 Comparison of GCA and Takayasu arteritis

	GCA	Takayasu's arteritis
Typical patient age (years)	>50	<40
Affected arteries	Extracranial carotid branches (temporal artery) Aorta also involved in a majority of cases	Aorta and major branches
Clinical features	Headache, fever, scalp tenderness and jaw claudication. Visual disturbance/blindness. Co-existent polymyalgia rheumatica	Systemic illness: sweats, fever, back pain, weight loss. 'Pulseless' disease due to occlusive arteritis
Diagnosis	Clinical and imaging: Doppler ultrasound arteriography, PET Temporal Artery Biopsy	Clinical PET Magetic resonance imaging (MRI) (rarely biopsy)

➕ **Clinical tip** Definitions of PUO

PUO was first defined as:

'A fever higher than 38.3°C (101°F) on several occasions, persisting without diagnosis for at least 3 weeks in spite of at least 1 week's investigation in hospital.' [6]

However, considering that most PUO patients are stable and investigations can be performed more quickly, the definition of the classical PUO was refined:

'A fever of 38.3°C or more that lasts for at least 3 weeks for which no cause can be found despite 3 days of inpatient investigation or 3 outpatient clinic visits.' [7]

Three further subtypes of PUO were also defined comprising nosocomial PUO, HIV PUO, and neutropenic PUO.

A more modern approach is to define PUO qualitatively, where a patient fits the definition only if no diagnosis is found after a minimum diagnostic workup [8]. It excludes patient with immunocompromise.

'A febrile illness of >3 weeks' duration, a temperature of >38.3°C on at least 2 occasions, without a diagnosis after standardized history taking, standardized physical examination, and obligatory investigations.'

Discussion

This case highlights the difficulties in diagnosing and prioritizing investigations in a patient with PUO. The patient had repeatedly visited her GP with non-specific symptoms that had not been recognized as anything more than the onset of the menopause. This resulted in a late referral, only after structural heart damage had already occurred. She had fever and evidence of a brisk inflammatory response (high CRP, neutrophilia, and later anaemia) and once infective endocarditis was excluded, she went on to have full PUO workup.

➕ Clinical tip Investigations in PUO

The most important aspects of management of PUO are a repeated detailed history and thorough examination. The next step is to verify the fever. Up to 35% of patients referred for PUO may not have a fever or may have fictitious fever [1].

The following is a summary of a diagnostic protocol described in the literature [8].

Step 1

Detailed history and examination, cessation/replacement of medication

Obligatory investigations:

- Full blood count
- Erythrocyte sedimentation rate (ESR)
- Complement-reactive protein (CRP)
- Liver function tests (LFTs): alkaline phosphatase (ALP), alanine transferase
- Electrolytes, creatinine
- Total protein
- Serum protein electrophoresis
- LDH
- Creatine kinase (CK)
- Antinuclear antibodies, rheumatoid factor
- Urinalysis and urine culture
- 3 sets of blood cultures
- Chest X-ray (CXR)
- Abdominal ultrasound or CT
- Tuberculin skin test (TST)

Step 2

With this complete, any potential diagnostic clues (PDCs) are followed with appropriate investigations. PDCs are 'all localizing signs, symptoms, and abnormalities potentially pointing toward a diagnosis.' If these do not result in an answer, or no obvious clues are present, patients should be tested for cryoglobulins. If there is still no diagnosis, FDG-PET should be performed and results pursued.

Step 3

If continuous fever persists and FDG-PET is normal or falsely positive, the following second-level tests can be performed:

- Bone marrow biopsy
- Temporal artery biopsy (age >55)
- Fundoscopy
- Abdominal and chest CT

If patients have only periodic fever, PET should be performed when the patient is symptomatic, and second-level tests requested only if there are PDCs suggestive of infection, vasculitis or malignancy, unless the patient is clinically deteriorating; full history and examination should be repeated.

Finally, if there is no diagnosis after this investigative protocol, stable patients may be followed up or treated symptomatically. Unstable patients may undergo further diagnostic workup, or consider therapeutic antimicrobial or steroid trials.

Other diagnostic tests, such as echocardiograms, specific microbial serology, lumbar puncture (LP), etc. are probably only helpful if clinical or investigative clues point towards relevant diagnoses.

❝ Expert comment

Despite the relatively low sensitivity of CXR, this simple low-cost diagnostic test remains obligatory in all patients with PUO. Abdominal imaging should also be performed in order to separate diseases that can be easily diagnosed from the true PUO cases. Abdominal ultrasound could be considered instead

(continued)

of abdominal CT, because of the relatively low cost, lack of radiation burden, and the absence of side effects. In particular, when FDG-PET/CT is performed at an earlier stage, abdominal CT may not be necessary. The diagnostic yield of echocardiography, X-rays of the sinuses, radiological or endoscopic evaluation of the GI tract, and bronchoscopy is very low when PDCs are absent, so these tests should not be performed as screening procedures.

There were many clues in the history and examination that led the team in multiple directions. The majority of clues in retrospect are associated with large vessel vasculitis (heart murmur, anaemia, back pain) but at the time suggested diagnoses as broad as infective endocarditis, GI tumour leading to blood loss, and osteomyelitis. Other clues were in retrospect 'red herrings' and suggested diverse conditions like cat scratch fever and chronic tooth abscess. There was the added pressure of time with a deteriorating structural heart defect—it was believed it would be better to delay surgery until a diagnosis was made, but this could not be postponed indefinitely.

⊕ Expert comment

The most important step in the diagnostic workup is a complete and repeated history taking, physical examination, and the obligatory investigations in a search for potentially diagnostic clues (PDCs). PDCs are defined as all localizing signs, symptoms, and abnormalities potentially pointing toward a diagnosis. Although often misleading, only with help of these PDCs can a limited list of probable diagnoses be made. As happened in this case, these clues should guide further diagnostic tests. In making a differential diagnosis it is important to remember that PUO is far more often caused by an atypical presentation of a rather common disease than by a very rare disease. I would have included vasculitis in the differential diagnosis earlier since this is a common cause of PUO in patients over 50 years old and it explained all signs and symptoms.

One of the important questions arising from this case is whether PET-CT—which proved to be diagnostic—ought to have been performed earlier and could have reduced the need for other investigations, saving radiation exposure, discomfort, time, and money.

PET scans assess for areas of increased metabolic activity. The benefit of PET-CT is that both structural abnormalities (CT) and areas with high metabolic activity (PET) can be assessed together. Due to the high sensitivity levels but slightly lower specificity, a positive result normally needs confirmation (e.g. with biopsy), but a negative result has been shown to have a good NPV [9]. In general, patients with no diagnosis do well [1]. In this case there was no structural vascular defect, but high FDG uptake localized the pathology to the aorta; the imaging was pathognomonic of large vessel vasculitis and further investigations were not necessary. Large vessel vasculitides can be difficult to diagnose due to lack of blood markers and diffuse symptoms, as in this case, and PET imaging has been shown to be particularly useful in diagnosis [10].

⊘ Evidence base   What is the sensitivity and specificity of PET/PET-CT in PUO?

One systematic review has pooled a number of studies to characterize the overall sensitivities and specificities [9].

Definitions
- True positive—abnormal findings that led to a focal diagnosis
- True negative—no abnormal findings with no focal diagnosis at follow-up
- False positive—abnormal findings with no relation to the final diagnosis/no diagnosis made
- False negative—no abnormal findings, but a focal cause was found by other means

Inclusion criteria

- Papers selected to exclude patients with immunocompromise, small cohort size, did not fit classic PUO definition
- 9 studies
- 5 using PET (4 retrospective and 1 prospective), 4 using PET-CT (3 retrospective and 1 prospective)
- Total of 388 patients
- PET
  - sensitivity 82.6% (95%CI 72.9–89.9)
  - specificity 57.8% (95% CI 48.8–66.5)

- PET-CT
  - sensitivity 98.2 (95% CI; 93.6–99.8)
  - specificity 85.9 (95% CI; 75.0–93.4)

Conclusions: Sensitivity was particularly high when the final diagnosis was infection, inflammation or neoplasm, but lower for miscellaneous diagnoses. The increased sensitivity and specificity of PET-CT might be due to better localization of abnormal tracer uptake, better definition of the diseased tissue, and better discrimination between physiological and pathological uptake [9].

There are two ways that PET can be used in the diagnosis of PUO. The first method, as in this case, is as a last resort due to availability of scanners and funding for this indication in the UK. There is limited information on how to choose patients for PET/PET-CT when other investigations have been exhausted. Studies have shown that factors that correlate with a useful PET/PET-CT are raised CRP, lymphadenopathy, and low haemoglobin level [11]. In the study by Bleeker-Rovers et al., PET was not useful in any of the 11 patients with normal CRP/ESR but was useful in 39% of the patients where these markers were elevated (p < 0.01) [2]. However, most patients with PUO do have an elevated CRP and so this does not narrow selection very much.

Another option is to use PET/PET-CT earlier in the PUO workup process before whole-body CT. Using PET at this early stage after basic routine tests (ultrasound abdomen and CXR) has been shown to be useful in 30% of cases in one diagnostic algorithm [2]. There are safety concerns over using PET-CT at an earlier stage because of the radiological dose. However, the dose is lower than that of CT thorax-abdomen-pelvis which is often used in the workup of PUO, and could be used as a substitute (Box 1.2). Further, due to PET's high sensitivity, other radiological/nuclear imaging may not be necessary.

✅ **Evidence base** A prospective multicentre study on fever of unknown origin. The yield of a structured diagnostic protocol [2]

Study design: A total of 73 patients with PUO were prospectively recruited from 1 university hospital and 5 community hospitals in the Netherlands between 2003 and 2005. Patients with immunosuppression were excluded. The mean age of the patients was 54 (range 26–87 years).

The modern definition of PUO was used, and patients were investigated according to the structure diagnostic protocol detailed in Clinical tip: Investigations in PUO.

Results: The cause of PUO was found to be infection 12 (16%), neoplasm 5 (7%), non-infectious inflammatory conditions 16 (22%), miscellaneous 4%, and no cause found 37 (51%). Of those with no diagnosis over a median of 12 months follow-up the fever subsided spontaneously in 16, resolved with NSAIDs or corticosteroids in 5, one died, and 15 remained with an undiagnosed fever.

(continued)

PDCs: On average 15 PDCs per person; 19% helpful but 81% not helpful. No case was diagnosed through PDCs alone and so 96% of patients went on to PET.

Usefulness of PET, chest, and abdominal computed tomography (CT) are compared (see Table 1.5).

Table 1.5 Usefulness of FDG-PET, chest CT, and abdominal CT

	No. performed (%)	Helpful (%)	False positive (%)	Sensitivity (%, 95% CI)	Specificity (%, 95% CI)
PET	70 (96)	23 (33)	10 (14)	92 (74–99)	78 (63–89)
Chest CT	46 (63)	9 (20)	8 (17)	82 (48–98)	77 (60–90)
Abdo CT	60 (82)	12 (20)	17 (28)	92 (64–100)	63 (48–77)

Source: Data from Chantal P Bleeker-Rovers et al, A prospective multi-centre study of the value of FDG-PET as part of a structured diagnostic protocol in patients with fever of unknown, *European Journal of Nuclear Medicine and Molecular Imaging*, Volume 34, Issue 5, pp. 694–703, Copyright © Springer-Verlag 2006.

Box 1.2 Public health

Clinicians have a responsibility to consider the long-term effects of radiological and scintigraphic tests on subjects, particularly for future risk of cancer.

In healthcare, effective radiation dose is given in millisieverts (mSv)—a calculation including consideration of the radiation dose to the organ, the relative biological effectiveness, and a tissue weighting factor. It is estimated that a dose of 1000 mSv gives a 5% lifetime chance of developing malignancy [12]. Comparative radiation doses are given in Table 1.6. Modern PET-CT scanners give relatively modest radiation doses (PET: 1.6 MBq/kg * 0.019 mSv/MBq = 0.0304 mSv/kg, and low dose CT = 1–3 mSv). A person of 70 kg would therefore receive a dose of around 5mSv, lower than for abdominal CT. Thus while PET-CT gives moderate doses, it is lower than the effective radiation dose of the standard CT-chest/abdomen/pelvis commonly used in investigation of PUO, and could be used instead of this test.

Table 1.6 Radiation dose of radiological investigations and other activities

Exposure	Effective radiation dose (mSv)
PET-CT	4–6
CT Chest	5–7
CT Abdomen-pelvis	8–11
1 Year in the sunshine	3.6
Return transatlantic flight	0.12

Source: Data from Heiko Schöder and Mithat Gönen, Screening for Cancer with PET and PET/CT: Potential and Limitations, *The Journal of Nuclear Medicine*, Volume 48, Number 1, Supplement pp. 4–18, Copyright © 2006 by the Society of Nuclear Medicine, Inc.

In summary, when managing a patient who has features of PUO, PET/PET-CT is a sensitive and specific test for detection of a range of focal pathologies. While it is expensive, it may well prove a cost-effective test. Used as part of a standardized diagnostic algorithm, it can provide early diagnosis in a range of conditions, and avoid further unnecessary investigations.

A final word from the expert

PUO was originally defined by Petersdorf and Beeson in 1961 to enable comparison of studies on this subject. The definition has been changed several times, for example, by excluding immunocompromised patients because this group needs an entirely different diagnostic and therapeutic approach. To enable the most optimal comparison of patients with PUO in different geographic areas, I prefer the definition using a qualitative criterion that requires a list of certain investigations to be performed to the quantitative criterion.

The etiology of PUO has changed over time as a result of changes in the broad spectrum of diseases causing PUO and the availability of new diagnostic techniques. In general, infection accounts for about one-quarter of cases of PUO, followed by non-infectious inflammatory diseases, and neoplasm. In the category non-infectious inflammatory diseases, GCA is the most important diagnosis, especially in elderly patients. The number of patients diagnosed with non-infectious inflammatory diseases will probably not decrease in the near future, because fever may precede more typical manifestations or other evidence by months in these diseases.

Although scintigraphic techniques do not directly provide a definitive diagnosis, i.e. a histological or a microbiological diagnosis, they often provide the anatomic localization where a particular metabolic process is ongoing and with the help of other techniques, such as biopsy and culture, can facilitate timely diagnosis and treatment. On the basis of the results of the literature and resulting from the favourable characteristics of FDG-PET, conventional scintigraphic techniques should be replaced by FDG-PET/CT in the investigation of patients with PUO in institutions where this technique is available. If a FDG-PET/CT had been performed instead of a CT scan of thorax-abdomen-pelvis and MRI, the diagnosis would have been reached immediately and a month-long admission would not have been necessary. Treatment would have been started earlier and the radiation exposure would have been much lower (4–6 mSv for FDG-PET/CT vs. >15 mSv). Performing a rather expensive FDG-PET/CT would also have resulted in fewer diagnostic tests and a shorter duration of admission for diagnostic purposes, ultimately reducing costs.

Although in this patient the cause of the fever was eventually found, recent PUO series have shown a high diagnostic failure rate of up to 50%. A diagnosis is more frequently reached before three weeks have elapsed because patients with fever tend to seek medical advice earlier and because better diagnostic techniques, such as CT and MRI, are widely available, leaving the more hard-to-diagnose cases to meet the definition of PUO. Empirical therapeutic trials with antibiotics, corticosteroids, or anti-tuberculous agents should be avoided except in patients whose condition is rapidly deteriorating. Empirical trials decrease the chance of reaching a diagnosis for which more specific and sometimes life-saving treatment might be more appropriate, such as malignant lymphoma.

References

1 Mackowiak PA, Durack DT. Fever of unknown origin. In: Mandel GL, Bennett JE, Dolin R. *Principles and Practice of Infectious Disease.* 7th Edition. Philadelphia, PA: Churchill Livingstone/Elsevier; 2009. p. 779–789.
2 Bleeker-Rovers CP, Vos FJ, Mudde AH et al. A prospective multi-centre study of the value of FDG-PET as part of a structured diagnostic protocol in patients with fever of unknown origin. *Eur J Nucl Med Mol Imaging* 2007; 34: 694–703.

3 Knockaert DC, Vanneste LJ, Bobbaers HJ. Fever of unknown origin in elderly patients. *J Am Geriatr Soc* 1993; 41: 1187–1192.

4 Seshadri N, Sonoda LI, Lever AM, Balan K. Superiority of 18F-FDG PET compared to 111In-labelled leucocyte scintigraphy in the evaluation of fever of unknown origin. *J Infect* 2012; 65: 71–79.

5 Meller J, Altenvoerde G, Munzel U et al. Fever of unknown origin: prospective comparison of [18F]FDG imaging with a double-head coincidence camera and gallium-67 citrate SPET. *Eur J Nucl Med* 2000; 27: 1617–1625.

6 Petersdorf RG, Beeson PB. Fever of unexplained origin: report on 100 cases. *Medicine (Baltimore)* 1961; 40: 1–30.

7 Durack DT, Street AC. Fever of unknown origin—reexamined and redefined. *Curr Clin Top Infect Dis* 1991; 11: 35–51.

8 Bleeker-Rovers CP, Vos FJ, De Kleijn EMHA et al. A prospective multicenter study on fever of unknown origin: the yield of a structured diagnostic protocol. *Medicine (Baltimore)* 2007; 86: 26–38.

9 Dong M, Zhao K, Liu Z, Wang G, Yang S, Zhou G. A meta-analysis of the value of fluorodeoxyglucose-PET/PET-CT in the evaluation of fever of unknown origin. *Eur J Radiol* 2011; 80: 834–844.

10 Treglia G, Mattoli MV, Leccisotti L, Ferraccioli G, Giordano A. Usefulness of whole-body fluorine-18-fluorodeoxyglucose positron emission tomography in patients with large-vessel vasculitis: a systematic review. *Clin Rheumatol* 2011; 30: 1265–1275.

11 Crouzet J, Boudousq V, Lechiche C et al. Place of (18)F-FDG-PET with computed tomography in the diagnostic algorithm of patients with fever of unknown origin. *Eur J Clin Microbiol Infect Dis* 2012; 31: 1727–1733.

12 Schöder H, Gönen M. Screening for cancer with PET and PET/CT: potential and limitations. *J Nucl Med* 2007; 48 Suppl 1: 4S–18S.

2 Neurological complications of Lyme borreliosis

Victoria Singh-Curry and Amber Arnold

ⓘ **Expert Commentary** Sue O'Connell

Case history

A 71-year-old right-handed man presented to his local emergency department in August with a 2-week history of progressive right arm numbness and weakness and more recent onset of confusion and fatigue.

Two months earlier, in June, he had sustained a tick bite to his right axilla while on holiday in a forested area of northern France. He had removed the tick himself but did not know how long it had been attached to his skin. Some days later he developed a large erythematous area around the site of the bite.

> **ⓘ Expert comment**
>
> In Europe hard ticks of the *Ixodes ricinus* group can carry pathogenic and non-pathogenic genospecies of *Borrelia burgdorferi* sensu lato (*Bbsl*) and other organisms including *Anaplasma phagocytophilum*, other rickettsias, *Babesia microti*, and tickborne encephalitis (TBE) virus. Co-infections of tick-transmitted pathogens can occur which may modify their clinical presentations.
>
> Ixodid tick blood meals last about 2–7 days depending on life-cycle stage. Ticks require high humidity; they frequently attach in skin folds such as groin, armpit, waistband area, and back of knee, and can easily remain unnoticed.
>
> Lyme borreliosis (LB) is by far the most common tick-transmitted infection in Europe, with well over 100,000 cases estimated to occur annually. TBE does not occur in the United Kingdom but is prevalent in parts of central Europe and Scandinavia and there are small foci in Switzerland.
>
> The erythematous area is very likely to be erythema migrans (EM) so even at this stage it is possible to say that the most likely diagnosis is LB. These events underline the importance of tick- and disease-awareness for both patients and clinicians in the prevention, early recognition, and appropriate management of LB. Avoidance of tick bites, use of insect repellent, and early removal of attached ticks are useful preventive measures, as infected ticks are unlikely to transmit borreliae within the first few hours of attachment. Post-tick bite antibiotic prophylaxis is not routinely recommended in Europe because the majority of ticks are not infected. The significance of the rash was not recognized at the time but early treatment would have prevented progression to later-stage disease. Recent studies have shown excellent short- and long-term outcomes for patients treated for EM [1].

One month later when the rash had resolved he developed pain in his right shoulder with radiation down to his right index finger. His right hand began to swell and became progressively weaker. He saw his general practitioner who gave him a prescription for codeine for the pain and arranged an urgent referral to the neurology department.

Over the next week he developed a mild headache, and fatigue, and noticed he had lost weight over the preceding month. The rash resolved. Before his outpatient appointment a week later he became confused and he presented to the emergency department.

The patient had no relevant past medical history or family history of note. He had a significant alcohol intake of about a bottle of wine per day, although at the time of admission he was not drinking. He was a non-smoker.

On admission he was afebrile and systemic examinations were normal. He appeared confused and scored 8/10 on the Abbreviated Mental Test, losing points on orientation and attention. There was no meningism and cranial nerve examination was unremarkable. He had normal tone in all four limbs and full power in the left upper limb and both lower limbs. In the right arm brachioradialis was weak. Wrist and finger flexion and extension were also weak. The triceps and brachioradialis jerks were diminished, with bilaterally flexor plantar responses. There was hyperaesthesia to light touch over the palm of the right hand with reduced sensation to pin-prick. Joint position and vibration sensation were normal.

To summarize, a 71-year-old man developed a subacute onset of right arm weakness and mild encephalopathy 2 months after a tick bite and subsequent erythematous rash. The subacute onset suggests inflammatory, infective, vasculitic, or compressive aetiologies. However, if the right arm symptoms and encephalopathy were caused by a common process, a compressive lesion would seem unlikely.

Blood tests on admission revealed a sodium level of 120 mmol/L, with the remainder of the renal function being normal. LFTs, bone profile, full blood count, CRP, thyroid function, cortisol, and vitamin B12 levels were normal. The red cell folate level was low at 96 ng/ML. An electrocardiogram (ECG) revealed normal sinus rhythm and a CXR showed minor apical thickening and scarring but was otherwise normal.

In view of the encephalopathy, an MRI of the brain was performed. This showed mild small-vessel disease and involutional change in keeping with the patient's age but no evidence of encephalitis. An electroencephalogram (EEG), performed a few days after admission, demonstrated mild diffuse and symmetrical excess of background activity in keeping with drowsiness or suggestive of low-grade encephalopathy.

⊕ **Clinical tip** Some major causes of encephalopathy (the list is not exhaustive)

Metabolic

- Hypoxia
- Hypoglycaemia
- Diabetic ketoacidosis
- Renal failure
- Liver failure
- Thyroid dysfunction
- Hyperpyrexia
- Systemic sepsis
- Porphyria
- Urea cycle enzyme defects
- Mitochondrial disorders

Infective

- **Viral:** herpes viruses: herpes simplex, varicella zoster, CMV, EBV
  - Human Immunodeficiency virus (HIV)
  - Enterovirus (including entero 71 and polio)
  - Measles, mumps, rubella
  - Influenza A
  - Rabies
  - Arboviruses (dependent on geography): TBE, West Nile, Japanese B encephalitis, eastern, western and Venezuelan equine encephalitis
- **Bacterial:** TB, *Mycoplasma pneumoniae*, listeriosis, brucellosis, *Nocardia* spp, *Salmonella* Typhi
- **Rickettsial:** Rocky Mountain spotted fever, typhus, Q fever, erlichiosis
- **Spirochaete:** LB, syphilis, leptospirosis
- **Fungal:** Cryptococcosis, histoplasmosis, candidiasis, aspergillosis, coccidiomycosis
- **Parasite:** *Falciparum* malaria (FM), toxoplasmosis, schistosomiasis
- **Prion**
- **Post-vaccination and post infectious encephalitis**

Toxic

- Alcohol: Wernicke-Korsakoff's syndrome
- Other drugs of abuse: cocaine, heroin
- Chemotherapeutic agents: methotrexate, cisplatin, vincristine, asparaginase, ifosfamide, 5-fluorouracil/levamisole
- Psychotropic medication: lithium, neuroleptics, tricyclics, fluoxetine, venlafaxine
- Anticholinergics: antiparkinsonian, antipsychotics, antihistamines, antiemetics, benzodiazepines
- Non-steroidal anti-inflammatory drugs
- Opioids
- Others: valproate, vigabatrin, penicillins, cephalosporins

Vascular

- Infarction
- Haemorrhage

Seizures

- Non-convulsive status
- Post-ictal

Possible causes of encephalopathy in this patient included metabolic derangements, including hyponatraemia, nutritional, particularly thiamine deficiency in the context of alcohol excess, and toxins including centrally acting medications such as strong analgesics and alcohol withdrawal. The patient received a course of parenteral followed by oral B vitamins and the codeine was withdrawn. The hyponatraemia resolved with rehydration. Infectious causes were also considered, especially LNB in view of the patient's history of travel, tick bite, and rash. Importantly LNB can be associated with hyponatraemia caused by the syndrome of inappropriate antidiuretic hormone (SIADH) secretion [3] (Box 2.1).

Box 2.1 LB ecology and microbiology [4]

LB is an infection caused by spirochaetes of the (*Bb*) group which are transmitted by hard ticks of the *Ixodes ricinus* complex during a blood meal. Larvae and nymphal ticks usually prey on small mammals and birds, which can be natural reservoir hosts of *Bb*. Adult ticks feed on larger animals including deer or sheep, which are not reservoir-competent but are important in helping to maintain the tick's reproductive cycle. Deer numbers have risen substantially in some regions, associated with increases in tick populations and LB incidence. The disease occurs in temperate regions of the northern hemisphere, mainly in forested, woodland, and heathland areas. The name comes from Lyme, Connecticut, where there was a geographic cluster of juvenile arthritis cases in 1977, initially termed Lyme arthritis. It later became apparent that this was a multi-system disease and that the same disease had been recognized in Europe for more than a century, where it is the most common tickborne infection. *B. burgdorferi* was identified in 1982 and was later cultured from the blood, cerebrospinal fluid (CSF), and skin of patients. At least 17 genospecies of *Bb* have been identified but currently only 5 are regarded as pathogenic. The only genospecies causing disease in North America, *Bb* sensu stricto, is arthritogenic and neurotropic. It also occurs focally in Europe but *B. afzelii* (strongly associated with skin manifestations and infrequently with neurological presentations) and *B. garinii*, which is strongly neurotropic, are the major European pathogenic genospecies. All can cause EM. Another genospecies, *B. valaisiana*, occurs widely in Europe but is apparently non-pathogenic. Geographic variations in European disease incidence and clinical presentations can be linked to variations in distribution of borrelial genospecies.

The signs and symptoms of LB most frequently appear in spring, summer, and early autumn, reflecting the life cycle of ixodid ticks (see Figure 2.1), which feed on blood just once in each of three stages (larva, nymph, and adult tick). Peak feeding periods are spring to midsummer with a secondary peak in autumn. Larvae can become infected with spirochaetes when feeding on an infected host. They then moult into nymphs and feed for a second time, usually from mid-April to late July. Most LB is acquired from nymphs as they are only the size of a poppy seed and are therefore difficult to notice compared to adult ticks, which can reach the size of a coffee bean after feeding.

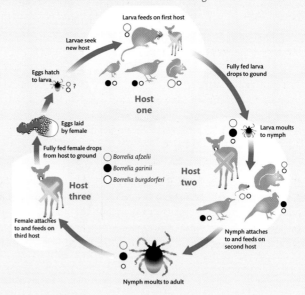

Figure 2.1 Life cycle of **Ixodes** tick

The *Ixodes* tick feeds on blood once in each of its three stages (larva, nymph, and adult tick). Larvae hatch in early spring and become infected with spirochaetes when attached to an infected host. They then moult into nymphs and from mid-April to late July feed for a second time. Before the meal, nymphs are only the size of a poppy seed and therefore difficult to notice. In late summer, the nymphs transform into adults and in autumn feed on a third host prior to reproducing. At this stage they are the size of an apple pip. It is during the second and third feeds that they may transmit *B. burgdorferi* spirochaetes. The size of the coloured closed circles indicates the relative involvement of different vertebrate reservoirs for the different genospecies. A cross indicates a non-reservoir host. Reprinted from *The Lancet*, Volume 379, Issue 9814, Stanek G et al., Lyme borreliosis, pp. 461–473, Copyright © 2012, with permission from Elsevier, http://www.sciencedirect.com/science/journal/01406736.

> ✅ **Evidence base** LB in the UK [4]
>
> Rates of LB diagnosis are increasing in the UK with 959 laboratory-confirmed cases reported in England and Wales in 2011 [5]. The reasons for the increase include increased awareness, better testing and reporting, as well as increased travel and recreational pursuits in areas where ticks are endemic. In the UK cases are most commonly contracted in the New Forest, Devon moors, the Scottish highlands, and Tayside but any area where ticks are present should be regarded as a possible risk area for LB. At least 15% of UK reported cases are contracted abroad, mostly in Europe and America.
>
> 'Neuroborreliosis in the South West of England' is a retrospective study of 88 serologically confirmed cases of LB cases acquired in South West England during the period 2000–2004 [4]. In this area around 600 tests were requested annually.
>
> **Results:** A total of 56 (64%) recalled having a tick bite, and EM (65%) and arthralgia/myalgia (27%) were the most common presenting complaints; 22 (25%) had neurological symptoms (excluding headache) including 14 with (unilateral or bilateral) facial palsy, 8 with confusion/drowsiness (exact cause not stated), 4 with meningism, 5 with radiculopathy, two with sixth nerve palsy. In the 22 neurological cases the median delay between symptoms (neurological or non-neurological) and serological testing was 20 days (IQR 10–32 days) and the median time from symptoms to treatment was 26 days (IQR 9–41). All patients received appropriate antibiotic treatment and had good resolution of symptoms.
>
> **Conclusion:** This study showed that neurological symptoms are common in patients with a diagnosis of LB in the southwest of England. The majority of cases suffered with radiculopathy, facial palsy, and acute meningitis. No cases of late Lyme encephalomyelitis, arthritis, or carditis were identified. Results are similar to the findings of other retrospective and prospective European studies [2].

In view of the patient's right arm problems, an MRI of the cervical spine was performed to exclude a structural cause or multi-radicular pathology. This revealed degenerative changes most marked in the lower cervical spine. There was bilateral foraminal narrowing at C4–C5 more marked on the right, in addition to bilateral foraminal narrowing at C5–C6 and C6–C7. No definite neural compression was seen and no myelitis. The patient's symptoms and signs could not be caused by compression of the right C5, 6, and 7 alone. Some of the muscles involved, as well as the areas of reduced sensation, are innervated by the C8 and T1 roots. These symptoms and signs could be caused by a combination of radial, median, and ulnar nerve involvement or a brachial plexus lesion. The patient underwent neurophysiological studies which revealed reduced sensory and motor action potentials confined to right median and ulnar nerve distributions. The corresponding 'F' responses were also absent, indicating a proximal lesion. There was no indication of conduction block at the common sites of entrapment (the elbow for the ulnar nerve and carpal tunnel for the median nerve). The findings were suggestive of high median and ulnar nerve palsies, indicating a mononeuritis multiplex or a lesion of the lower brachial plexus.

> ➕ **Clinical tip**
> Differential diagnosis of mononeuritis multiplex
>
> **Metabolic:** Diabetes mellitus
> **Infective:** LNB, hepatitis A, C, parvovirus B19, HIV, leprosy
> **Vasculitides:** Wegener's granulomatosis, GCA, cryoglobulinaemia, polyarteritis nodosa, rheumatoid arthritis, Sjögren's disease
> **Other:** sarcoid, amyloidosis, para-neoplastic syndromes

The CXR excluded the presence of a cervical rib and the history was not suggestive of an abscess or haematoma. In view of the patient's history, mononeuritis multiplex (or partial brachial neuritis) secondary to Lyme disease was high on the list of differential diagnoses.

> ➕ **Clinical tip** LNB: Summary of potential historical, clinical, and laboratory findings [6]
>
> **History**
> - Endemic area exposure with time spent outdoors
> - *Ixodid* tick exposure or bite
> - Engorged attached tick
> - EM, or rash suspicious of EM, preceding onset of neurological symptoms
>
> (continued)

- Flu-like symptoms preceding neurological symptoms
- Neurological syndrome with associated systemic symptoms (arthralgia, fatigue, myalgia, palpitations)

Examination

- Systemic involvement (skin, musculoskeletal, cardiovascular, ocular)
- Neurological manifestations, including:
  - Cranial neuropathy, in particular unilateral/bilateral facial nerve palsy
  - Radiculopathy
  - Brachial or lumbar plexopathy
  - Mononeuritis multiplex
  - (Aseptic) meningitis/meningoencephalitis/myelitis

Laboratory

- Serum anti-*B. burgdorferi* antibodies
- Elevated acute phase reactants, LFTs (early infection)
- CSF abnormalities (intrathecal anti-*B. burgdorferi* antibodies, mononuclear pleocytosis, elevated protein)
- Neurophysiology consistent with multifocal radiculopathy, plexopathy, neuropathy
- Abnormal cognitive function tests
- Encephalopathic EEG
- Abnormal ECG (conduction block)

The patient underwent further blood tests and an LP for CSF examination. HIV and syphilis serology were negative. CSF analysis revealed a WCC of 13/mm^3 (predominantly mononuclear cells) and a red cell count of 136/mm^3. The protein level was high at 1.29 g/L with glucose in the normal range at 3.5 mmol/L (serum 5.1 mmol/L). Viral PCR tests for herpes simplex virus (HSV), varicella zoster, and enterovirus were negative, as was TB culture.

A serum sample was sent for *Bb* antibody tests, but as there was a high clinical suspicion of LNB, the patient commenced treatment with intravenous ceftriaxone while results were pending. Serological results revealed that the immunoglobulin M (IgM) immunoblot was positive and immunoglobulin G (IgG) was equivocal, consistent with the clinical history of a recently acquired infection. Unfortunately the CSF sample sent to microbiology was insufficient to enable *Bb* testing.

Expert comment

European LNB is associated with elevated cell count in the CSF, typically 10–1000 leucocytes/mm^3, mainly mononuclear cells. A substantial number of patients have elevated CSF protein and oligoclonal IgG bands [6].

Clinical tip European Federation of Neurological Societies (EFNS) suggested case definitions for LNB [6] (Box 2.2)

Box 2.2

Definite neuroborreliosis	Possible neuroborreliosis*
All three criteria fulfilled	Two criteria fulfilled

1 Neurological symptoms suggestive of LNB without other obvious reasons
2 CSF pleocytosis
3 Intrathecal *B. burgdorferi* antibody production

* If criterion 3 is absent, after a duration of 6 weeks, *Bb* antibodies must be found in the serum. CSF, cerebrospinal fluid.
Reproduced from Å Mygland et al, EFNS guidelines on the diagnosis and management of European Lyme neuroborreliosis, *European Journal of Neurology*, Volume 17, Issue 1, Copyright © 2009 The Author(s). Journal compilation © 2009 EFNS, with permission from John Wiley and Sons Ltd.

⭐ **Learning point** Serological testing in the diagnosis of LB

Borrelial culture and DNA detection methods have a low clinical diagnostic yield and are applied mainly in research settings. Serology is the mainstay of laboratory diagnostic support. The antibody response takes several weeks to evolve and serological tests are not routinely recommended for the diagnosis of EM, which is made primarily on clinical findings, as antibody tests are likely to be negative at this early stage [7]. Laboratory supporting evidence is required for the diagnosis of suspected disseminated manifestations, including LNB. Early-generation enzyme immunoassay (EIA) tests for *Bb* antibodies were poorly specific and led to many misdiagnoses; hence supplemental immunoblot (Western blot) tests were introduced as a second step, allowing more detailed assessment of reactions to *Bb*-specific antigens to improve overall specificity. Sensitive new-generation EIAs based on recombinant antigens are now widely available. They have higher but not perfect specificity, so second-stage immunoblots from reference laboratories remain useful, particularly in cases with difficult clinical features.

The diagnostic sensitivity of ELISA screening assays is around 70–95% in early disseminated LB, depending on disease duration. If an initial test is negative in a patient with suspected early disseminated infection (e.g. facial palsy) a second sample taken 2–3 weeks later should be tested for evidence of seroconversion. Virtually all patients with late-stage manifestations will have detectable antibodies [6,7]. In cases of suspected neuroborreliosis the EFNS guidelines recommend that CSF be evaluated for intrathecal antibody production, in addition to cell count, protein, and oligoclonal bands [6].

The clinical significance of antibody test results must be interpreted carefully in the light of the patient's presentation. Background seroprevalence can range from <1% to over 20% in some European populations [7]. False-positive IgM results are not uncommon in patients with conditions such as rheumatoid arthritis and other inflammatory conditions, and IgM tests should not be used in patients with prolonged duration of symptoms. Positive IgM results in the absence of detectable IgG are highly likely to be false-positive in this setting. Other tests that have poor specificity and have frequently contributed to misdiagnoses include lymphocyte transformation tests (LTTs), live blood microscopy, and unorthodox Western blot methods [2,6,7].

➕ **Clinical tip**

Due to the relatively low specificity of the serological tests for antibodies to *Bb*, testing should be confined to those individuals with a history of potential exposure to ticks in the context of appropriate clinical symptoms.

⭐ **Learning point** Treatment of LB [2]

Evidence-based guidelines and consensus statements for the treatment of Lyme disease have been published by numerous American and European expert groups. The following oral agents are recommended as first-line treatments for all non-neurological presentations: doxycycline, amoxicillin, phenoxymethylpenicillin, or cefuroxime [2]. European Federation of Neurological Sciences guidelines [6] recommend that oral doxycycline is as effective as intravenous ceftriaxone in patients with early LNB confined to the meninges, cranial nerves, nerve roots, or peripheral nerves. They recommend intravenous ceftriaxone for patients with early LNB with encephalitis, myelitis, or vasculitis (2 weeks' treatment) and for late neuroborreliosis (3 weeks). No guidelines recommend prolonged, open-ended, or multiple treatment courses for patients with persistent symptoms following appropriately treated infections.

✅ **Evidence base** Oral doxycycline versus intravenous ceftriaxone for European LNB: a multicentre, non-inferiority, double-blind, randomised trial [8]

Study design: This landmark trial took place across 9 hospitals over 3 years in Norway. It was a randomized doubled blind study of 102 adults with LNB who were randomized to receive 200 mg of oral doxycycline once daily (od) or 2 g of intravenous ceftriaxone for 14 days.

Inclusion criteria: Neurological symptoms suggestive of LNB without any other obvious cause plus one of: CSF WCC of over 5/mL, intrathecal production of specific *B. burgdorferi* antibodies, or acrodermatitis chronicum atrophicans (a late-stage skin condition with associated peripheral neuropathy). All patients were given a composite clinical score (range 0 to 64, 0 = best) based on interview and neurological examination. The primary outcome was reduction in clinical score at 4 months. A clinical score was also obtained at day 13 of treatment and LP for CSF analyses were also obtained and assessed at day 0, day 13, and 4 months. Analysis was per protocol.

(continued)

Results: Results are displayed in Table 2.1. No difference was seen between groups in improvement of clinical score, numbers reporting complete recovery, numbers reporting continuing symptoms, or CSF parameters. When outcomes at 13 days were compared to 4 months they showed that improvement continued after completion of the antibiotic course to 4 months. None of the patients in either group required further antibiotic courses.

Table 2.1 Clinical and laboratory findings

	Doxycycline (n=54)	Ceftriaxone (n=48)
Tick bite recalled	30 (56%)	26 (54%)
EM recalled	17 (31%)	5 (10%)
Mean duration of symptoms (weeks)	10)	8)
Mean CSF WCC	194	178
Bannwarth's syndrome (lymphocytic CSF, radiculopathy, cranial neuropathy)	18 (33%)	12 (25%)
Facial palsy	12 (22%)	9 (19%)
Other cranial neuropathies	2 (4%)	3 (6%)
Radiculopathy	13 (24%)	18 (38%)
Arm paresis	1 (2%)	1 (2%)
Cognitive deficiency	0 (0%)	1 (2%)
Only subjective complaints (incl. memory problems)	4 (7%)	4 (8%)
Mean clinical score improvement at 4 months (difference between groups p = 0.84 not significant)	4.5 (95% CI 3.6–5.5)	4.4 (95% CI 3.4–5.4)
Total number to report full recovery at 4 months (difference between groups p = 0.13 not significant)	26 (48%)	16 (33%)
Residual symptoms at 4 months (difference between groups p = 0.13 not significant)	28% (52%)	32 (67%)

Source: Data from *Lancet Neurology*, Volume 7, Issue 8, Ljostad U., et al., Oral doxycycline versus intravenous ceftriaxone for European neuroborreliosis: a multi-centre non-inferiority, double-blind randomised trial, pp. 690–695, Copyright © 2008 Elsevier Ltd. All rights reserved.

Additional follow-up studies of patients enrolled in this trial have continued to show non-inferiority of oral doxycycline versus parenteral ceftriaxone and that severity, CSF WCC, and longer duration of illness prior to treatment are predictors of poorer outcome [9].

How this study relates to our patient

The results suggest that a patient with radiculopathy due to LB contracted in Europe could be treated with oral doxycycline rather than parenteral ceftriaxone. Furthermore, although the results are not significantly different between groups, there is a trend for better results with doxycycline.

Our patient had some encephalopathic features which might have been directly caused by borrelial CNS infection, therefore we followed the EFNS guidelines [6], which recommend parenteral ceftriaxone in the management of encephalitis as there are insufficient clinical trial outcome data currently available on doxycycline in Lyme encephalitis or encephalomyelitis.

The trial results show that improvement can be slow, suggesting that our patient may continue to improve over the next few months.

> **⊕ Clinical tip**
>
> There is a potential risk of Jarisch-Herxheimer reaction when antibiotic treatment is commenced for LB. It occurs within the first few hours of treatment and is thought to be triggered by release of spirochaetal lipoproteins. The patient can have fever, rigors, hypotension, tachycardia, flushing, hyperventilation, myalgia, headache, and exacerbation of skin lesions. It is self-limiting, usually lasting 12–24 hours. Some practitioners choose to treat prophylactically with aspirin (e.g. 4-hourly for 1–2 days) or prednisolone, particularly if treatment is commenced in the outpatient setting.

The patient improved clinically with a 3-week course of ceftriaxone 2 g daily. His headache resolved and the encephalopathy improved, although there was still some impairment in concentration. A repeat EEG 10 weeks following treatment revealed a mild excess of background non-specific slow wave activity, which might reflect a degree of residual cerebral dysfunction.

He had improvement in power at the elbow and wrist, although there was continued significant weakness of the intrinsic muscles of the hand and he had ongoing neuropathic pain, requiring pregabalin. He continues to take pregabalin but his requirements are reducing and he has been referred to the physiotherapy department for further rehabilitation of his hand.

Discussion

This patient presented with subacute onset of mononeuritis multiplex and encephalopathy, with a history of a tick bite sustained 2 months previously in an area endemic for LB. He satisfied the clinical and laboratory criteria for a diagnosis of possible LNB due to the lack of data on CSF *Bb* antibodies. He received intravenous ceftriaxone treatment for LNB, with some improvement in all of the clinical features. LB can be associated with a wide array of neurological features localizing particularly to the peripheral nervous system including radiculopathy, plexopathy, and neuropathy, especially mononeuritis multiplex as in the case presented here. Cranial neuropathies are also common, especially the facial nerve, which may be affected bilaterally. All are usually associated with a CSF pleocytosis.

The central nervous system can also be affected by LNB in various ways. Lymphocytic meningitis occurs frequently, but meningoencephalitis and other manifestations are less common. Encephalomyelitis occurs in approximately 0.1% of infected, untreated patients [9]. MRI may reveal white matter changes resembling those seen in multiple sclerosis. Regardless of the antimicrobial agent used, recovery may be incomplete, especially if severe damage has occurred prior to treatment.

Some patients with disseminated LB experience difficulties with memory and information processing, but have normal neurological examinations, imaging, and CSF findings. This seems to be similar to toxic-metabolic encephalopathies seen in other systemic inflammatory conditions, probably mediated by the entry of cytokines and other neuro-immunomodulators into the CNS, and may have been a feature of our patient's presentation. It usually resolves gradually after appropriate antimicrobial therapy [10,11]. Our patient had several possible factors contributing to his encephalopathic features. In the case this had little consequence except that he was cautiously treated with intravenous ceftriaxone rather than oral doxycycline with all the risks associated with intravenous administration.

Most patients with features of early LB, such as EM, facial palsy, and other manifestations of early LNB, do not present particular difficulties in diagnosis and management as long as a tick exposure risk is sought and the possibility of *Bb* infection is recognized. A group of patients providing more difficult clinical challenges are those who have been referred with a diagnosis of 'chronic Lyme disease'. This term is applied to quite varying patient groups [12,13], including those with untreated late-stage infection or permanent damage despite treatment—usually late LNB or peripheral neuropathy associated with ACA—and to patients with persistent subjective symptoms following treatment ('post-Lyme syndrome' (PLS)).

Prospective studies of patients treated for EM have shown excellent short- and long-term outcomes, with no excess of subjective symptoms when compared to matched controls [1]. Following disseminated LB some patients experience persistent symptoms including fatigue, arthralgia, myalgia, headache, paraesthesia, sleep disturbance, irritability, and concentration difficulties, and termed PLS. These symptoms usually resolve over a period of months. It is not uncommon to develop a post-infective fatigue syndrome following other systemic infections, where the severity of the fatigue syndrome may be predicted by the severity of the acute illness [14]. Occurrence rates of PLS are similar to those of post-infective fatigue syndrome in other infections. Furthermore, trials of prolonged antibiotic treatment in patients with persistent symptoms following LB have failed to show sustained benefit or laboratory evidence for persisting infection [12,13]. Reflecting this, no set of guidelines recommends prolonged, open-ended or multiple treatment courses for patients with persistent symptoms following appropriately treated infections.

The term 'chronic Lyme disease' is also incorrectly applied to patients with a prior history of Lyme disease who have a current medical condition wrongly attributed to Lyme and to some patients with no clinical or laboratory evidence of either current or past infection. One study of 240 patients diagnosed with 'chronic Lyme disease' referred to a specialist centre demonstrated that just 19% had active Lyme disease and 10% had PLS [15]. The remainder of the cohort, 71%, had no evidence for current or prior infection. Despite this, over 65% of these patients had received at least one course of antibiotics, with some receiving multiple courses of parenteral antibiotics over months or years. Factors leading to misdiagnoses included the use of unorthodox and poorly specific clinical case definitions and of unreliable tests or laboratories. It is important to consider the potential harm of multiple courses of unnecessary parenteral antibiotics, in addition to the effect of failure to address the true cause of an individual's symptoms. It is also important to remember that patients in all categories will require time and discussion as they are likely to have accessed misleading and sometimes distressing information on the internet.

The patient presented here made substantial clinical improvement following an appropriate course of treatment for early LNB. Further improvement would be expected with time and supportive and symptomatic treatment, including physiotherapy and occupational therapy.

A final word from the expert

Extensive research into LB has been carried out over the past 40 years, and the natural history of the disease, its diagnosis, and clinical management are well established. This case usefully illustrates several practical points related to LB.

Awareness of the risks associated with tick bites and the measures needed for preventing them remains low in the UK. The significance of EM rashes is often unrecognized and the opportunity for early and highly effective treatment can be missed. Each year about 20% of laboratory-confirmed cases of LB in the UK are known to have been acquired abroad, usually recreationally, underlining the importance of assessing a patient's travel and tick exposure risk history.

Peripheral nerve lesions are a common feature of LNB but Lyme is frequently overlooked in the differential unless the patient lives in a Lyme-endemic area, where there is greater clinical awareness of the condition. Delayed diagnosis and treatment can result in prolonged pain and delayed or incomplete neurological recovery, especially in older patients.

Rare presentations of LNB include a chronic encephalomyelitis which can clinically resemble multiple sclerosis. Patients characteristically have CSF pleocytosis and strongly positive Bb IgG reactions in CSF and serum. Antibiotic treatment is effective in eradicating infection but clinical recovery can be slow and incomplete in severely affected patients, again underlining the importance of early diagnosis and treatment in preventing progression to this severe complication.

Further research into PLS could lead to improvements in its management and might be useful in the understanding of causative mechanisms of post-infection syndromes in general.

References

1 Stupica D, Lusa L, Ruzic-Sabljic E, Cerar T, Strle F. Treatment of erythema migrans with doxycycline for 10 days versus 15 days. *Clin Infect Dis* 2012; 55: 343–350.

2 Stanek G, Wormer GP, Gray J, Strle F. Lyme borreliosis. *Lancet* 2011; 379: 461–473.

3 Perkins MP, Shumway M, Jackson WL. Lyme neuroborreliosis presenting as syndrome of inappropriate antidiuretic hormone secretion. *Med Gen Med* 2006; (8)3: 71.

4 Health Protection Agency. Epidemiology of Lyme borreliosis http://www.hpa.org. uk/Topics/InfectiousDiseases/InfectionsAZ/LymeDisease/EpidemiologicalData/ lymLymeepidemiology/. Accessed 04 March 2014.

5 Lovett JK, Evans PH, O'Connell S, Gutowski NJ. Neuroborreliosis in the South West of England. *Epidemiol Infect* 2008; 136: 1707–1711.

6 Mygland Å, Ljøstad U, Fingerle V, Rupprecht T, Schmutzhard E, Steiner I. EFNS guidelines on the diagnosis and management of European Lyme neuroborreliosis. *Eur J Neurol* 2010; 17: 8–16.

7 Wilske B, Fingerle V, Schulte-Spechtel U. Microbiological and serological diagnosis of Lyme borreliosis. *FEMS Immunol Med Microbiol* 2007; 49: 13–21.

8 Ljostad U, Skogwall E, Eikeland R et al. Oral doxycycline versus intravenous ceftriaxone for European neuroborreliosis: a multi-centre non-inferiority, double-blind randomised trial. *Lancet Neurol* 2008; 7: 690–695.

9 Eikeland R, Myland A, Herlofson K, Ljostad U. Risk factors for a non-favourable outcome after treated European neuroborreliosis. *Acta Neurol Scand* 2013; 127: 154–160.

10 Halperin JJ. Nervous system involvement. In: Halperin JJ. Ed. *Lyme disease; an evidence-based approach*. CAB International 2011: pp208–220.

11 Halperin JJ, Baker P, Wormser GP. Common misconceptions about Lyme disease. *Am J Med* 2013; 126: 264.e1–7.

12 O'Connell S. Lyme borreliosis: current issues in diagnosis and management. *Curr Opin Infect Dis* 2010; 23: 231–235.

13 Marques A. Chronic Lyme disease: a review. *Infect Dis Clin N Am* 2008; 22: 341–360.

14 Hickie I, Davenport T, Wakefield D et al. Post-infective and chronic fatigue syndromes precipitated by viral and non-viral pathogens: prospective scohort study. *BMJ* 2006; 333: 575–581.

15 Hassett AL, Radvanski DC, Buyske S, Savage SV, Sigal SH. Psychiatric comorbidity and other psychological factors in patients with 'chronic Lyme disease'. *Am J Med* 2009; 122: 843–850.

Leptospirosis and its complications

Nicholas Easom and Amber Arnold

⟨⟨ Expert commentary David Moore

Case history

A 30-year-old woman born in the United Kingdom presented to the emergency department with a 3-day history of fever and rigors. She also described a headache with retro-orbital pain, myalgia with severe lower back pain, abdominal pain in the morning, and nausea with a single episode of vomiting. She had noticed that her left eye had become red a day before. There was no history of rash, diarrhoea, urinary symptoms, or cough.

She had returned 6 days earlier from a 2-week holiday in Laos, Vietnam, and Thailand, travelling with a friend who was well. They had spent most of their time on beaches and in cities but had also swum in a river and had been caving.They did not have any animal contacts or tick bites.

> **⟨⟨ Expert comment**
>
> Conditions associated with fever and freshwater exposure in Asia include Katayama fever (*Schistosoma* spp), melioidosis (*Burkholderia pseudomallei*), and leptospirosis (*Leptospira interrogans*). A history of freshwater exposure in a patient with undifferentiated fever should prompt consideration of leptospirosis but the absence of such a history should not discourage the diagnosis where the clinical picture is consistent. With growing recognition of the wide epidemiological scope of this disease, the resulting increase in the number and range of patients being tested (and diagnosed) starts to blur the conventionally crisp image of leptospirosis.

The patient had no significant past medical history and was not taking medications other than malarone for malaria prophylaxis, which she had tolerated well and taken as prescribed. The woman reported smoking on holiday but not when she was in the UK.

On examination the patient was noted to appear unwell. Observations revealed a temperature of 36.8°C, blood pressure 104/62, respiratory rate 20 breaths/min, oxygen saturations 98%, and she was tachycardic at 110 bpm. Clinical examination was unremarkable except that conjunctival injection was observed. Her chest was clear and there were no other localizing signs on examination of other systems. An ECG showed a sinus tachycardia. She was admitted to the ID ward.

> **⊕ Clinical tip**
>
> Despite normal chest examination and no reported respiratory symptoms all patients with an undifferentiated fever should have a chest X ray as part of their workup.

Routine blood tests including blood cultures and an urgent malaria film were performed. Urine dipstick tests were clear for leucocytes and nitrites; a urine sample was not sent to the laboratory for culture. A pregnancy test was negative. The malaria film was also negative. The clinical impression at this point was of likely dengue fever or typhoid. The patient, however, felt too unwell to go home and the raised inflammatory markers were a concern and so she was admitted to hospital for overnight observation (Table 3.1).

Table 3.1 Blood results on admission

Hb	13.3 g/dL	Sodium	139 mmol/L
WCC	8.42 × 10⁹/L	Potassium	4.3 mmol/L
Neutrophils	7.58 × 10⁹/L	Urea	4.7 mmol/L
Lymphocytes	0.42 × 10⁹/L	Creatinine	67 µmol/L
Eosinophils	0.15 × 10⁹/L	ALP	95 iu/L
Platelet count	153 × 10⁹/L	ALT	83 iu/L
ESR	106 mm/h	Bilirubin	13 µmol/L
		Albumin	38 g/L
		CRP	312.5 mg/L

➕ **Clinical tip** Differential diagnosis and liaison with local and reference laboratories

Differential diagnosis

- Viral: influenza, dengue, HIV seroconversion
- Bacterial: UTI, community acquired/atypical pneumonia, tonsillitis, typhoid, melioidosis
- Parasite: malaria, Katayama fever (acute schistosomiasis)
- Rickettsial: scrub typhus
- Spirochaete: Lyme disease, secondary syphilis

Pick up the phone! In cases such as this with a broad differential and where many of the key diagnostic tests (dengue serology) are sent to a reference laboratory, it is always helpful to contact both the local and reference laboratories directly. Once the microbiologists are interested in your case it is often possible for them to perform tests more quickly, help you with the differential diagnosis and suggest further tests, and to convey the results back as soon as they become available.

The patient deteriorated overnight and was found to have a fever of 39°C, a pulse rate of 130 bpm, and oxygen saturations on air of 83%. The nursing team instigated high flow oxygen and the medical team were called urgently. On examination bilateral coarse crepitations were heard on auscultation of the chest with decreased air entry at

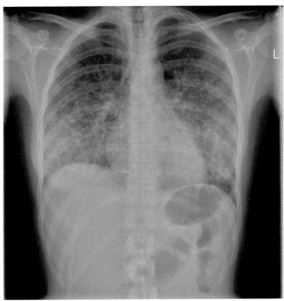

Figure 3.1 Chest radiograph performed on the second day of admission which demonstrates bilateral patchy infiltrates.

the right lung base. Arterial blood gas analysis confirmed hypoxia with a pO_2 of 6.85 kPa. The pH was normal at 7.4 but there was a mild metabolic acidosis with a base excess of -3.8 mmol/L. The chest radiograph demonstrated widespread bilateral intra-alveolar shadowing more confluent in both mid and lower zones (Figure 3.1). Oxygen saturations improved with high flow oxygen, and intravenous cefuroxime and clarithromycin and IV fluids were commenced as per the local protocol for severe pneumonia.

⊕ **Clinical tip** Causes of bilateral airspace shadowing on CXR

Non-infective

- Pulmonary oedema, e.g. intravenous fluid overload, cardiac failure
- Adult respiratory distress syndrome (ARDS)
- Pulmonary haemorrhage: vasculitis, Wegener's granulomatosis, microscopic polyangiitis, connective tissue disorders
- Sarcoidosis
- Pulmonary embolus
- Malignancy

Infective

- Bacterial: *Mycoplasma* and *Legionella* pneumonia, Gram-negative pneumonias (e.g. *K. pneumoniae*, staphylococcal pneumonia*
- Mycobacteria: TB
- Viral: influenza*, respiratory syncytial virus, varicella zoster virus, dengue*, adenovirus, CMV, HSV, Hantavirus pulmonary syndrome*
- Fungal: PCP, disseminated candidiasis, invasive *Aspergillus*
- Spirochaetes: leptospirosis*
- Parasite: malaria*

* Infectious agents which may cause diffuse airspace shadowing via pulmonary haemorrhage in immunocompetent adults.

The next morning the patient became increasingly hypoxic with a pO_2 of 7.98 on 35% inspired oxygen. Blood tests also deteriorated with a rise in creatinine level to 192 μmol/L. The patient was transferred to the intensive care unit (ICU). The intensive care physicians discussed with the microbiologist on call whether to change the antibiotics. At this stage a severe community-acquired pneumonia was still the principal clinical differential diagnosis. Before escalating antibiotics an urgent legionella antigen and HIV test were perfomed, which were negative, and so neither a fluoroquinolone nor PCP treatment was added. Doxycycline was added for the possibility of rickettsial infection. A long discussion about whether to escalate the cefuroxime to ceftazidine or meropenem to cover melioidosis was initiated but, as the patient was improving on the ICU, it was decided to hold off this change.

❝ **Expert comment**

Management of patients with undifferentiated fever should always take account of reported prior epidemiological exposures. Specific additional diagnoses to consider in travellers returning from Asia include scrub typhus (and other rickettsial diseases), melioidosis (highly endemic in focal areas, particularly well described in northern Thailand, but rare in travellers), and a range of arboviral (e.g. dengue, chikungunya) and other viral (e.g. influenza) infections. Addition of empiric doxycycline to a broad-spectrum antibiotic regimen is often justified in sick patients where rickettsial disease is a possibility.

The microbiologist suggested sending nasopharyngeal swabs for respiratory viral PCR and serology for mycoplasma, coxiella, chlamydia, and leptospirosis. A pneumococcal urinary antigen test was negative.

Over the following days the patient improved and was discharged from the ICU after 2 days. On the sixth day of her admission the leptospira reference laboratory reported the leptospira IgM result by telephone, which was positive at 1:640 on the admission sample, confirming a diagnosis of severe leptospirosis. At this point the antibiotics were narrowed to intravenous benzyl penicillin to complete a 10-day course. She was discharged home on day 10. On discharge the patient explained that she was a keen swimmer and took part in triathlons where she had to swim in lakes and rivers. The patient was concerned whether she should continue this activity and asked about the risk from swimming in rivers in the UK. The senior house officer who discharged her said she would look it up and they would discuss it at her clinic appointment in a week's time (Box 3.1).

Learning point Time course and microbiological diagnosis of leptospirosis

Following exposure to *L. interrogans* there is an incubation period of between 1 week and 1 month before the onset of symptoms, usually beginning with sudden onset of fever. Myalgia (lumbar area and calves) and headache are the most common symptoms in this early 'septicaemic' phase. Nausea, vomiting, and conjunctival suffusion are also common.

After a few days the symptoms resolve as antibody responses develop. The illness may end there or may progress after 3–10 days to the immunological phase (see Figure 3.2), with return of fever and myalgia and the sudden onset of complications including renal failure, jaundice, pulmonary haemorrhage, and aseptic meningitis. There may be two distinct phases, or the phases may run together as in this case.

Diagnosis is possible by a variety of methods at different stages of illness. Direct visualization of leptospires by dark-field microscopy of blood (first week) or urine (from the second week) can be performed but has a low sensitivity and specificity. PCR assays have been developed and applied to a range of bodily fluids pre- and post-mortem. These are not yet well evaluated in the clinical setting but offer the promise of early diagnosis, when treatment is likely to be of greatest benefit (see Evidence base: Penicillin in late-stage leptospirosis—a randomized controlled trial (RCT)), and diagnosis of fulminant disease, where death occurs before seroconversion. Culture of leptospires from blood and CSF is possible, but requires special media and growth may take several weeks. Cultures must be taken within the first 10 days. Leptospires can be cultured from urine after the first week of illness but urine must be collected and processed within 1 hour as leptospires survive poorly in acidic environments.

Most diagnoses are made by the microscopic agglutination test (MAT) or IgM serology. A positive MAT requires a four-fold increase in titre between acute and convalescent serum. The MAT uses a panel of serogroups, so in the convalescent phase it is possible to infer the infecting serogroup. A single titre of 1:800 or greater in the context of a compatible illness is strongly suggestive of recent infection. Up to 10% of patients have delayed seroconversion of 30 days or more, and false-positives are possible with a number of conditions including HIV and the spirochaetes responsible for syphilis and Lyme disease. IgM can be detected by ELISA after 5–7 days from the onset of illness, and is more sensitive than MAT early in the illness. It is also a simpler test to perform, but unlike the MAT cannot offer information about the infecting serogroup.

Discussion

This case represents the major challenges of diagnosis and management of a patient with fever due to leptospirosis returning from Asia. Leptospirosis is a multi-system disease with a variety of presentations and can be very difficult to diagnose, especially in mild disease or early stages [5]. There is scant evidence to guide ideal management, and although antibiotics are recommended there is no clear data to suggest they make a significant difference to the outcome [6,7,8].

Box 3.1 Infection control

In the UK there are about 30–60 confirmed cases each year (~1 per million population). In 2010 there were 39 confirmed cases of which 17 were acquired overseas and 14 of these were acquired in South East Asia (including Thailand). Most were associated with water sports or accidental water contact rather than contact with animals. Of the 22 that were acquired in the UK, 10 were occupationally acquired: 7 had direct contact with cattle, sheep, or other mammals (4 farmers, 2 abattoir workers, 1 game keeper) and 3 were in contact with water (1 carpenter, 1 builder, 1 rowing instructor). The others were related to non-occupational activities: 4 had contact with rivers (1 canoeist and 3 recreational fishermen) and the others had contact with rats, mice, or contaminated sewers [1].

Immunity is largely serovar-specific and so the patient would be at risk of reinfection by different serovars in the UK. The risk of acquiring infection in UK rivers is low. Stagnant water, warmer weather, and heavy rains increase the risks. In a case–control study of an outbreak after a triathlon in Springfield, USA, swallowing water was the main risk factor for infection [2]. It is also thought that open cuts and abrasions increase the risk, and cuts should prevented by wearing footwear in the water or be covered with water-resistant protection if present before entering the water. Showering after exposure is also recommended. One trial of antibiotic prophylaxis in soldiers suggests that 200 mg of doxycycline once a week is effective [3]; however, this finding has not been replicated in another trial in residents in an endemic area. A recent Cochrane review did not show definite benefit [4]. There is also no evidence that secondary prophylaxis is effective [4]. However, early treatment should be sought if the patient were to become unwell 7–14 days after entering the water. There is no vaccine available in the UK.
Since 2010 leptospirosis is no longer a notifiable disease.

⊕ **Learning point** Epidemiology

Leptospirosis is a globally distributed zoonosis caused by *Leptospira interrogans*, a spirochaete. The leptospires are excreted in the urine of usually asymptomatic carrier mammals, and infect humans through contact with animal urine or indirect contact with contaminated water. Leptospires enter the body through mucous membranes, intestinal tract, conjunctiva, and broken skin. Some serovars are widespread, most notably serovar *icterohaemorrhagiae*, which is ubiquitous and causes most infection in the UK. This serovar is associated with the *Rattus* species of rat as well as other mammals. In Asia serovar *lai* is common. No association has been found between illness course or mortality and serovar type.

Leptospirosis is primarily a disease of tropical and subtropical regions due to increased survival of the leptospires in warmer climates as well as poor quality drinking and washing water [9]. Outbreaks in the tropics are more likely after heavy rainfall. In one case series in the Peruvian Amazon city of Iquitos, leptospirosis accounted for 20–30% of presentations of acute undifferentiated fever [5]. The disease is less common in temperate regions but is more common in the summer or autumn when water temperatures are higher.

✓ **Evidence base** Leptospirosis—prognostic factors associated with mortality

A retrospective analysis of 68 patients with serology-confirmed severe leptospirosis admitted to the Teaching Hospital of Pointe-a-Pitre in the French West Indies between 1989 and 1993 [10]. Leptospirosis was diagnosed by serology.

Method: Admission symptoms, chest radiography, ECG, and laboratory findings for the 56 survivors (82%) were compared to those of the 12 non-survivors (18%) and risk factors for death established. Multivariate logistic regression was used to establish risk factors independently associated with death.

Results: Death was due to myocarditis (4 patients), irreversible septic shock (2), acute respiratory failure (2), single organ failure (2), and multiple organ failure (2).

A total of 17 features were found to be significantly different in the non-survivors compared to the survivors including higher bilirubin, creatinine kinase, aspartate transaminase (AST), and lactate ranges. However, only five factors were independently associated by multivariate logistic regression: these were dyspnoea, oliguria, high white blood cell count, repolarization abnormalities on ECG, and alveolar infiltrates on chest radiography.

This case illustrates the broad differential in the early, 'septicaemic' phase as well as in the immunological phase of leptospirosis (Figure 3.2).

The early differential includes influenza, dengue, other acute viral illness, malaria, typhoid, and rickettsial infections. In terms of clinical findings only conjunctival suffusion, which has been reported to occur in 30–99% of hospitalized cases in the developing world but only 16% in a French case series, is specific to leptospirosis [11,12]. The other symptoms of myalgia and headache are common to all the differential diagnoses. As in our case, routine blood results are also not very helpful in discriminating between these diagnoses. In our case there is a mildly raised ALT but this finding is common in viral infections as well as typhoid and malaria. The renal function is normal, which is common in early leptospirosis. The platelets are at the lower end of normal; however, again, this could fit with viral infection including dengue or malaria. Significant levels of thrombocytopenia can occur in leptospirosis and again this finding would not differentiate dengue [10,12]. The leucocyte count may or may not be elevated in most of these infections. These non-specific clinical and laboratory findings emphasize the importance of the history of exposure.

In this case the patient was admitted for observations at the early stage and was not immediately given antibiotics. One question that arises from the case is whether she might not have deteriorated if she had been given antibiotics sooner. Although current WHO guidelines [13] recommend treating severe leptospirosis with benzylpenicillin and mild disease with doxycycline or another appropriate oral antibiotic, there have been few trials that show that antibiotics improve outcome. In a recent meta-analysis of seven trials (four comparing penicillin to placebo and three comparing different antibiotics with each other) no significant mortality benefit was found in the groups receiving antibiotics compared to placebo. All of the trials were judged to contain a significant risk of bias, and in only two of the four trials comparing antibiotic against placebo were there any deaths, making a true comparison of outcomes very difficult. There was a trend towards decreased duration of illness of around two days in the patients receiving antibiotics [6].

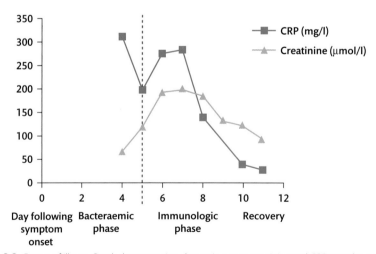

Figure 3.2 Course of illness. Graph demonstrating change in serum creatinine and CRP over the course of the illness. The patient underwent a marked deterioration in clinical condition on the fifth day of her illness (the second day following admission) with marked hypoxia, bilateral CXR changes, and worsening renal impairment despite fluid resuscitation. This is typical of the immunological phase of leptospirosis.

Our patient was eventually treated the next day with cefotaxime. Would penicillin have been a better option if leptospirosis had been considered earlier? One trial included in the Cochrane review demonstrated no difference between penicillin G and cefotaxime [8].The Cochrane review found no difference between antibiotic regimens including penicillins, cephalosporins, doxycycline, or azithromycin although increased risk of adverse events (GI upset) was found in one of the doxycycline trials.

In our case a CXR was performed relatively late in the patient's admission. Considering that the patient had a raised respiratory rate at presentation and she was admitted with no diagnosis, a CXR should have been performed earlier. Respiratory complications in leptospirosis are common [14] in the immunological stage of leptospirosis and have been found to be associated with poor prognosis [15]. Considering that the main complications from leptospirosis are thought to arise in the immunologically mediated stage, steroids have been considered as adjunct to antibiotics. In a large case series from an outbreak in Sri Lanka, high death rates prompted the hospital to treat severe cases with a bolus of methylprednisolone. Mortality rates improved but it is unclear what other changes in management were instituted over the same time period [16]. A recent randomized, open-label, multicentre trial from Thailand with three arms—standard care plus dexamethasone, standard care plus desmopressin, and a control arm—showed no significant difference in mortality (although numbers were low and there was a trend towards increased mortality in the desmopressin arm) but did demonstrate a significant increase in nosocomial infection in the dexamethasone group [17].

⭐ **Learning point** Leptospirosis and the lung

Pulmonary involvement is common in both icteric and anicteric leptospirosis, with rates of respiratory symptoms in the range 30–70% and radiographic changes noted in a similar percentage [11,14]. Symptoms include dyspnoea, cough, and pulmonary haemorrhage. The most common radiographic changes are bilateral patchy alveolar infiltrates in the lower lobes. Both dyspnoea and alveolar infiltrates are poor prognostic features of severe leptospirosis (Evidence base: Leptospirosis—prognostic factors associated with mortality). The exact pathophysiology of pulmonary involvement is not known but on post-mortem the lungs show areas of haemorrhage [14].

One retrospective study suggested that smoking history (>20 per day) is a risk factor for pulmonary involvement [18]. It may be possible to identify patients at high risk of pulmonary haemorrhage by use of a prediction model that combines clinical features and laboratory tests but the published scoring systems are cumbersome and so are unlikely to be used in routine practice [19]. Therefore clinically all patients suspected of leptospirosis should have a CXR and careful monitoring with transfer to ICU if decline in respiratory function is observed. Management is supportive.

✅ **Evidence base** Penicillin at the late stage of leptospirosis—a RCT [6]

Study design: An unblinded RCT of penicillin treatment in 253 patients admitted to hospital with late-stage leptospirosis in Brazil from 1997–1999. Late-stage was defined as more than 4 days from symptom onset.

Inclusion criteria: Eligible participants had more than 4 days of symptoms and scored 26 points or more on the WHO probability score for leptospirosis. Diagnosis was confirmed with the macroscopic slide test, the microagglutination test (MAT), and *Leptospira* blood cultures.

Method: Participants were randomized to the penicillin treatment (n= 125) or control (n = 128) arms. Patients in the treatment arm received penicillin at a dose of 1 million units 4-hourly. Baseline characteristics of the two groups were similar except with regard to leucocyte count on admission. Logistic regression was used to adjust for baseline differences in leucocyte count.

Results: There were 23 deaths, 14 (60.9%) due to renal failure, 1 (4.3%) due to respiratory failure, and 8 (34.8%) due to multi-organ failure. Ten deaths (44%) occurred in the first 3 days following admission. All of the patients who died were jaundiced.

There were 15 deaths in the penicillin arm and 8 in the control arm, giving an odds ratio (OR) for death in the treatment arm of 2.04 (95% confidence interval (CI) 0.83–5.01, p= 0.118). Length of hospital stay was very similar in the two groups: 9.4 ± 3.5 and 9.0 ± 3.4 days in the penicillin and control groups, respectively.

Conclusion: This is the largest trial of antibiotic use in leptospirosis and does not support the use of antibiotics in late-stage leptospirosis.

⊕ **Clinical tip** Complications of leptospirosis

Clinical manifestations of leptospirosis range from a mild, self-limiting febrile illness (90% of cases) to severe disease with life-threatening manifestations [11]. Consider this diagnosis in any patient with an appropriate exposure history (incubation 5–14 days) and any of the following complications:

- Jaundice (5–10%)
- Pulmonary involvement (30–70%)
- Acute renal impairment (16–40% renal tubular necrosis and interstitial nephritis)
- Shock (rare)
- Meningitis (≤25% higher rates in children)
- Cardiac involvement (myocarditis or conduction defects) (rare)
- Weil's syndrome (jaundice, renal failure and haemorrhagic pneumonitis) (5%)
- Uveitis (2%–40%; can present weeks, months, or years afterwards)
- Death (4–20%)

Most cases are probably asymptomatic and percentages relate to case series of severe cases.

The patient in the case improved and was discharged home despite having risk factors for a poor outcome. Mortality rates in severe disease are in the range 0–20% depending on the location of the series and which patients are classified as severe [10,12,15,20]. There is some evidence to suggest that the outcomes in the developed world are improved; however, it is unclear which interventions (renal support, transfusion of blood and blood products, high flow oxygen and ventilatory support, invasive monitoring, and cardiovascular support) contribute to improved mortality [12].

A final word from the expert

The fact that infections with *Leptospira* sp. may pass largely unnoticed—either asymptomatic or as a mild self-limiting febrile illness—is evidenced by the high seroprevalence reported in many populations living in daily contact with contaminated freshwater. However, the spectrum of disease extends from acute, undifferentiated fever through to severe, life-threatening, multi-organ failure in the eponymous (and rare) Weil's disease.

There is no doubt that leptospirosis is enormously underdiagnosed—the relative frequency of disease severity can be viewed as a pyramid with probably the vast majority of infections causing only trivial symptoms, if any at all (at the pyramid base), a smaller proportion leading to illness sufficient to provoke contact with healthcare services, a minority requiring hospital admission, and a tiny tip to the pyramid representing the infrequent, serious, sometimes fatal cases.

Respiratory complications, particularly haemorrhage, are increasingly recognized and may occur in the absence of jaundice, which lessens the chance that leptospirosis may be considered in the differential diagnosis. In general leptospire numbers in lung tissue are considerably lower than in liver or blood, prompting hypotheses that pulmonary damage may be toxin or immune mediated.

Management of patients with undifferentiated fever should always take account of reported prior epidemiological exposures. Many patients with leptospirosis can recall freshwater exposure but this history is often only elicited on direct questioning—if you don't ask you won't be told—and a lack of such reported exposure does not rule out the diagnosis.

The lack of a rapid, point-of-care diagnostic test and very limited access to laboratory testing means that empiric treatment with presumptive or, at best, retrospective serological diagnosis is the rule.

Since leptospirosis is usually self-limiting, the need for specific antibiotic therapy is debated, though in serious disease the restrictive approach is less easily taken. Organisms are susceptible to most antibiotic classes—penicillins and doxycycline are most commonly used.

References

1 Health Protection Agency. *Leptospira infections in 2010*. Published 2011. Available from http://www.hpa.org.uk/Topics/InfectiousDiseases/InfectionsAZ/Leptospirosis/EpidemiologicalData/lepto005EpiData2010/ (accessed 9 Oct 2013).

2 Morgan J, Bornstein SL, Karpati AM et al. Outbreak of leptospirosis among triathlon participants and community residents in Springfield, Illinois, 1998. *Clin Infect Dis* 2002; 34: 1593–1599.

3 Takafuji ET, Kirkpatrick JW, Miller RN et al. An efficacy trial of doxycycline chemoprophylaxis against leptospirosis. *N Eng J Med* 1984; 310: 497–500.

4 Brett-Major DM, Lipnick RJ. Antibiotic prophylaxis for leptospirosis. *Cochrane Database Syst Rev* 2009, Issue 3. Art. No.: CD007342. DOI: 10.1002/14651858.CD007342.pub2.

5 Bharti AR, Nally JE, Ricaldi JN et al. Leptospirosis: a zoonotic disease of global importance. *Lancet Infect Dis* 2003; (3): 757–771.

6 Brett-Major DM, Coldren R. Antibiotics for leptospirosis. *Cochrane Database Syst Rev* 2012, Issue 2. Art. No.: CD008264. DOI: 10.1002/14651858.CD008264.pub2.

7 Costa E, Lopes AA, Sacramento E et al. Penicillin at the late stage of leptospirosis: a randomised controlled trial. *Rev Inst Med Trop S. Paulo* 2003; 45: 141–145.

8 Panaphut T, Domrongkitchaiporn S, Vibhagool A et al. Ceftriaxone compared with sodium penicillin for treatment of severe leptospirosis. *Clin Infect Dis* 2003; 36: 1507–1513.

9 Pappas G, Papadimitriou P, Siozopoulou V et al. The globalisation of leptospirosis: worldwide incidence trends. *Int J Infect Dis* 2008; 12: 351–357.

10 Dupont H, Dupont-Perdrizet D, Perie JL et al. Leptospirosis: Prognostic factors associated with mortality. *Clin Infect Dis* 1997; 25: 720–724.

11 Levett PN. Leptospirosis. *Clin Microbiol Rev* 2001; 14: 296–326.

12 Abgueguen P, Delbos V, Blanvillain J et al. Clinical aspects and prognostic factors of leptospirosis in adults. Retrospective study in France. *J Infect* 2008; 57: 171–178.

13 World Health Organization. *Human Leptospirosis: Guidance for Diagnosis, Surveillance and Control* (2003) www.who.int/csr/don/en/WHO_CDS_CSR_EPH_2002.23.pdf

14 Segura ER, Ganoza CA, Campos K et al. Clinical spectrum of pulmonary involvement in leptospirosis in a region of endemicity, with quantification of leptospiral burden. *Clin Infect Dis* 2005; 40: 343.

15 Doudier B, Garcia S, Jarno P et al. Prognostic factors associated with severe leptospirosis. *Clin Microbiol Infect* 2006; 12: 299–300.

16 Kularatne SAM, Budagoda BDSS, de Alwis VKD et al. High efficacy of bolus methylprednisolone in severe leptospirosis: a descriptive study in Sri Lanka. *Postgrad Med J* 2011; 87: 13–17.

17 Niwattayakul K, Kaewtasi S, Chueasuwanchai S et al. An open randomised controlled trial of desmopressin and pulsed dexamethasone as adjunct therapy in patients with pulmonary involvement associated with severe leptospirosis. *Clin Microbiol Infect* 2010; 16: 1207–1212.

18 Martinez Garcia MA, de Diego Damia A, Menendez Villanueva R et al. Pulmonary involvement in Leptospirosis. *Eur J Clin Microbiol Infect Dis* 2000; 19: 471–474.

19 Marotto PCF, Ko AI, Murta-Nascimento C et al. Early identification of leptospirosis-associated pulmonary haemorrhage syndrome by use of a validated prediction model. *J Infect* 2010; 60: 218–223.

20 Esen S, Sunbul M, Leblebicioglu H et al. Impact of clinical and laboratory findings on prognosis in leptospirosis. *Swiss Med Wkly* 2004; 134: 347–352.

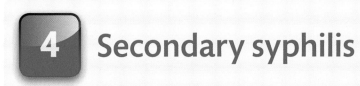

Secondary syphilis

Angela Houston

Expert commentary Patrick French

Case history

A 50-year-old man presented to the emergency department with a headache associated with a widespread rash covering his entire body. The rash first appeared 2 weeks ago. It was non-pruritic and started on his abdomen. Over the course of a week it spread to involve his entire body. He had seen his general practitioner 4 days ago after developing a headache, and at the time was diagnosed with a viral exantham and was advised to take regular paracetamol. Despite this, he complained that his headache had become worse during the last 2 days and this triggered his presentation. The headache was not associated with any neck stiffness or photophobia. He had not vomited but felt very nauseated. He had no history of fevers, night sweats, or weight loss. His only past medical history included hypertension, for which he took amlodipine 10 mg daily. He was allergic to penicillin, which caused a drug rash.

He had no foreign travel in the past 6 months but had returned to visit family in Jamaica 9 months previously. He had grown up in Jamaica and moved to the United Kingdom 25 years ago. He had no pets at home and no exposure to animals. He denied any illicit drug use and was a non-smoker. He drank approximately 20 units of alcohol a week. He did admit to having a new male partner he met 2 months ago. Before that he had no regular sexual partner. His last sexual health screen including an HIV test was performed 2 years ago when he was told he was HIV negative.

On examination he was a well-nourished man. He had a widespread symmetrical non-pruritic maculopapular rash which was also present on his palms and the soles of his feet. The lesions were purplish in colour and well circumscribed. He had widespread non-tender lymphadenopathy. There was no oral or genital ulceration, his joints were not swollen or tender, and his chest was clear with an audible first and second heart sound and no murmurs. His abdomen was soft and non-tender with no evidence of organomegaly.

He had no neck stiffness or meningism and Kernig's sign was negative. Cranial nerves I–XII were all intact and there was no evidence of any focal neurological deficit. In view of the rash and headache the emergency department started high-dose cefotaxime even though he did not have any objective signs of meningism. A CXR, blood tests, and blood cultures were undertaken and he was seen by the ID registrar who requested an urgent HIV test. Blood results revealed a marginally raised CRP at 12 mg/L, normal haematological indices, and normal LFTs.

The differential diagnosis at this point included bacterial meningitis which was thought to be unlikely as his headache had been present for 4 days and he was not meningitic; it could be a viral meningitis as he was not overtly septic; acute HIV seroconversion illness with the rash, lymphadenopathy and headache; or syphilitic meningitis.

Table 4.1 Results

Opening pressure	15 cm CSF
WCC	30 cells/µL
Differential	95% lymphocytes
RBC	<3 cells/µL
Protein	0.55 g/dL
CSF glucose	3.2 mmol/dL
Serum glucose	6.3 mmol/dL
India Ink	Negative
Viral PCR	Negative for HSV1, HSV2, and enteroviruses
CSF RPR	positive titre of 1 in 8
Further results	
CD4 lymphocyte count	556 cells/mm^3 (36%)
HIV viral load (VL)	18,000 copies/mL
Syphilis EIA IgG/IgM	Positive
TPPA	Positive
RPR	1:32
Cryptococcal antigen (CrAg) test	Negative
Blood cultures	No growth at 5 days

Tuberculous or cryptococcal meningitis (CM) were also a possibility although it would be hard to explain the rash in this context. His CXR was unremarkable. He underwent an enhanced CT scan of his head which was reported as normal with no evidence of any space-occupying lesions and so the decision was made to undertake an LP.

Two hours after receiving the dose of cefotaxime he became increasingly unwell with a worsening of the rash and headache and development of myalgia and a low-grade fever (see Table 4.1).

⊕ **Clinical tip**

Remember to think about endemic treponemal infections when positive syphilis serology is seen in a patient from an endemic area.

This patient comes from Jamaica where the infection, yaws, used to be hyperendemic and sporadic cases do still occur. Yaws is caused by *Treponema pallidum* subspecies *pertunue*. The disease is usually acquired in childhood and leads to chronic skin ulceration, usually (but not always) on the lower legs. Yaws became rare in the Caribbean after the WHO Mass Eradication Programme in the 1950s but worldwide it is estimated that 500,000 new cases of yaws occur per year.

Yaws, pinta, and bejel are all endemic treponemal infections (Table 4.2). These infections are transmitted person-to-person by skin or mucous membrane contact. They all cause similar localized primary lesions which often ulcerate before disseminating to the mucous membranes, bone, or cartilage. CNS and congenital infections do not occur. Most people do not know they have been infected; however, previous childhood infections can manifest as circular scars on the lower legs.

Table 4.2 Causes of endemic treponemal infections

Pathogen	Disease	Distribution
T. pallidum subsp. *pallidum*	Syphilis	Worldwide
T. pallidum subsp. *pertenue*	Yaws	Hot, humid, rural areas
T. pallidum subsp. *endemicium*	Bejel	Hot, dry, and arid, rural area. N Africa, SE Asia and E Mediterranean
T. carateum	Pinta	South America and the Caribbean

Source: Data from *Microbes and Infection*, Volume 4, Issue 2, Antal et al, The endemic treponematoses, pp. 83–94, Copyright © 2002 Éditions scientifiques et médicales Elsevier SAS. All rights reserved.

(continued)

You should always examine the whole skin for evidence of previous infection in someone from an endemic area. These infections cause serological changes identical to syphilis [1]. Although the RPR/VDL is low in most cases of yaws it is usually not possible to exclude active or latent syphilis, and most clinicians manage patients who have these infections as though they have syphilis, while ensuring that patients are aware of the limitations and diagnostic uncertainties of treponemal serology.

As his CSF demonstrated a lymphocytic pleocytosis with a mildly elevated protein, normal glucose, and normal peripheral WCC, it was thought bacterial meningitis was unlikely so the cefotaxime was stopped. The HIV test was reported as positive and confirmed with a second blood test the next day. His CD4 count was 556 (36%). In view of his positive syphilis EIA and TPPA blood serology, raised CSF protein, WCC and positive RPR, it was thought his diagnosis was most likely secondary syphilis with symptomatic syphilitic meningitis (meningovascular syphilis).

⊗ **Learning point** Secondary syphilis

Approximately 2–3 months after acquisition of syphilis, patients can develop a systemic illness characterized by a rash, constitutional symptoms, and generalized lymphadenopathy. Most patients who have a rash with secondary syphilis have a maculopapular rash (often including the palms and soles of the feet and usually not pruritic), often mucocutaneous ulceration, and generalized lymphadenopathy. Rarer symptoms of secondary syphilis include patchy alopecia, hepatitis, condylomata, splenomegaly, periosteitis, and glomerulonephritis. The CNS may become involved, as in our case; in up to 2–5% of patients with meningitis (presenting as headache), cranial nerve palsies (usually the vestibulocochlear nerve [VIII]) or anterior and posterior uveitis being the most common events.

His serum CrAg was negative and his viral PCR on the CSF was negative, which helped to confirm the diagnosis. He was sent the next day for a full genitourinary screen which was otherwise unremarkable. His partners were contact traced by the health advisers at the local genitourinary medicine (GUM) department. In view of his penicillin allergy his antibiotics were changed to doxycycline 200 mg twice a day for 28 days.

In retrospect, the worsening headache, myalgia, and worsening rash after receiving cefotaxime was likely caused by a Jarisch-Herxheimer reaction from a release of pro-inflammatory cytokines (TNF, IL-1, IL-6) driven by the action of treponemal antigens released as a result of antimicrobial chemotherapy.

⊕ **Clinical tip**

Classically the rash of secondary syphilis is non-pruritic and affects all the skin including the palms and soles. It maybe macular, papular, or macular/papular. However in many patients it can be atypical including rashes which are localized in the palms and soles, or may spare the palms and soles, and can range from very mild to florid or pruritic, which is particularly the case in people with dark skin.

❝ **Expert comment**

Although doxycycline in high dose should treat neurosyphilis adequately, the evidence to support its use is weak. Some clinicians and some national guidelines such as those from the US Centers for Disease Control (CDC) recommend that all patients with neurosyphilis who report penicillin allergy should receive penicillin desensitization followed by high-dose parenteral penicillin.

⊕ **Clinical tip**

The Jarisch-Herxheimer reaction can occur in 70–90% of people treated for secondary syphilis. This manifests itself as a low-grade fever, myalgia, headaches, and malaise which begins within a few hours of starting treatment. In most people this will last 3–12 hours and is self-limiting. Treatment is with antipyretics. All patients should be warned about this before starting treatment. It is sometimes difficult to differentiate this clinically from a drug reaction [2]. A study of the Jarisch-Herxheimer reaction in HIV-infected patients with neurosyphilis concluded that risk factors included a high RPR titre, early syphilis, and prior penicillin use.

The reaction is thought to result from the large release of treponemal lipopolysaccharide from dying spirochaetes. This release causes an increase in circulating anti-tumour necrosis factor alpha (TNF-α) and interleukin (IL) 6 and 8. There is no clear role for steroids in the prevention or treatment of the Jarisch-Herxheimer reaction in early syphilis although an open small study showed that high-dose steroids can prevent Jarisch-Herxheimer reaction occurring in early syphilis. However, some clinicians do cover the first days of the treatment of late syphilis with steroids to prevent the Jarisch-Herxheimer reaction occurring in vital organs such as coronary arteries or cranial nerves.

His headache and rash resolved over the next few days but he complained of blurring of his vision on day 3. He was seen urgently in the eye clinic as there was some concern that he might be developing uveitis. An ophthalmologist performed a slit lamp examination and could find no evidence of inflammation in the eye and his acuity remained 6/6 on the Snellen chart in both eyes. His visual symptoms resolved after 24–48 hours and on follow-up remained normal. On discharge, outpatient follow-up was arranged and he was monitored over the next year with syphilis serology performed monthly for the first 3 months. The RPR fell four-fold (1 in 8) at 16 weeks and became negative 12 months after treatment. He remained symptom-free and was monitored for his HIV infection.

❝ Expert comment
Epidemiology of syphilis in the UK

Between 1985 and 1997 syphilis was no longer endemic in the UK as an ID, with occasional sporadic cases, imported cases, and cases of late infection only. In 1997, however, it re-emerged as an important disease particularly among men who have sex with men (MSM) and this remains the most important group affected by syphilis. The majority of individuals who are infected with syphilis in the UK are MSM, and the MSM are disproportionately HIV positive.

Discussion

Here we have a case of an HIV-positive man presenting with secondary syphilis associated with acute meningovascular syphilis causing meningitis.

Neurosyphilis simply means a syphilitic infection in the central nervous system and usually presents with one of three main syndromes (Box 4.1).

Box 4.1 Signs and symptoms of neurosyphilis

Parenchymal infection
General paresis/cortical involvement
- Changes in personality, affect, intellect, insight, and judgement
- Hyperactive reflexes
- Speech disturbances
- Pupillary disturbances (Argyll Robertson pupils)

Tabes dorsalis/spinal cord involvement
- Shooting or lightning pains into lower back or lower legs
- Ataxia
- Romberg's sign
- Pupillary disturbances (Argyll Robertson pupils)
- Cranial nerve involvement (II–VII)
- Peripheral neuropathy
- incontinence of bladder and bowel
- Impotence

Meningovascular infection
- Seizures
- Aphasia
- Hemiplegia or hemiparesis

✪ Learning point Neurosyphilis pathophysiology early and late and natural history early and late

During the secondary stage of syphilis the treponemes become disseminated throughout the body and enter the CNS. *T. pallidum* can be isolated in CSF of 25–40% of patients with early syphilis but, in the vast majority of cases, patients are not aware of this invasion of the CNS (asymptomatic meningitis) and the infection is cleared by the host's immune system via opsonized macrophages. However, 2–5% of patients will present with symptomatic meningitis ranging from simple meningitis to cranial neuropathies. This results from a failure to clear the organism from the CSF and persistent infection can develop into late neurosyphilis [3].

Late CNS infection can be divided into meningovascular disease which classically occurs 2–7 years after infection, leading to ischaemic symptoms (consider in stroke in a young person); and parenchymal

(continued)

disease where there is destruction of the neurones usually within the cortex or spinal cord and leads to general paresis and tabes dorsalis. Spinal cord involvement usually involves demyelination of the posterior columns, resulting in problems of proprioception, and loss of vibration sense and ability to balance. Classically patients develop lightning-like pains in their arms and legs caused by a sensory neuropathy.

In historical studies 80% of people who were diagnosed with general paresis died within 4 years of the diagnosis. Although sometimes cited as an important cause of dementia, general paresis is rare. In a large meta-analysis of over 5,000 patients attending memory clinics, infection was found to contribute to memory decline in only 0.3% of cases of which the majority were attributed to syphilis. However, these patients were from a self-selected population in a memory clinic so there may have been cases of patients with late latent syphilis who had already been treated after diagnosis before referral to specialist services [4].

✅ **Evidence base** The Oslo study of the natural history of untreated syphilis [5]

Most of our knowledge on the natural history of syphilis comes from turn-of-the-century studies from Oslo when a Norwegian venereologist, Boeck, described the evolution of infection in more than 1,400 patients with primary and secondary syphilis between 1891 and 1910. Because he believed that the available therapies at the time were highly toxic and of little benefit, patients received no treatment and were instead hospitalized until their symptoms had fully resolved (1–12 months, average 3.6 months) and they no longer posed any public health risk. His work was completed by his successor, Bruusgaard, who reported on the 25-year follow-up of 473 of these patients, published in 1929.

A total of 27.7% of males and 24% of females developed clinical relapse (secondary or tertiary syphilis) within 5 years of leaving hospital (Table 4.3) [5].

Table 4.3 Outcome of untreated syphilis

	Males	Females	Onset of post-primary infection
Gummatous disease	14.4%	16.7%	1–46 years (average 15 years)
Cardiovascular disease	13.6%	7.6%	20–30 years
Neurosyphilis			
• Meningovascular	9.4%	5%	5–7 years
• Tabes dorsalis	3.6%	1.7%	10–20 years
• General paresis	2.5%	1.4%	10–20 years
	3.0%	1.7%	

Source: Data from *Journal of Chronic Diseases*, Volume 2, Issue 3, Clark, E.G. and N. Danbolt, The Oslo study of the natural history of untreated syphilis; an epidemiologic investigation based on a restudy of the Boeck-Bruusgaard material; a review and appraisal, pp. 311–344, Copyright © 1955 Published by Elsevier Inc.

Early meningovascular syphilis as seen here presents acutely and primarily affects the meninges or cerebral/spinal cord vasculature causing a basal meningitis and cranial nerve lesions. This is the most common form of neurosyphilis you are likely to see in modern medical practice.

This man did not have clear neurological signs but did have a chronic headache which would be consistent with a basal meningitis, a rash, and serological evidence of secondary syphilis. The doctor decided to perform an LP as the differential diagnosis when he presented to the emergency department was wide and included acute HIV seroconversion along with other opportunistic infections (OIs) associated with HIV. The diagnosis of neurosyphilis was based on the identification of CSF inflammation, including a lymphocytic pleocytosis that is typically >10 cells/µL, an elevated protein concentration that is usually >100 mg/dL, and a reactive CSF-VDRL (Venereal Disease Research Laboratory) or RPR (rapid plasma reagin).

⭐ **Learning point** Syphilis serology

Because no *in vitro* culture of *Treponema pallidum* is possible and direct tests (dark-ground microscopy and PCR) are not widely available, the most commonly used tests to diagnose syphilis are serological. These are divided into specific treponemal tests which can be used to look for evidence of treponemal-specific antibody production as a screening test, and the non-specific cardiolipin tests which are useful in monitoring disease activity.

The specific treponemal serological tests include: treponemal enzyme-linked immunoassay (EIA) which can detect any combination of IgG, IgG plus IgM, or IgM alone, or *T. pallidum* haemagglutination assay (TPHA) and *T. pallidum* particle agglutination assay (TPPA).

The combined IgG/IgM EIA is a good screening test as IgM is usually detected towards the end of the second week and IgG by week 4 post-infection. This is a relatively easy test to do on a standard automated platform in the virology laboratory. A positive test should always be repeated on a second sample and confirmed with a second treponemal-specific test.

Non-treponemal cardiolipin tests include the VDRL and RPR tests. Although these are non-specific they are useful in monitoring disease activity and response to treatment. If syphilis is suspected with a positive EIA/TPHA or TPPA test, take a RPR/VDRL titre on the day treatment starts to act as a baseline value to monitor response to treatment. False-negative results can occur as the result of a prozone effect if the titres in the plasma are extremely high. However, laboratories routinely dilute RPR-tested sera in patients with positive treponemal tests in order to avoid the false-negative of the prozone effect (Table 4.4, Figure 4.1).

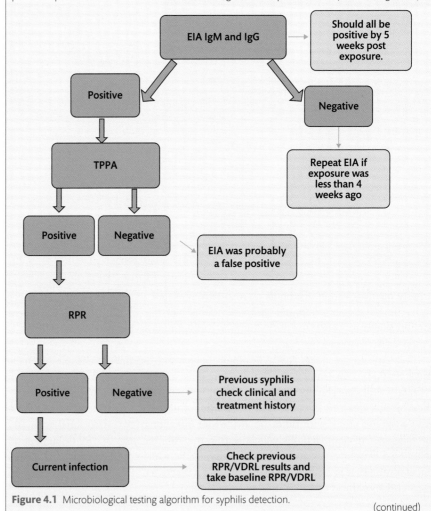

Figure 4.1 Microbiological testing algorithm for syphilis detection.

(continued)

Table 4.4 Syphilis serology

	Primary (all tests maybe negative)*	Secondary	Tertiary/late syphilis	Treated syphilis
EIA (IgM/IgG) (screening test)	Positive	Positive	Positive	Positive/negative
TPPA/TPHA (confirmation test)	Positive	Positive	Positive	Positive
RPR/VDRL (test for disease activity)	Positive	Positive (usually more than 1 in 8)	Positive/negative	Negative

* Don't forget in very early syphilis the TPPA/TPHA can be negative and in late syphilis the RPR/VDRL can be negative, which can be similar to treated syphilis. If any confusion, refer to an expert to discuss.

✚ Clinical tip CSF findings in neurosyphilis

Acute (secondary) neurosyphilis normally affects the CSF, meninges, and vasculature whereas late syphilis affects the brain parenchyma and spinal cord, which is why the CSF findings can be different (Table 4.5).

Table 4.5 Typical CSF findings in neurosyphilis

	Meningovascular syphilis	Tertiary neurosyphilis (tabes dorsalis)	Tertiary neurosyphilis (general paresis)
WCC	>5	>5 or normal	>5
Differential	Lymphocytes	Lymphocytes	Lymphocytes
Protein	Raised	Raised	Raised
Glucose			
VDRL/RPR	Positive	Positive/negative	Positive

In the case syphilis was diagnosed on the basis of a lymphocytosis, raised protein, and positive RPR in the CSF with positive serum TPPA and RPR. There can be some difficulty in interpreting the CSF results in someone with HIV, as HIV alone can cause a CSF lymphocytosis and elevated protein.

❝ Expert comment Syphilis serology

It is difficult to use the RPR titre as a guide to staging syphilis; however, patients with secondary syphilis usually have an RPR titre greater than 1:8.

Syphilis must always be considered in patients presenting with a rash and headache but neurosyphilis can be difficult to rule out, because mild CSF pleocytosis and elevated protein could have been caused by the HIV itself [6] (Table 4.4). The important point is to consider syphilis as a cause of meningitis, particularly in patients with risk factors. If the diagnosis is uncertain, the case should be discussed with an expert.

Patients with early meningovascular syphilitic meningitis often complain of headache, and visual acuity may be impaired if there is concomitant uveitis, vitritis, retinitis, or optic neuritis. Anterior uveitis can occur in 5–10% of patients with secondary syphilis and an active surveillance programme to identify new cases of syphilitic anterior uveitis reported 35 new cases between September 2009 and December 2010 in the UK and Ireland [7]. Anterior uveitis may be more common in HIV co-infected individuals. Our case did not have uveitis but this was considered when he complained of visual disturbance. Other important signs to consider include cranial neuropathies, particularly of the optic, facial, or auditory nerve resulting in hearing loss with or without tinnitus. Optic and auditory symptoms are part of the neurosyphilis spectrum but are not always associated with other signs of syphilitic meningitis. Sensorineural hearing loss and visual problems can present as a separate entity [8].

Rarely, meningovascular neurosyphilis can present later in the course of infection with symptoms caused by an infective arteritis. Although now unusual, this later form of meningovascular syphilis presents with localized ischaemia, thrombus or infarction of the brain or spinal cord, classically presenting as an ischaemic stroke in a young person. Such patients can present with a prodromal period when they complain of headache, dizziness, or personality changes, for days or weeks before the onset of ischaemia or stroke. The middle cerebral artery and its branches are most commonly affected. Less commonly the anterior spinal artery and its branches are involved, which causes spinal cord infarction.

The other two main syndromes are caused by infection in the CNS parenchyma leading to destruction of the neurones within the cortex or spinal cord. General paresis presents with progressive dementia and personality change and tabes dorsalis presents with spinal cord involvement.

☼ Learning point Indications to undertake an LP in syphilis for neurosyphilis

CSF abnormalities are common in people with primary or secondary syphilis and can be found in up to 30% of patients, the majority of whom do NOT go on to develop any clinical evidence of neurosyphilis.

The UK guidelines suggest the minimum standards for any HIV-infected patient with positive syphilis serology is that they should have a full neurological examination. If they have any neurological signs or symptoms including papillodoema they should have a CT scan of their head followed by an LP, which is also required to exclude other OIs.

There is ongoing debate about the need for LP to exclude CNS involvement in patients with latent syphilis who remain asymptomatic, particularly if they are HIV positive. It is now only thought necessary to perform LP if there are neurological signs or symptoms, or evidence of treatment failure [11]. A negative serum VDRL/RPR usually rules out neurosyphilis; however, some patients, particularly those with late neurosyphilis and otosyphilis, may have negative serum RPR tests. If the TPHA or TPPA is negative in the CSF, it virtually excludes neurosyphilis as a diagnosis. However, many patients will have a positive TPPA/TPHA in the CSF irrespective of whether they have neurosyphilis. A positive CSF-VDRL/RPR test result, needs to be interpreted with caution as any condition that causes inflammation to the blood–brain barrier may allow serum immunoglobulins to leach into the CSF and cause a false-positive result (i.e. it lacks specificity); for an accurate assessment, the CSF should not be contaminated with blood. Neurosyphilis is also more likely if the CSF TPHA is >320 or TPPA titre >640.

⊕ Clinical tip

In contrast to asymptomatic patients, all patients with neurological symptoms or signs and positive syphilis serology should have an LP; however, the chances of having neurosyphilis if the patient has a serum RPR of 1 in 4 or less is remote.

⊕ Clinical tip

Current up-to-date treatment options for the different manifestations of syphilis are available in the UK and European guidelines [10,11].

Tabes dorsalis classically affects the posterior columns, which causes a sensory ataxia with lightning-like pains in the extremities or face, bowel and bladder dysfunction, and rarely Argyll Robertson pupil and optic atrophy. There are always a few unusual manifestations of neurosyphilis which don't fall into these broad syndromes. After all, syphilis has always been known as the great imitator. There are case reports of people who have presented with signs and symptoms akin to herpes encephalitis, acute confusion and MRI changes consistent with temporal lobe encephalitis which resolved with treatment for neurosyphilis [8]. This is probably a result of meningo-vascular syphilis but with inflammation in an atypical vascular domain. It is therefore wise to always consider syphilis in any patient who presents with neurological signs and symptoms.

There is still controversy about the role of HIV with syphilis. Certainly HIV seems to modify the course of early syphilis.

❝ Expert comment HIV and syphilis

Of early syphilis cases identified in the UK, 30–40% are HIV-positive individuals. In primary syphilis the initial chancres are more likely to be multiple, large, and painful (in comparison to the classical single, painless chancre). These chancres are also more likely to persist and be present when secondary syphilis occurs. There is debate about the impact of HIV infection on the development of late syphilis. Case reports have suggested that more rapid progression to neurosyphilis after early syphilis, and treatment

(continued)

failure with benzothine penicillin in early syphilis, are more common in HIV-infected people; however, this has not been confirmed by larger studies or controlled studies. There is some evidence that neurological involvement of syphilis (as diagnosed by CSF abnormalities) is commoner among people who are HIV positive, and response to treatment of neurosyphilis by CSF assessment is slower in HIV-positive individuals. The importance of this and the impact this has on clinical disease is uncertain [9].

It is important to closely monitor patients with neurosyphilis during and following treatment to look for evidence of treatment failure or relapse of infection. In cases of early syphilis this means checking the RPR/VDRL at months 1, 2, 3, 6, and 12 and then 6-monthly until the RPR/VDRL becomes negative or stable (serofast) at low titre. In patients presenting with later forms of syphilis the RPR/VDRL should be checked 3-monthly until it is negative or stable (serofast) at low titre. The expected response to treatment is a fall in RPR/VDRL fourfold by 6–12 months following adequate treatment. All patients with neurosyphilis should have a repeat LP 6 months after treatment to check that the CSF WCC has normalized and the CSF RPR/VDRL titre has declined.

As there is concern that HIV can cause increase in the relapse rates in syphilis, patients who are HIV positive should continue to undergo at least an annual RPR/VDRL check in clinic. Sexually active HIV patients should have syphilis testing at each routine blood monitoring visit. A fourfold increase in the RPR/VDRL is suggestive of re-infection or treatment failure. Specific treponemal tests (TPPA/TPHA) will remain positive for life so it is important to document this clearly so there is no confusion at a later date.

❝ Expert comment

Some patients with fully treated syphilis do not achieve a negative serum RPR after curative treatment. This is more likely to happen in patients with late infection, repeat infection, or HIV. If standard therapy has been used, there has been a satisfactory initial RPR decline, and there is no evidence of re-infection, the patient can be discharged with a low titre RPR that is stable (i.e. the same titre 3 months apart). This is called a serofast titre and is the level from which re-infection is judged.

A final word from the expert

Over the past 10 years syphilis has once again become endemic in the UK. Most people with syphilis are MSM and they are disproportianately HIV positive. Primary syphilis should be considered as part of the differential diagnosis in all individuals with mouth or anogenital ulceration, and secondary syphilis should be considered in all those with rash and consititutional symptoms. This case illustrates how meningovascular syphilis may present, and neurosyphilis should be considered in patients with almost any neurological presentation.

The key to managing syphilis is considering the diagnosis in the first place! Screening for syphilis is easy and cheap using the new IgG/IgM tests and these are always positive in patients with syphilis, apart from the rare individuals with incubating or very early primary infection who are unlikely to be seen in general medical settings.

Once a positive test result comes back you can obtain advice on further investigations and management from your local STI clinic. Infectious syphilis remains a relatively uncommon infection, with about 3,500 new cases per year in the UK. Syphilis is an STI and the STI clinic will ensure that your patient's sexual partners are traced, tested, and treated.

References

1 Antal GM, Lukehart SA, Meheus AZ. The endemic treponematoses. *Microb Infect* 2002; 4: 83–94.
2 Yang CJ, Lee NY, Lin YH et al. Jarisch-Herxheimer reaction after penicillin therapy among patients with syphilis in the era of the HIV infection epidemic: incidence and risk factors. *Clin Infect Dis* 2010; 51: 976–979.
3 Ghanem KG. Review: Neurosyphilis: a historical perspective and review. *CNS Neurosci Ther* 2010; 16: e157–e168.

4 Clarfield A. The decreasing prevalence of reversible dementias: An updated meta-analysis. *Arch Intern Med* 2003; 163: 2219–2229.

5 Clark EG, Danbolt N. The Oslo study of the natural history of untreated syphilis: An epidemiologic investigation based on a restudy of the Boeck–Bruusgaard material a review and appraisal. *J Chron Dis* 1955; 2: 311–344.

6 Marra C, Maxwell CL, Collier AC, Robertson KR, Imrie A. Interpreting cerebrospinal fluid pleocytosis in HIV in the era of potent antiretroviral therapy. *BMC Infect Dis* 2007; 7: 37.

7 Goh B, et al. O3-S1.01 British Ocular Syphilis Study (BOSS): National Surveillance Study of intraocular inflammation secondary to infectious syphilis. *Sex Transm Infect* 2011; 87(Suppl 1): A69.

8 Marra C. Neurosyphilis. *Curr Neurol Neurosci Rep* 2004; 4: 435–440.

9 Marra CM, Maxwell CL, Tantalo L et al. Normalization of cerebrospinal fluid abnormalities after neurosyphilis therapy: does HIV status matter? *Clin Infect Dis* 2004; 38: 1001–1006.

10 French P, Gomberg M, Janier M et al., IUSTI. 2008 European Guidelines on the management of syphilis. *Int J STD AIDS* 2009; 20: 300–309.

11 Kingston M, French P, Goh B et al. UK National Guidelines on the Management of Syphilis 2008. *Int J STD AIDS* 2008; 19: 729–740.

HIV-associated multicentric Castleman's disease

5

Michael Rayment

⏀ **Expert commentary** Mark Bower

Case history

A 47-year-old white man presents to his HIV outpatient clinic with a 3-week history of flu-like symptoms, comprising fevers, night sweats, malaise, and myalgia. He is a gay man diagnosed with HIV-1 infection 8 years before on a routine sexual health screen, whereupon his CD4 count was 654 cells/µL and his HIV VL 1287 copies/mL. He remains naïve to antiretroviral therapy (ART), with a recent CD4 count of 399 cells/µL and VL of 338,000 copies/mL. Three months earlier, he had developed symptoms of proctitis, secondary to *Lymphogranuloma venereum* infection of the rectum. An iron-deficiency anaemia was also identified at the same time [haemoglobin 10.5 g/dL (normal range (NR) 12.5–17.0 g/dL); mean corpuscular volume (MCV) 82.7 fL (NR: 83.0–101.0 fL); iron 8 µmol/L (NR 9–29 µmol/L); transferrin saturation 16% (NR 20–45%)]. The symptoms of colitis had settled after 3 weeks' treatment with doxycycline, but the iron-deficient anaemia had persisted.

At presentation, no other symptoms of intercurrent or focal infection are identified, and systems enquiry is otherwise unremarkable.

He is noted to be febrile (38.1°C) with widespread, non-tender, mobile lymph nodes (0.5–1 cm) palpable in cervical, axillary, and inguinal regions. Examination of the cardiovascular and respiratory systems is unremarkable, but splenomegaly is clinically apparent. A chest radiograph is normal. Blood tests taken at the initial screening visit show a microcytic anaemia with iron deficiency and a mild reticulocytosis, elevated bilirubin, and elevated inflammatory markers (see Table 5.1). Lactate dehydrogenase levels are normal. Serology for syphilis, EBV, CMV, parvovirus, leishmania, and toxoplasma is undertaken, plus immunoglobulins, protein electrophoresis, direct antiglobulin testing (DAT), and serum human herpes virus-8 (HHV-8) VL.

The patient proceeds to CT, which confirms splenomegaly and size-significant lymphadenopathy in the axillary, mediastinal, para-aortic, common iliac, and inguinal chains suggestive of lymphoma. On ultrasound scanning of the inguinal nodes prior to attempted aspiration, the nodes are demonstrated to have normal fatty hila and normal morphology, mitigating against lymphoma, and aspiration is not attempted.

One week later, the patient's HHV-8 VL is reported at 283,000 DNA copies/mL. All other serological investigations are unremarkable. Polyclonal hypergammaglobulinaemia is noted, and the DAT supports auto-immune haemolysis (see Table 5.1). The patient remains symptomatic with high fevers and malaise, new-onset nasal congestion, and remains anaemic. He is treated with transfusions of packed red cells.

In light of the high HHV-8 VL, symptomatology, splenomegaly with lymphadenopathy, and haemolytic anaemia, a diagnosis of HIV-associated multicentric Castleman's disease (HIV-MCD) is suspected.

Table 5.1 Blood results at presentation

Haematology	Value	Biochemistry	Value	Serology	Result
Haemoglobin	9.6 g/dL	Urea and electrolytes	Normal	Syphilis	EIA negative
WCC	4.9×10^9/L	Bilirubin	26 µmol/L	Toxoplasma	Negative
Platelets	206×10^9/L	Alanine aminotransferase (ALT)	16 iu/L	CMV	IgM negative
ESR	94 mm/h	ALP	98 iu/L	Parvovirus	IgM negative
Reticulocytes	74.20×10^9/L	Corrected calcium	2.25 mmol/L	Hepatitis C	IgG negative
Reticulocytes %	2.40%	Albumin	30 g/L	Hepatitis B	sAg negative
Iron	8 µmol/L	Lactate dehydrogenase	193 iu/L	EBV	IgM negative
Transferrin saturations	16%	CRP	62.2 mg/L	Leishmania	IgG negative
Ferritin	1163 microgram/L	Immunoglobulins	Marked polyclonal increase in gamma globulins	HHV-8 VL	283,000 DNA copies/mL
DAT	Positive				

> ⭐ **Learning point** The pathophysiology of HIV-associated multicentric Castleman's disease (MCD)
>
> HHV-8 (or Kaposi's sarcoma-associated herpesvirus; KSHV) is a human lymphotropic virus. The virus is thought to be transmitted by saliva—from mother to child (MTCT), or by sexual contact, particularly sex between men. The seroprevalence of HHV-8 in MSM is approximately 20% in HIV-negative MSM, and up to 60–80% in HIV-positive MSM. HHV-8 is aetiologically linked with Kaposi's sarcoma (KS), primary effusion lymphoma (PEL), and HIV-MCD. Virtually all patients with HIV-MCD are HHV-8 seropositive, and nearly all have detectable levels of HHV-8 DNA. The correlation between the levels of HHV-8 and symptomatology, and symptom remission after administration of therapy, provides evidence of its critical role in HIV-MCD.
>
> HHV-8 encodes a number of proteins implicated in human cell cycle regulation and cytokine signalling. Perhaps most important among these is a viral homologue of the human cytokine IL-6. Viral IL-6 (vIL-6) exhibits high homology with its human counterpart, particularly that part involved in receptor binding, and thus it binds to human IL-6 receptors with high affinity. IL-6 is a cytokine produced by a number of cell types, particularly T cells and B cells. It induces the differentiation and proliferation of these cells, drives the synthesis of acute-phase reactant proteins, and has been shown to be associated with many of the constitutional symptoms (fever, malaise, etc.) associated with several inflammatory disorders.
>
> A simplified model for the pathophysiology of HIV-MCD is that HHV-8-infected cells, particularly plasmablasts, secrete vIL-6. The consequent vIL-6 excess then drives lymphocyte proliferation and inflammatory systemic symptoms. Vascular proliferation of tumour cells, which is a key histopathological finding of HIV-MCD, may also be driven by secretion of vascular endothelial growth factor, a downstream result of high IL-6 levels [1].
>
> Understanding the pathophysiology of HIV-MCD has facilitated the development of therapies. The use of the anti-CD20 monoclonal antibody (mAb) rituximab may work by targeting and destroying CD20+ mature B lymphocytes, which act as a sanctuary site for HHV-8 replication and also produce large volumes of IL-6. Many HHV-8 infected cells do not express CD20, however, and rituximab has also been shown to be effective in the treatment of HIV-negative Castleman's disease, so the mechanism
>
> (continued)

by which it works may be more complex than this model. The use of anti-IL-6 therapies has been shown to produce symptomatic and biochemical remission of the disease, but only for as long as treatment is continued.

⊗ **Learning point** Clinching the diagnosis: histology, and the role of the French Agence Nationale de Recherche sur le SIDA 117 CastlemaB trial group scoring system

The diagnosis of HIV-MCD is based on the presence of histopathological features, and histological diagnosis must be pursued actively in patients in whom the diagnosis of HIV-MCD enters the differential. The optimum sample is a full lymph node excision, guided by FDG avidity on PET-CT. A fine needle aspiration (FNA) should not be relied upon to rule out the disease, and as such an excisional biopsy should be attempted as first line. Owing to the remitting and relapsing nature of HIV-MCD, clinical features should also be present to confirm a diagnosis of active disease [2].

While there are no evidence-based criteria for establishing a diagnosis of active HIV-MCD, the French Agence Nationale de Recherche sur le SIDA 117 CastlemaB trial group have described criteria to define an attack of HIV-MCD [3]. Patients require a fever, a raised serum CRP more than 20 mg/L in the absence of any other cause, and three of 12 additional clinical findings: peripheral lymphadenopathy, splenomegaly, oedema, pleural effusion, ascites, cough, nasal obstruction, rash, xerostomia, jaundice, central neurological symptoms, and autoimmune haemolytic anaemia. The incidence of each of these criteria is not described in the CastlemaB trial, but has been described in retrospective cohort analyses from London, with good sensitivity and specificity [4].

---

❻ **Expert comment** IL-6 targeted treatments for HIV-VE MCD

Although the biological mechanisms underlying MCD are not yet fully understood, recent advances mainly related to the role of HHV-8 and IL-6 and other chemokines have led to the development of promising targeted therapies. HIV seronegative patients with HHV-8 negative MCD may be treated with mAbs to IL 6 (siltuxima) or its receptor (tocilizumab). However, this looks less promising in HIV-MCD because the HHV-8 homologue of IL-6 only shares 25% sequence homology with human IL-6 and can use alternative receptors.

❻ **Expert comment** Rare conditions

Like many uncommon conditions, establishing the diagnosis of MCD is crucial as it allows life-saving treatment. Rare diagnoses are only made if clinicians think of wide differential diagnoses and perform the appropriate investigations.

The patient is referred for PET-CT. This shows avid FDG uptake within lymph nodes at multiple sites (particularly in the axillae) and diffuse uptake in the enlarged spleen (see Figure 5.1), supporting the diagnosis.

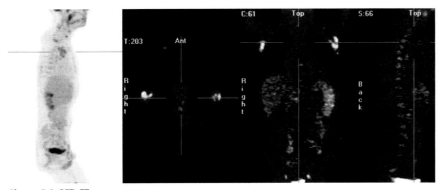

Figure 5.1 PET-CT
Positron emission computed tomography (PET-CT) showing avid FDG uptake within enlarged lymph nodes at multiple sites (most notably the axillae), and diffuse uptake in an enlarged spleen.

➕ Clinical tip Use of positron emission tomography

PET is a nuclear medicine imaging technique based on the detection of gamma rays emitted by a positron-emitting radionuclide bound to a biologically active molecule. Three-dimensional images of tracer concentration within the body are then constructed using simultaneous CT. Most commonly, the molecule used is the glucose analogue FDG. The concentrations of tracer imaged thus measure tissue metabolic activity, in terms of regional glucose uptake. Lymph nodes involved in HIV-MCD have been shown to have avid FDG uptake on PET-CT, and PET-CT has greater sensitivity in detecting disease than conventional CT, which can detect enlarged nodes only [5].

A surgical lymph node excision of two axillary nodes is performed. The histological examination of the excised nodes confirms a diagnosis of HIV-MCD. The lymph node shows a follicular pattern with expanded mantle zones. Larger lymphoid cells (plasmablasts) are present within the mantle zones. These cells express HHV-8-LANA-1 and IgM, and show lambda light chain restriction. There are no features of microlymphoma or KS (Figures 5.2 and 5.3).

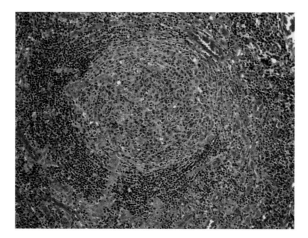

Figure 5.2 Histology of excised axillary lymph node
The lymph node shows a follicular pattern with expanded mantle zones. Larger lymphoid cells (plasmablasts) are present within the mantle zones.
Courtesy of Prof K. Naresh, Imperial College London.

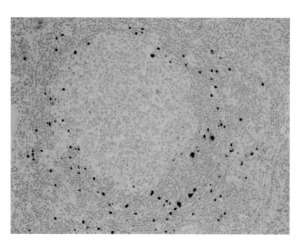

Figure 5.3 Histology of excised axillary lymph node
On immunohistochemistry, the large lymphoid cells with nucleoli (so-called 'plasmablasts') harbour HHV-8 virus as demonstrated by the presence of HHV-8 latent nuclear antigen-1 (LANA-1).
Courtesy of Prof K. Naresh, Imperial College London.

⊕ Clinical tip Considering HIV-MCD and KS

KS is caused by the same viral agent thought to be responsible for HIV-MCD, and thus the coexistence of the two pathologies is frequently observed. Nodal KS is often diagnosed histologically alongside MCD.

This is of clinical relevance, as several case series have described the progression of coexisting KS in patients treated with rituximab-based regimens [3,6]. There is no published evidence of KS appearing *de novo* following rituximab treatment in HIV-MCD patients without previous or coexisting KS, however. In the literature, the majority of KS exacerbations were mild, and required conservative management with continued ART, although systemic chemotherapy with liposomal anthracyclines has sometimes been indicated.

❝ Expert comment Histology

Histological confirmation of MCD is required prior to starting treatment and the characteristic features include large hyperplastic germinal centres, vascular proliferation, and sheets of plasmablastic lymphoid cells in the interfollicular regions. These plasmablasts express high levels of light-chain restricted IgM and contain HHV-8 (identified by immunohistochemical staining for HHV-8-associated latent nuclear antigen 1—LANA-1).

The patient commences four cycles of weekly etoposide and rituximab chemotherapy. He commences ART with raltegravir (RAL) and Truvada™, and starts full OI chemoprophylaxis.

❝ Expert comment The role of HAART in MCD

It is generally accepted that the use of combination antiretroviral therapy (cART) is an important complement to therapy in HIV-MCD, as for other HIV-associated malignancies. However, there is scant evidence for any direct effect of cART against HIV-MCD, unlike the effect of cART on KS. It is well documented that the survival of patients with HIV-MCD has improved since the era of cART, although this temporal improvement also coincides with the development of rituximab-based approaches to treating HIV-MCD. There is indirect support for the theory that cART play a relatively minor role in this improvement in survival. Epidemiological evidence suggests that neither nadir CD4 cell count nor use of cART influences the risk for HIV-MCD. Moreover, a high proportion of patients develop HIV-MCD while on fully suppressive cART with a good CD4 cell count and an undetectable (UD) plasma HIV VL. The failure of cART to control HIV-MCD is also supported by case reports, which include a description of acute deterioration of MCD while starting cART. Nevertheless, antiretroviral treatment is important in the management of HIV-MCD because it may limit the fall in CD4 cell count with chemoimmunotherapy and may reduce the reactivation of KS related to the immunotherapy.

Chemotherapy is well tolerated, and the patient is symptomatically better at completion. The haemolysis resolves, and inflammatory markers have settled. Four weeks post-completion, CT shows complete regression of lymphadenopathy and a normal-sized spleen. An HHV-8 VL is UD. Three months post-completion, the patient remains well. Both HIV and HHV-8 VLs are UD and the CD4 count has risen to 500. The patient continues on successful ART. He will be monitored long term for signs of clinical, radiological, and biochemical relapse.

✔ Evidence base The relationship between the quantity of HHV-8 in peripheral blood and HHV-8 associated diseases [7]

Quantitative measurement of HHV-8 in blood (both plasma and peripheral blood mononuclear cells; PBMCs) is of value in all HHV-8-associated diseases, but there are important differences in the utility of this test in each disease.

In this retrospective study of 107 patients, 105 blood samples and four lymphomatous effusion fluid samples (pleural or peritoneal) were analysed. DNA was extracted from PBMCs and was subjected to a real-time PCR assay that quantified both HHV-8 (ORF73) and human albumin genes. The number of viral copies was calculated by dividing the number of ORF73 copies by half the number of albumin gene copies. The study design was cross-sectional and each patient contributed only one sample. A total of 71 patients had presented with KS (of which 48 were HIV-positive and 23 were

(continued)

HIV-negative), 28 had presented with HIV-MCD, and eight patients had presented with PEL (of which six were HIV-positive and two were HIV-negative). Patients with KS and HIV-MCD had either active disease or disease in remission.

Among patients with active disease, the highest HHV-8 DNA levels were observed in effusion fluid samples from patients with PEL (7.2 $\log_{10}$ copies/150,000 cells), followed by blood samples from patients with HIV-MCD and PEL (4.86 and 3.83 $\log_{10}$ copies/150,000 cells, respectively). The lowest levels were observed in blood samples from patients with KS (2.63 $\log_{10}$ copies/150,000 cells).

HHV-8 DNA levels were higher in patients with active KS or HIV-MCD than in those with KS or HIV-MCD in remission. The levels of HHV-8 in active KS vs. KS in remission, while statistically significantly different, were low in both groups, precluding the use of this test to monitor disease activity or response to therapy in this group. Conversely, the difference in HHV-8 level in active HIV-MCD vs. HIV-MCD in remission was very great: thus, HHV-8 VL can be used to monitor response to therapy and relapse in this group.

Because the three diseases can occur consecutively or simultaneously in a given patient, measurement of the HHV-8 DNA level can be used as a discriminatory diagnostic tool in a patient with one known HHV-8 associated disease. As the authors suggest, in a patient presenting with KS and pleural effusion, a high level of HHV-8 DNA in the pleural fluid (approximately 7 $\log_{10}$) could suggest a concomitant diagnosis of PEL. In a patient presenting with KS, fever, and lymph node enlargement, a high blood level of HHV-8 DNA (approximately 4–5 $\log_{10}$) may suggest that the patient has HIV-MCD.

⊕ **Clinical tip** HIV-MCD occurs at all stages of HIV infection

HIV-MCD has a vastly increased incidence in people living with HIV infection. Importantly, however (and in contrast to most acquired immunodeficiency syndrome (AIDS)-defining malignancies, such as non-Hodgkin's lymphoma), epidemiological studies have demonstrated *no* correlation with CD4 count or the use of ART [8]. Indeed, there is a suggestion that the incidence of HIV-MCD is increasing in the post-ART era (although case identification bias may play a role), and that it appears to occur more frequently in older HIV-positive individuals with well-preserved immune function. A systematic review of all 72 cases of HIV-MCD published up to 2007 found that 64% of the 48 patients diagnosed with HIV-MCD in the ART era were already on ART at the time of HIV-MCD diagnosis [9].

Always consider HIV-MCD in the differential if a patient presents with symptomatology consistent with the diagnosis, regardless of their stage of HIV infection, the CD4 count, and whether or not the patient is on ART.

✪ **Learning point** Use of ART in patients with HIV-MCD

The incidence of HIV-MCD appears to be unrelated to CD4 count and HIV VL, with many patients developing the disease while on successful ART (see Clinical Tip: HIV-MCD occurs at all stages of HIV infection). The role of ART in patients with HIV-MCD remains unclear. Case reports suggest the use of ART alone has failed to control (and paradoxically can worsen) symptoms of HIV-MCD in ART-naïve individuals with the disease [10]. The initiation or continuation of ART in combination with cytotoxic chemotherapy in patients with HIV-associated lymphoproliferative disorders (predominantly non-Hodgkin's lymphoma) remains contentious, but has been shown in several studies to improve outcomes, despite overlapping toxicities and the potential for drug–drug interactions [11,12]. Many of these interactions relate to the enzyme-inhibiting effects of protease inhibitors (PIs) on the cytochrome P450 system and p-glycoprotein, usually increasing the exposure to cytotoxic agents metabolized by these pathways, and thus increasing the likelihood of toxicity, such as cytopenias. Conversely, non-nucleoside reverse transcriptase inhibitors (NNRTIs) may reduce the exposure to cytotoxic agents through induction of these pathways and limit efficacy. Nevertheless, use of ART in the setting of HIV-MCD treated with chemotherapy may benefit the patient in terms of limiting the precipitous fall in CD4 count often observed with the use of chemotherapy, and by preventing the exacerbation of pre-exisiting KS after chemotherapy.

Our patient was ARV naïve at presentation with a wild-type virus. Newer antiretroviral agents are now available which do not act on the cytochrome P450 systems. The integrase inhibitor (INI), RAL, is metabolized by glucuronidation, and results in minimal drug–drug interactions while conferring excellent virological control and immunological recovery. Use of the CCR5 antagonist maraviroc (MVC) could also be considered in a patient with an R5-tropic virus, but this agent is metabolized by the CYP3A4 isoenzyme, and dose adjustments may be necessary if co-administered with chemotherapy. Thus, we elected to use RAL with a nucleoside backbone of Truvada™ in this patient, with prompt virological suppression. There are limited published data to support this approach beyond case reports [13], but there is sound pharmacodynamic reasoning behind this regimen. Switching to an alternative (od) regimen could be considered once the HIV-MCD is in remission and no further chemotherapy is planned.

Discussion

Treatment of HIV-associated MCD

The gold-standard treatment for HIV-MCD remains unclear, and research is hampered by the rarity of the condition. Much evidence is derived from small series, open-label trials and expert opinion. In the pre-ART era, cytotoxic chemotherapy was shown to induce rapid remission of the disease in the majority, but relapses occurred frequently and the progression-free interval was brief [14].

The introduction of ART and the addition of the anti-CD20 mAb rituximab to the therapeutic options have resulted in a change in approach and improved outcomes. Numerous case series and two open-label studies have used rituximab. One study of 21 patients with newly diagnosed HIV-MCD reported a radiological response rate of 67%, and the overall and disease-free survival rates at 2 years were 95% and 79%, respectively [6]. In a second prospective study of 24 patients, use of rituximab induced a sustained remission of 1 year's duration in 17 of 24 (71%) patients and the 1-year overall survival was 92% [3].

⊘ **Evidence base** Rituximab in HIV-associated multicentric Castleman disease [3]

This open-label, phase II trial was designed to investigate the efficacy and safety of the anti-CD20 mAb, rituximab, as initial monotherapy in patients with HIV-MCD, and to correlate clinical outcomes with immune subset, plasma cytokine, and HIV and HHV-8 virological variables.

Patients were recruited from three HIV oncology centres. Over 3 years, 21 consecutive patients (18 men) with newly diagnosed HIV-MCD were treated prospectively in a non-randomized fashion with a standard dose of rituximab (375 mg/m²) at weekly intervals. All biopsy specimens had been reviewed and confirmed to be plasmablastic variants of HIV-MCD with no evidence of microlymphoma.

Plasma HHV-8 measurements were undertaken at diagnosis, and at months 1 and 3 after rituximab therapy. Progression-free and overall survival rates were assessed using the Kaplan-Meier method. Changes in haematological, biochemical, immunological, virological, and radiological outcomes during and after therapy were assessed.

For the 21 patients, the median follow-up was 12 months. One patient died before completing therapy. Twenty achieved remission of symptoms, and 14 (67%) achieved a radiological response. The overall and disease-free survival rates at 2 years were 95% (95% CI 86–100%) and 79% (95% CI 49–100%), respectively.

Plasma acute phase proteins, immunoglobulins, and HHV-8 VL all decreased significantly after rituximab therapy. All patients were started on effective ART, and there were no meaningful adverse effects of rituximab on HIV outcomes. The main adverse effect was reactivation of KS.

Rituximab monotherapy was shown to fail in both trials in patients with aggressive disease and evidence of end-organ failure. A stratified approach may therefore be appropriate: patients with evidence of severe disease (as defined by performance status and the presence of end-organ failure) may benefit from combination therapy with rituximab plus cytotoxic agents. Most experience is with rituximab given with intravenous etoposide.

In a large London case series of more than 50 patients with HIV-MCD, the use of rituximab or rituximab plus etoposide on a risk stratification basis has improved outcomes. The overall survival was 94% at 2 years and 90% at 5 years, compared with 42% and 33% in twelve patients treated before introduction of rituximab [4]. Our case study patient received combination rituximab/etoposide therapy, as he had end-organ disease manifest by severe haemolytic anaemia.

It is important to remember that HIV-MCD is a relapsing and remitting disease. In the same case series, eight of 46 patients who achieved clinical remission suffered symptomatic, histologically confirmed HIV-MCD relapse. The median time to relapse was 2 years. The 2- and 5-year progression-free survival rates for all 49 patients treated with rituximab-based therapy were 85% and 61%, respectively. All patients have been successfully retreated with rituximab-based therapy.

HIV-MCD relapses may occur at any CD4 cell count and are not prevented by effective HIV viral suppression. The optimum therapy for relapse prevention and treatment remains to be defined. Some centres have used maintenance rituximab therapy. However, in one trial of periodic rituximab therapy to maintain disease remission in patients with HIV-associated lymphomas (*not* HIV-MCD), there was evidence of excess respiratory infection-related deaths among patients who received maintenance rituximab [15]. Some antivirals, such as cidofovir, ganciclovir, and foscarnet, have been shown to have effective anti-HHV-8 activity. None has been of clinical use in treatment of acute HIV-MCD, but the use of oral agents (such as valganciclovir, which is highly effective against HHV-8 [16]) in maintenance therapy is promising, but lacks evidence currently.

> **❝ Expert comment** The role of antiherpes drugs in MCD
>
> Like KS, HIV-MCD is attributed to HHV-8 infection and in the case of HIV-MCD a high proportion of infected plasmablasts harbour lytic phase HHV-8. This lytic replication theoretically confers greater sensitivity to anti-herpesvirus agents and several anti-herpetic agents (ganciclovir, valganciclovir, cidofovir, and foscarnet) have been reported to show activity against HHV-8 *in vitro*. However, these antiherpesvirus drugs have had very limited success *in vivo* in HIV patients with MCD. None of seven patients responded to cidofovir, only two of four achieved remission with foscarnet, whereas ganciclovir and its oral derivative, valganciclovir, induced remission in one patient and reduced the frequency of relapse in a further two patients. In a multicentre retrospective study 12 patients were treated with various antiherpesvirus therapies with or without cytotoxic therapy (but no rituximab), and only four obtained a sustained clinical response including only three of eight treated with valganciclovir. One possible explanation for the poor results with valganciclovir is that it acts at a relatively late step in the lytic cycle of HHV-8 and may not be expected to suppress production of vIL-6, which is an early lytic gene product.

The follow-up of patients with successfully treated HIV-MCD likewise remains uncertain. It is prudent to monitor patients for clinical and biochemical relapse (with periodic HHV-8 DNA measures) but for how long is unclear. The risk of non-Hodgkin's lymphomas (many of which are HHV-8 associated) in patients with previous HIV-MCD is much higher than in matched controls, and it may be beneficial to monitor patients for early disease.

⊗ **Learning point** HHV-8 VL testing and other quantitative markers of disease activity

In addition to histopathology and clinical features, the only other investigation of value in routine clinical practice in establishing the diagnosis of HIV-MCD is quantitative measurement of HHV-8 DNA levels in plasma or PBMC. HHV-8 DNA is almost always detectable in the blood of patients with active HIV-MCD, and levels appear to correlate with symptomatic disease [7]. In patients with KS, HHV-8 DNA is only rarely detectable and, if detected, the levels are substantially lower—see Evidence base: The relationship between the quantity of HHV-8 in peripheral blood and HHV-8 associated diseases [7]. Plasma levels are comparable to levels detected within PBMC, so either may be used in management [17].

In our patient, levels of HHV-8 were high at presentation and UD at the end of chemotherapy. Levels may be measured longitudinally to detect relapse of HIV-MCD, but must always be interpreted within the clinical context (for example, whether the patient has become symptomatic of the disease once more). Rising levels may predict the likelihood of a subsequent attack [18].

Levels of plasma cytokines (notably IL-6 and IL-10, which are implicated in the pathogenesis of HIV-MCD; see Discussion) may rise and fall in association with disease activity, but their role in routine clinical care remains to be established.

CRP levels have also been shown to correlate closely with disease activity levels and are closely related to HHV-8 levels, and may be used longitudinally. Figure 5.4 shows receiver operating characteristic curves of serum CRP and plasma HHV-8 DNA in distinguishing active vs. remission of HIV-MCD, and the close relationship between them.

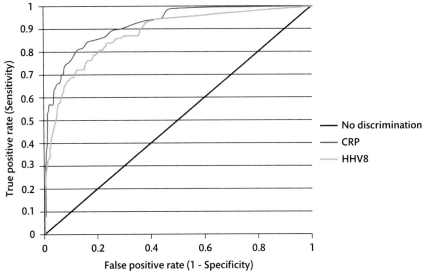

Figure 5.4 Receiver operating characteristic curves of serum CRP and plasma HHV-8 DNA in distinguishing active or remission of HIV-MCD, and the close relationship between them. A total of 471 matched CRP and HHV-8 DNA samples were available from 45 patients with HIV-MCD either in clinical remission (332) or during an active episode (139) of HIV-MCD.
Reproduced with permission from Mark Bower, How I treat HIV-associated multicentric Castleman disease, *Blood*, Volume 116, Number 22, pp. 4415–4421, Copyright © 2010 by The American Society of Hematology.

A final word from the expert

The advances in the clinical management of MCD is one of the apotheoses of HIV medicine in the post-HAART era. The combination of pathophysiology-based diagnostics and rational targeted therapy has dramatically improved survival. Prior to the introduction of mAb therapy, nearly half of all patients with HIV-MCD died within a year, while nowadays over 90% are alive 5 years following the diagnosis.

References

1 El-Osta HE, Kurzrock R. Castleman's Disease: From basic mechanisms to molecular therapeutics. *Oncologist* 2011; 16: 497–511.
2 Du MQ, Bacon CM, Isaacson PG. Kaposi sarcoma-associated herpesvirus/human herpes-virus 8 and lymphoproliferative disorders. *J Clin Pathol* 2007; 60: 1350–1357.
3 Gerard L, Berezne A, Galicier L et al. Prospective study of rituximab in chemotherapy-dependent human immunodeficiency virus associated multicentric Castleman's disease: ANRS 117 CastlemaB Trial. *J Clin Oncol* 2007; 25: 3350–3356.
4 Bower M, Newsom-Davis T, Naresh K et al. Clinical features and outcome in HIV-associated multicentric Castleman's disease. *J Clin Oncol* 2011; 29: 2481–2486.
5 Barker R, Kazmi F, Stebbing J et al. FDG-PET/CT imaging in the management of HIV-associated multicentric Castleman's disease. *Eur J Nucl Med Mol Imaging* 2009; 36: 648–652.
6 Bower M, Powles T, Williams S et al. Brief communication: Rituximab in HIV-associated multicentric Castleman disease. *Ann Intern Med* 2007; 147: 836–839.
7 Marcelin AG, Motol J, Guihot A et al. Relationship between the quantity of Kaposi sarcoma-associated herpesvirus (KSHV) in peripheral blood and effusion fluid samples and KSHV-associated disease. *J Infect Dis* 2007; 196: 1163–1166.
8 Powles T, Stebbing J, Bazeos A et al. The role of immune suppression and HHV-8 in the increasing incidence of HIV-associated multicentric Castleman's disease. *Ann Oncol* 2009; 20: 775–779.
9 Mylona EE, Baraboutis IG, Lekakis LJ, Georgiou O, Papastamopoulos V, Skoutelis A. Multicentric Castleman's disease in HIV infection: a systematic review of the literature. *AIDS Rev* 2008; 10: 25–35.
10 Dupin N, Krivine A, Calvez V, Gorin I, Franck N, Escande JP. No effect of protease inhibitor on clinical and virological evolution of Castleman's disease in an HIV-1-infected patient. *AIDS* 1997; 11: 1400–1401.
11 Ribera J-M, Oriol A, Morgades M et al. Safety and efficacy of cyclophosphamide, Adriamycin, vincristine, prednisone and rituximab in patients with human immunodeficiency virus-associated diffuse large B-cell lymphoma: results of a phase II trial. *Br J Haematol* 2008; 140: 411–419.
12 Spina M, Jaeger U, Sparano JA et al. Rituximab plus infusional cyclophosphamide, doxorubicin, and etoposide in HIV-associated non-Hodgkin lymphoma: pooled results from 3 Phase 2 trials. *Blood* 2005; 105: 1891–1897.
13 Fulco P, Hynicka L, Rackely D. Raltegravir-based HAART regimen in a patient with large B-cell lymphoma. *Ann Pharmacother* 2010; 44: 377–382.
14 Oksenhendler E, Duarte M, Soulier J et al. Multicentric Castleman's disease in HIV infection: a clinical and pathological study of 20 patients. *AIDS* 1996; 10: 61–67.

15 Kaplan LD, Lee JY, Ambinder RF et al. Rituximab does not improve clinical outcome in a randomized phase III trial of CHOP with or without rituximab in patients with HIV-associated non-Hodgkin's lymphoma: AIDS-malignancies consortium trial 010. *Blood* 2005; 24: 1538–1543.

16 Casper C, Krantz EM, Corey L et al. Valganciclovir for suppression of human herpesvirus-8 replication: a randomized, double-blind, placebo-controlled, crossover trial. *J Infect Dis* 2008; 198: 23–30.

17 Tedeschi R, Marus A, Bidoli E, Simonelli C, De Paoli P. Human herpesvirus 8 DNA quantification in matched plasma and PBMCs samples of patients with HHV8-related lymphoproliferative diseases. *J Clin Virol* 2008; 43: 255–259.

18 Stebbing J, Adams C, Sanitt A et al. Plasma HHV8 DNA predicts relapse in individuals with HIV-associated multicentric Castleman disease. *Blood* 2011; 118: 271–275.

6 HIV and prevention of mother-to-child transmission

Aseel Hegazi

⊕ Expert commentary Phillip Hay

Case history

A 26-year-old Nigerian lady presented with a week-long history of worsening fever, cough, and shortness of breath. She was 28 weeks into her first pregnancy, which had otherwise been uneventful and had included a negative routine antenatal test for HIV at 12 weeks' gestation.

There was no significant past medical history and she was a lifelong non-smoker. She had been working in the UK as a cleaner for 8 years and had last travelled abroad 2 years previously. She reported that she and her partner had both tested negative for HIV a year previously.

On examination she was tachypnoeic and was found to be hypoxic with a pO_2 of 7.1 kPa on air. CXR showed bilateral perihilar infiltrates. Other initial investigations and observations are shown in Table 6.1.

Specimens were sent for further investigations including an urgent HIV test.

> **⊕ Clinical tip**
>
> Repeat HIV testing in the third trimester should always be considered in pregnant patients who are in a 'high-risk' group regardless of the reported sexual history, especially since partners are not routinely tested during antenatal screening. There is some evidence that a high level of progesterone upregulates the expression of CCR5 HIV-1 co-receptor, resulting in an increased risk of HIV acquisition in pregnancy. A substantial proportion of residual vertical HIV transmissions that occur despite routine antenatal screening may be from subsequent maternal seroconversion during pregnancy or breastfeeding.

This test showed a positive p24 antigen with a negative HIV antibody test, confirming a diagnosis of acute HIV seroconversion. HIV-1 VL was 1.74×10^7 copies/mL and her CD4 count was 199 cells/μL (12%).

Table 6.1 Routine blood tests and observations on admission

Haematology		Biochemistry		Observations	
Hb	10.2 g/dL	Na	135 mmol/L	HR	95 bpm
WCC	6.4×10^9/L	K	3.9 mmol/L	BP	125/80 mmHg
Neutrophils	5.9×10^9/L	Urea	2.0 mmol/L	Temperature	38°C
Lymphocytes	0.5×10^9/L	Creatinine	45 mmol/L	O_2 sats	93% on air
Platelets	270×10^9/L	Bilirubin	35 μmol/L	Respiratory rate	33 bpm
Clotting	Normal	ALT	141 iu/L		
Malaria films	Negative	ALP	98 iu/L		
		GGT	290 iu/L		
		CRP	32 mg/L		

> ⊕ **Clinical tip**
>
> Symptoms of HIV seroconversion are non-specific and the diagnosis is often missed at initial presentation. During acute infection a 'window period' exists during which patients typically have very high HIV RNA levels with negative or indeterminate HIV antibody test results. About 7 days later, results of tests to detect p24 antigen (a viral core protein that transiently appears in the blood during and before the development of detectable HIV antibodies) become positive. Although fourth-generation HIV tests which detect both p24 antigen and HIV antibody have reduced the window period considerably, VL and repeat testing should always be carried out if initial HIV testing is negative and seroconversion is suspected.

The baseline HIV resistance test showed wild-type virus. Plasma CMV VL was UD. A CT scan of the chest showed patchy areas of upper lobe ground-glass shadowing and a diagnosis of *Pneumocystis* pneumonia (PCP) was confirmed from an induced sputum sample.

> ⊕ **Expert comment**
>
> The differential diagnosis of a respiratory presentation in young adults is wide, with community-acquired pneumonia with *Pneumococcus* or atypical pathogens most common. Pregnant women are particularly vulnerable to certain infections such as varicella zoster. Always consider CMV disease in any immunocompromised patient. CMV pneumonitis is characterized by fever, dyspnoea, hypoxia, and diffuse pulmonary infiltrates on CXR. CMV can also cause a hepatitis such as that seen here. The absence of a peripheral CMV viraemia does not completely exclude end-organ disease. The X-ray changes and hypoxia in this case are suggestive of PCP in someone known to be HIV-positive. PCP was reported in about 3% of symptomatic seroconverters in a series from Argentina, and acute presentations were associated with very high plasma VLs, as in this case [1].
>
> The admitting team did well to organize an immediate HIV test as it would have been easy to dismiss the possibility, knowing that she and her partner had tested negative recently. We cannot assume that the reported partner is necessarily the only one. A recent review reported that rates of paternal discrepancy vary between studies from 0.8% to 30% (median 3.7%, n = 17), which must under-represent rates of partner change not resulting in conception, before and during pregnancy [2].

She was treated with high-dose co-trimoxazole and oral prednisolone. Three days into her PCP treatment she was started on ART consisting of Truvada™ (emtricitabine (FTC) and tenofovir (TDF)), RAL, and boosted atazanavir (ATV). Two weeks later she was discharged from hospital having made a rapid clinical recovery. Her VL had dropped to 17,400 copies/mL and CD4 count had increased to 427 cells/µL (31%). A full screen for sexually transmitted infections (STIs) was negative.

> ⊕ **Clinical tip**
>
> Remember to screen for and treat any genital tract infections in HIV-infected pregnant women. Infections such as bacterial vaginosis and *Trichomonas vaginalis* have been associated with premature rupture of membranes and may increase the risk of HIV MTCT. Ulcerative STIs such as HSV and syphilis are associated with increased HIV genital tract shedding and onward transmission of the virus. *Chlamydia trachomatis* and *Neisseria gonorrhoeae* can be acquired during passage through the birth canal, causing neonatal complications, and untreated syphilis can also cause severe paediatric disease. Don't forget to screen and treat the partners!

At 36 weeks' gestation she experienced premature rupture of the membranes. She received a stat dose of nevirapine and an emergency lower segment caesarean section

(CS) was carried out under intravenous (IV) zidovudine (ZDV) cover. Delivery VL was 870 copies/mL. She delivered a healthy baby girl who received 4 weeks of postnatal antiretroviral prophylaxis with nevirapine, ZDV, and lamivudine (3TC) and tested negative for HIV up until the age of 18 months (Box 6.1).

❝ Expert comment

Babies exposed to HIV perinatally are tested for proviral DNA in PBMCs. If the first sample, taken shortly after birth, is positive this implies that infection was acquired *in utero*. If the second sample at 6 weeks old is positive this suggests perinatal acquisition. The third sample at 12 weeks and final HIV-antibody test at 18 months of age provide further reassurance if all tests are negative. Anecdotally, a few late seroconversions after 18 months of age have been seen in the UK. It is thought that breastfeeding may have occurred, but it is difficult to determine the route of transmission definitively in such cases.

Discussion

This case highlights the challenges faced in preventing MTCT when a late diagnosis of HIV is made. This situation is now rare in the UK due to the widespread uptake of routine antenatal testing. A small number of HIV-infected women remain undiagnosed at the time of delivery, resulting in potentially preventable cases of vertical transmission. A proportion of these women will have tested HIV negative antenatally and subsequently seroconverted while pregnant or breastfeeding. Acute HIV infection is usually associated with very high HIV VLs and maternal acquisition of HIV during pregnancy is associated with higher MTCT rates [3].

MTCT of HIV-1 can take place *in utero*, intrapartum, or postnatally through breast-feeding. In the absence of medical intervention, the HIV-1 perinatal transmission rate is between 10% and 45% in non-breastfeeding women [4]. Around one-third of these transmissions occur during gestation with the remaining two-thirds occurring during delivery [4]. Breastfeeding is an additional contributor to rates of HIV-1 MTCT and the cumulative probability of transmission via this route increases with the duration of breastfeeding (from 1.6% at 3 months of age to 9.3% at 18 months of age) [5].

With the exception of the avoidance of breastfeeding, the first medical intervention demonstrated to significantly reduce the risk of HIV-1 MTCT was ZDV mono-therapy. The ACTG 076 study [6] randomized pregnant women to receive antepartum ZDV orally plus intrapartum IV ZDV with their infants receiving a 6-week course of oral ZDV. A reduction in the perinatal HIV-1 transmission rate from 25.5% to 8.3% was observed. Subsequent studies demonstrated the benefit of planned CS which was shown to reduce the risk of MTCT by a further 50% [7]. HAART may also have a protective effect compared with ZDV monotherapy which appears to be independent of its influence on HIV-1 VL [8].

Single-dose nevirapine (200 mg) given to the mother at the onset of labour followed by a single oral dose given to the neonate 72 hours after birth was also demonstrated to be highly effective at reducing HIV-1 MTCT, with results suggesting a 50% reduction in transmission during the first 14–16 weeks of life in breastfed infants [9]. While single-dose nevirapine continues to be used in resource-limited settings, it is no longer a recommended intervention because of widespread NNRTI resistance that subsequently develops in women treated with this regimen [1].

In the HAART era, the additional benefit conferred by elective CS in mothers with a fully suppressed HIV-1 VL remains uncertain (Tables 6.2 and 6.3). While most guidelines recommend that the majority of HIV-1 infected women should receive HAART in pregnancy, ZDV monotherapy with planned CS remains an option for some women.

Table 6.2 HIV-1 MTCT rates in the UK and Ireland 2000–2006 from the National Study of HIV in Pregnancy and Childhood (NSHPC) [10]

	MTCT rate (%)	95% CI	Number infected	Total
HAART + elective CS	0.7	(0.4–1.2)	17	2337
HAART + planned vaginal delivery	0.7	(0.2–1.8)	4	565
HAART + emergency CS	1.7	(1.0–2.8)	15	877
ZDV mono + elective CS	0.0	0.0 (0.0–0.8)	0	467

Source: Data from Townsend CL et al, Low rates of mother-to-child transmission of HIV following effective pregnancy interventions in the United Kingdom and Ireland, 2000–2006, *AIDS*, Volume 22, Issue 8, pp. 973–281, Copyright © 2008 Lippincott Williams & Wilkins.

Table 6.3 HIV-1 MTCT rates in women receiving HAART in the UK and Ireland 2000–2006 from the National Study of HIV in Pregnancy and Childhood (NSHPC) [10]

	MTCT rate (%)	95% CI	Number infected	Total
HAART	1.0	(0.7–1.3)	40	4120
HAART from conception	0.1	(0.0–0.6)	1	928
HAART + VL <50 copies/ml	0.1	(0.0–0.4)	3	2117

Source: Data from Townsend CL et al, Low rates of mother-to-child transmission of HIV following effective pregnancy interventions in the United Kingdom and Ireland, 2000–2006, *AIDS*, Volume 22, Issue 8, pp. 973–281, Copyright © 2008 Lippincott Williams & Wilkins.

Learning point Guidelines for using ART in pregnancy [1]

Women conceiving on an effective HAART regimen should continue this. Exceptions are PI monotherapy (which should be intensified) and stavudine (D4T) or didanosine which should not be prescribed.

Women not on HAART who require it for their own health should start treatment as soon as possible. Truvada™, Combivir™, or Kivexa™ are acceptable nucleoside backbones. The third agent should be EFV or nevirapine (if the CD4 count is <250 cells/mL) or a boosted PI.

Women not on HAART who do not require it for their own health should start temporary HAART by the 24th week of pregnancy. Patients with a VL >30,000 copies/mL should start by the beginning of the second trimester. Truvada™, Combivir™, or Kivexa™ are acceptable nucleoside backbones. A boosted PI is recommended as a third agent (NNRTIs are not recommended because of their long half-life and the risk of developing resistance if ART is abruptly stopped). Other options include:

- A triple nucleoside regimen (Trizivir™) in patients with a baseline VL <100,000 copies/mL.
- ZDV monotherapy in women planning a CS who have a baseline VL <10,000 copies/mL and a CD4 count >350 cells/μL.

Women presenting after 28 weeks who are not already on treatment should start HAART without delay. If the VL is unknown or >100,000 copies/mL a three- or four-drug regimen that includes RAL is suggested.

Untreated women presenting in labour at term should receive a stat dose of nevirapine (200 mg) and commence Combivir™ and RAL. A stat dose of Truvada™ (2 tablets) should also be considered. Intravenous ZDV should be infused for the duration of labour and delivery.

Expert comment

The latest BHIVA pregnancy guidelines (2012) contain several amendments to previous advice [1].

The UK and Ireland audit showed a rate of transmission of approximately 1/1,000 (three transmissions from 2,117 women) when maternal VL was fully suppressed at <50 copies/mL between 2000 and 2006 [10]. Two of these transmissions occurred *in utero* rather than at delivery [10]. This, and the data about the importance of early treatment to achieve an UD VL at delivery, have led to the recommendation for treatment to start early in the second trimester more frequently than was done previously [11].

Pregnant women often experience nausea with PIs. Allowing the use of EFV which has a low rate of GI side effects is useful. The prospective registry has been essential in generating safety data about the lack of neural tube defects in babies exposed to EFV *in utero*. In contrast to PIs, NNRTIs have not so far been associated with preterm birth.

Learning point Antiretroviral Pregnancy Registry

The Antiretroviral Pregnancy Registry is a voluntary collaborative project designed to record data on prenatal exposure to antiretroviral drugs for the purpose of assessing potential teratogenicity. Observational data is collected prospectively on congenital birth defects in babies exposed to antiretroviral drugs in the first trimester of pregnancy and rates are compared to those of the background population and those only exposed to the same drug in the second and third trimesters. Over 16,000 pregnant women are so far included on the database, of whom around 80% are based in the USA. Interim data from the study is published on the registry website every 6 months.

To date, the prevalence of birth defects among women with first trimester antiretroviral exposure has not differed significantly from that of either the background population, or that of women exposed in later trimesters. With sufficient power to detect a rate greater than 1.5-fold higher than the general population, no increase in birth defects has been associated with first trimester exposure to ZDV, 3TC, FTC, lopinavir (LPV), nevirapine, ritonavir, TDF, or nelfinavir. For abacavir, efavirenz (EFV), DRV, ATV, didanosine, indinavir, and D4T a rate greater than two fold higher than the general population has been excluded.

Source: data from the Antiretroviral Pregnancy Registry, available from www.apregistry.com

Maternal HAART has been shown to significantly reduce the risk of HIV transmission from breastfeeding and reductions of up to 93% in MTCT rates have been observed in some African settings [12]. Complete avoidance of breastfeeding, however, totally eliminates the risk of transmission by this route and remains recommended in settings where it is safe and affordable.

Maternal VL at delivery is the strongest determinant of risk of HIV MTCT [13] and achieving virological suppression by that time is a key aim for those starting HAART in pregnancy. The likelihood of achieving an UD VL by the time of delivery is partly determined by the VL at the start of treatment and the timing of HAART initiation. Around 54% of women with an HIV VL > 32,640 copies/mL who commence HAART after 20 weeks' gestation will fail to achieve an UD VL by the time of delivery [11].

✔ Evidence base The Women and Infants Transmission Study [13]

The Women and Infants Transmission Study (WITS) cohort study was among the first to provide evidence of the importance of maternal HIV VL in predicting HIV MTCT. WITS was a North American multicentre prospective longitudinal study examining the natural history of HIV infection in pregnant women and their babies. The study began recruiting before highly active antiretroviral therapy (HAART) became available.

A total of 552 mother-and-baby pairs were enrolled between 1990 and 1995 in a study examining the relationship between maternal plasma HIV-1 VL and the risk and timing of MTCT. Antiretroviral usage was at the discretion of the managing clinician and the use of ZDV in the cohort increased over the time as evidence for its benefit in preventing mother-to-child transmission of HIV emerged. Around 80% of babies in the cohort were delivered vaginally.

An overall transmission rate of 20.6% was observed which declined over the course of the study as ZDV use became more common. Maternal plasma HIV-1 VL was found to be strongly associated with the risk of transmission even after adjustment for other factors. Prolonged rupture of membranes (>4 hours) and low infant birth weight (<2,500 g) were also independently associated with transmission risk. Treatment with ZDV was seen to reduce the vertical transmission rate of HIV, an effect which did not solely occur as a result of reduced maternal HIV-1 RNA levels.

Transmission rates were highest in mothers with HIV-1 VLs greater than 50,000 copies/mL, with the highest rates (63.3%) seen in women with VLs greater than 100,000 copies/mL who had not received ZDV. On the other hand, no transmissions were seen in the 56 patients whose VL was below 1,000 copies/mL at the time of delivery.

Many factors are taken into consideration when deciding when to start new HAART in pregnancy. It is often preferred not to start new drugs in the first trimester in order to avoid complications due to pregnancy-induced nausea and vomiting. Although emerging safety data on antiretroviral drugs in pregnancy is reassuring, minimizing foetal exposure to drugs in early pregnancy is also sometimes favoured. In general, women starting HAART in pregnancy to prevent MTCT should begin treatment by the 24th gestation week at the latest. Those with higher VLs (> 30,000 copies/mL) should start by the beginning of the second trimester.

✔ Evidence base PIs and preterm labour

Some studies have reported an increased risk of preterm delivery (<37 weeks gestational age) with ritonavir-boosted PIs whereas others have not found this association. Much of the evidence for an association comes from cohort studies, and confounding due to other factors associated with preterm

(continued)

labour (e.g. ethnicity, smoking, recreational drug use, obstetric history, and disease stage) is difficult to control for.

The European Collaborative Study [14] was among the first to report an association. Among 3,920 mother-and-baby pairs, of whom only 896 were receiving ART, women receiving PI-based HAART were more than twice as likely to deliver prematurely than those who were untreated (AOR 2.60; 95% CI 1.43–4.75). **The French Perinatal Cohort** [15] enrolled 13,271 women between 1990 and 2009 in a study examining prematurity. Of these, 1,253 women were included in a sub-study investigating factors associated with preterm birth among patients starting PI-based ART during pregnancy; 85% of these women were taking ritonavir-boosted PIs, the majority of whom were prescribed LPV. The most frequently used non-boosted PI was nelfinavir (92% of those not on LPV). Boosted PI use was significantly associated with preterm birth compared with unboosted PIs (aHR 2.03; 95% CI 1.06–3.89; p =.03). However, 61% of premature deliveries occurred due to spontaneous rupture of membranes and this did not seem to be related to boosted PI use. **The Botswana Mma Bana Trial** [16] compared rates of preterm delivery between 267 pregnant women randomized to receive a boosted PI-based regimen and 263 women randomized to receive a triple nucleoside reverse transcriptase (NRTI) inhibitor regimen. The PI-based regimen was significantly associated with preterm delivery in the study, with a twofold higher rate of preterm delivery compared with the triple NRTI-based regimen (AOR 2.02; 95% CI 1.25–3.27).

Other large observational studies and meta-analyses, however, have failed to find any significant association between PI use and prematurity [17]. In the **International Maternal Paediatric Adolescent AIDS Clinical Trials Group** [18] women initiating PI-based HAART in pregnancy were directly compared with those initiating non-PI-based regimens and no association was found between the ART regimen used and the risk of preterm delivery.

In the absence of a specifically designed randomized study, the data regarding PIs and preterm delivery remain equivocal. PI-based HAART, however, remains a crucial component of PMTCT (prevention of mother-to-child transmission) and any potential risks must be balanced against safety, efficacy, and tolerability.

⭐ **Learning point** Key points in obstetric management [1]

Vaginal delivery is recommended for women on HAART with a HIV VL <50 HIV copies/mL plasma at gestational week 36, in the absence of any obstetric contraindications. Obstetric management in these women should follow the same general principles as the HIV uninfected population. Vaginal delivery is also recommended for elite controllers.*

Elective CS is recommended for all women with a VL > 400 copies/mL at week 36. Elective CS is also recommended for all women taking ZDV monotherapy, regardless of delivery VL (with the exception of elite controllers).

Elective CS carried out primarily for PMTCT should usually be carried out between 38 and 39 weeks' gestation. This contrasts with the optimal timing for CS planned for obstetric reasons, which is between 39 and 40 weeks' gestation.

Immediate CS is recommended for all patients experiencing pre-labour spontaneous rupture of membranes at term who have a VL ≥1,000 copies/mL. If maternal VL is <50 copies/mL then immediate induction of labour is recommended.

Intrapartum IV ZDV infusion is recommended for all women where VL is unknown or >10,000 copies/mL. An infusion can also be considered in women on zidovudine monotherapy or in women on HAART with a VL between 50 and 10,000 copies/mL regardless of mode of delivery.

*Elite controllers are a small subset of HIV-infected individuals who maintain an UD plasma VL without ART.

Seroconversion in late pregnancy was complicated in this case by an OI, *Pneumocystis jirovecii* pneumonia (PCP). Like many other infections, PCP usually has a more aggressive course during pregnancy. Additionally, it has been associated with preterm labour and other adverse foetal outcomes [19]. First-line treatment for PCP is 21 days of high-dose co-trimoxazole, and this recommendation does not differ in pregnancy [20]. Steroids should also be used for patients with a pO_2 < 9.3 kPa. Early initiation of HAART (within 2 weeks of PCP treatment) has not been associated with an increased risk of immune reconstitution inflammatory syndrome (IRIS) and drug interactions are usually manageable [20].

Patients presenting in the third trimester of pregnancy with a high VL (> 100,000 copies/mL) should be treated with a three- or four-drug HAART regimen that includes RAL [1]. The HIV-1 INI RAL has been shown to have rapid antiretroviral activity with shorter times to achieving virological suppression when used in combination treatments than conventional cART. Like most antiretroviral drugs, RAL is unlicensed in pregnancy; however, the speed of virological decay observed makes it a highly attractive option in late pregnancy.

A dramatic 4.9 log drop in HIV VL within 8 weeks of starting ART was seen in the patient in this case. It is possible that magnitude of this drop may have been partly exaggerated by the natural course of acute HIV infection. However, the use of RAL is likely to have significantly contributed to the extent and rapidity of this virological response, and similarly rapid declines in HIV VL in patients with established HIV infection have been observed in late pregnancy.

Four weeks of antiretroviral post-exposure prophylaxis (PEP) is recommended for all infants born to HIV-infected mothers and three-drug HAART is advised for those born to mothers with a detectable VL [1]. Infant PEP should start as soon as possible within 72 hours of delivery. For most babies requiring triple therapy, a regimen of ZDV, 3TC, and nevirapine is used.

HIV infection is associated with an increased risk of preterm labour and preterm neonates may be at increased risk of acquiring HIV vertically [14]. Absorption of orally administered drugs in preterm neonates is unpredictable due to the immaturity of their GI tract. There may also be delays in starting enteral feeding in those who are very preterm because of the risk of necrotizing enterocolitis. Parenteral antiretroviral drugs that can be used in preterm neonates unable to take oral medication are limited to IV ZDV and IV enfuvirtide (ENF) (T20). Intravenous ENF is unlicensed and has not yet been subjected to formal neonatal pharmacokinetic studies.

An additional option is preloading the infant transplacentally. A 200 mg stat dose of oral nevirapine given to the mother at least 2 hours before delivery is the most common drug used in this way, and effective therapeutic nevirapine concentrations (> 100 ng/mL) can be maintained in the neonate for up to 6 days [21]. RAL and double dose Truvada™ (TDF + FTC) also cross the placenta rapidly and have been used to load infants transplacentally; their use should always be considered in any situation where the infant is anticipated to have difficulty receiving oral PEP [22]. Drug elimination is likely to be more prolonged in preterm neonates compared to term babies, probably due to immature hepatic metabolism pathways [21,23].

HIV seroconversion in late pregnancy poses a number of management difficulties and allows minimal time for the patient to adjust to the diagnosis or make informed choices. The patient's co-operation and adherence to treatment in this case was critical to the success of all the medical interventions implemented, and input from multidisciplinary HIV, obstetric, and paediatric team members is invaluable. This case illustrates some of the complexities that can arise when managing HIV in pregnancy and how developments in our understanding of antiretroviral pharmacology can play an important role in the prevention of HIV MTCT.

A final word from the expert

There were many challenges presented by this case, not least considering the diagnosis of HIV seroconversion as well as PCP, which is uncommon during seroconversion. If clinically indicated to confirm a diagnosis a CT scan can be performed in pregnancy; and guidelines for the use of CT are becoming available. Some mothers have reported feeling that they were treated as vehicles of potential infection by clinicians focusing on reducing the risk of MTCT, so it is important to manage the mother for her own sake.

Nevertheless, rapid reduction of VL is likely to reduce the risk of MTCT *in utero* and at delivery. INIs have a unique role in the rapid reduction in VL. RAL does not, however, have a high genetic barrier to resistance (GBR) so quadruple therapy including two nucleoside analogues and a boosted protease inhibitor (bPI) should be initiated while awaiting the baseline resistance test in case of transmitted resistance. An additional consideration is that if the baby is born prematurely RAL and nevirapine, given as a single dose, will maintain therapeutic levels for at least a few days even in very premature neonates who may not absorb oral drugs adequately. Double-dose TDF will also be effective in preloading, if the mother is not already on a TDF-containing regimen.

All units managing HIV-positive pregnant women should be encouraged to report to the prospective pregnancy registry to help increase information about the safety of antiretroviral treatment in pregnancy: http://www.apregistry.com. In the UK, HIV-positive women are strongly encouraged not to breastfeed. This means that they return to fertility rapidly. It is important to plan postnatal contraception during the pregnancy to avoid an unplanned further pregnancy.

References

1 Taylor GP, Clayden P, Dhar J et al. British HIV Association guidelines for the management of HIV infection in pregnant women 2012. *HIV Med* 2012; 13(suppl 2): 87–157.

2 Bellis MA, Hughes K, Hughes S, Ashton JR. Measuring paternal discrepancy and its public health consequences. *J Epidemiol Community Health* 2005; 59: 749–754.

3 Birkhead GS, Pulver WP, Warren BL, Hackel S, Rodríguez D, Smith L. Acquiring human immunodeficiency virus during pregnancy and mother-to-child transmission in New York: 2002–2006. *Obstet Gynecol* 2010; 115: 1247–1255.

4 De Cock KM, Fowler MG, Mercier E et al. Prevention of mother-to-child HIV transmission in resource-poor countries. *JAMA* 2000; 283: 1175–1182.

5 Read JS. Late postnatal transmission of HIV-1 in breast-fed children: an individual patient data meta-analysis. *J Infect Dis* 2004; 189: 2154–2166.

6 Connor EM, Sperling RS, Gelber R et al. Reduction of maternal–infant transmission of human immunodeficiency virus type 1 with zidovudine treatment. *N Eng J Med* 1994; 331: 1173–1180.

7 Read J, Scherpbier H, Boer K. The mode of delivery and the risk of vertical transmission of human immunodeficiency virus type 1: a meta-analysis of 15 prospective cohort studies: the International Perinatal HIV Group. *N Eng J Med* 1999; 340: 977–987.

8 Cooper ER, Charurat M, Mofenson L et al. Combination antiretroviral strategies for the treatment of pregnant HIV-1-infected women and prevention of perinatal HIV-1 transmission. *J Acquir Immune Defic Syndr* 2002; 29: 484–494.

9 Guay LA, Musoke P, Fleming T et al. Intrapartum and neonatal single-dose nevirapine compared with zidovudine for prevention of mother-to-child transmission of HIV-1 in Kampala, Uganda: HIVNET 012 randomised trial. *Lancet* 1999; 354: 795–802.

10 Townsend CL, Cortina-Borja M, Peckham CS, de Ruiter A, Lyall H, Tookey PA. Low rates of mother-to-child transmission of HIV following effective pregnancy interventions in the United Kingdom and Ireland, 2000–2006. *AIDS* 2008; 22: 973–981.

11 Read PJ, Mandalia S, Khan P et al. When should HAART be initiated in pregnancy to achieve an undetectable HIV viral load by delivery? *AIDS* 2012; 26: 1095–1103.

12 Marazzi MC, Nielsen-Saines K, Buonomo E et al. Increased infant human immunodeficiency virus-type one free survival at one year of age in sub-saharan Africa with maternal use of highly active antiretroviral therapy during breast-feeding. *Pediatr Infect Dis J* 2009; 28: 483–487.

13 Garcia PM, Kalish LA, Pitt J et al. Maternal levels of plasma human immunodeficiency virus type 1 RNA and the risk of perinatal transmission. Women and Infants Transmission Study Group. *N Eng J Med* 1999; 341: 394–402.

14 European Collaborative Study; Swiss Mother and Child HIV Cohort Study. Combination antiretroviral therapy and duration of pregnancy. *AIDS (Lond)* 2000; 14: 2913–2920.

15 Sibiude J, Warszawski J, Tubiana R et al. Premature delivery in HIV-infected women starting protease inhibitor therapy during pregnancy: role of the ritonavir boost? *Clin Infect Dis* 2012; 54: 1348–1360.

16 Powis KM, Kitch D, Ogwu A et al. Increased risk of preterm delivery among HIV-infected women randomized to protease versus nucleoside reverse transcriptase inhibitor-based HAART during pregnancy. *J Infect Dis* 2011; 204: 506–514.

17 Kourtis AP, Schmid CH, Jamieson DJ, Lau J. Use of antiretroviral therapy in pregnant HIV-infected women and the risk of premature delivery: a meta-analysis. *AIDS* 2007; 21: 607–615.

18 Patel K, Shapiro DE, Brogly SB et al. Prenatal protease inhibitor use and risk of peterm birth among HIV-infected women initiating antiretroviral drugs during pregnancy. *J Infect Dis* 2010; 201: 1035–1044.

19 Ahmad H, Mehta NJ, Manikal VM et al. *Pneumocystis carinii* pneumonia in pregnancy. *Chest* 2001; 120: 666–671.

20 Nelson M, Dockrell D, Edwards S. British HIV Association and British Infection Association guidelines for the treatment of opportunistic infection in HIV–seropositive individuals 2011. *HIV Med* 2011; 12: 1–5.

21 Mirochnick M, Fenton T, Gagnier P et al. Pharmacokinetics of nevirapine in human immunodeficiency virus type 1-infected pregnant women and their neonates. *J Infect Dis* 1998; 178: 368–374.

22 TEmAA, ANRS 12109 Study Group, Arrivé E, Chaix M, Nerrienet E et al. Tolerance and viral resistance after single-dose nevirapine with tenofovir and emtricitabine to prevent vertical transmission of HIV-1. *AIDS (Lond)* 2009; 23: 825–833.

23 Hegazi A, Mc Keown D, Doerholt K, Donaghy S, Sadiq ST, Hay P. Raltegravir in the prevention of mother-to-child transmission of HIV-1: effective transplacental transfer and delayed plasma clearance observed in preterm neonates. *AIDS* 2012; 26: 2421–2423.

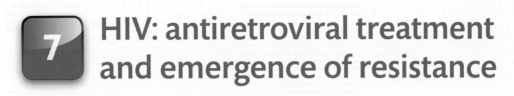

7 HIV: antiretroviral treatment and emergence of resistance

Daniel Bradshaw and Amber Arnold

Expert commentary Andrew Carr

Case history

A 35-year-old homosexual male was diagnosed at routine testing with subtype B HIV-1 infection in 2007. There was a history of depression in 2001. He took no regular medications or recreational drugs and had never received HIV PEP. His last negative HIV test had been 1.5 years previously. His CD4 count was 460 (27%) cells/mm^3 and VL 23,000 copies/mL. Viral genotypic resistance testing (genotyping) showed the reverse transcriptase (RT) mutation T215C.

⊕ Learning point Resistance testing

High production rates and lack of proof-reading ability in RT lead to high mutation rates and many quasi-species of virus within each individual.

The presence of an antiretroviral drug in a non-suppressive regimen will exert a selective pressure favouring expansion of pre-existing antiretroviral-resistant quasi-species. Sufficient potency to suppress viral replication to UD levels has traditionally required at least three fully active agents.

Three methods for determining drug susceptibility are used: genotype, phenotype, and virtual phenotype testing.

1. Genotypic testing (e.g. Trugene) is the most widely used method for detecting drug resistance. This method involves identification of nucleotide sequences at key regions of the genome known to be associated with antiviral resistance. Results are interpreted in the context of known phenotypic effects of resistance mutations from previous phenotypic assays. The main advantage is that this is a quick and relatively cheap process. However, the main disadvantage is that quasi-species at <20% of the total population cannot be detected in most routine assays and these assays are not very sensitive with low VLs (e.g. <500–1,000 copies/mL). The other disadvantages are that in patients with multiple resistances it is difficult to predict how all the mutations will interact; and that new mutations may be identified for which there are no phenotypic data and the relevance difficult to determine.
2. Phenotypic testing (e.g. Antivirogram) involves culturing virus in different concentrations of drug and looking for the concentration required to inhibit viral replication by 50% (IC50). Phenotyping assays are less commonly used than genotypic testing as they are slower, more expensive, and involve handling live virus. They are useful, however, in multidrug-resistant (MDR) HIV where resistance may be difficult to predict from the genetic analysis, given the complex pattern of mutations. Phenotypic testing is reported as fold change (FC) in the IC50 relative to a control wild-type virus. Different cut-offs are used for FCs to define whether or not a virus is susceptible to a particular drug.
3. Virtual phenotyping can be thought of as the interpretation phase of genotypic testing. The genotype is compared to a large database of genotype–phenotype pairs which have been previously sequenced and phenotyped. A predicted FC is reported. Genotypic assays are the most commonly used due to ease and cost. The BHIVA guidelines suggest performing genotypic testing on newly diagnosed patients, those with a slow response to initial therapy, and for those thought to be failing ART, to help guide a new drug regimen [1]. Resistance testing should be undertaken while the patient is still on the failing regimen or within weeks of stopping the regimen to ensure that mutations will be identified.

> ➕ **Clinical tip** How to interpret a genotypic resistance assay result
>
> As in the case described, each time a sample is submitted for resistance testing a list of mutations will come back from the laboratory. Mutations are routinely listed as a codon number preceded by a letter representing the amino acid in wild-type virus and followed by a letter representing the amino acid that has been substituted; e.g. M184V means that at codon 184 methionine has been replaced by valine. If two letters are seen at the end it indicates a mix; e.g. M184M/V represents a mix of wild-type methionine and new-type valine.
>
> Most laboratories will interpret the results for you. If you want to check the interpretations you can always key in the mutations to a database yourself. There are many online databases which can be used to predict phenotypic drug sensitivities from known genotypic information. The most popular of these is HIVdb, developed by Stanford University Medical Center, which is rapidly updated in the light of evidence from new studies (hivdb.stanford.edu). Other databases accessible to the public are maintained by the Agence Nationale de Recherche sur le Sida (ANRS) (www.anrs.fr) and Rega Institute for Medical Research (www.kuleuven.be/rega/rei).
>
> A single resistance profile may not identify all the resistance mutations potentially present. Mutations may be at levels lower than those detected by conventional sequencing and if there have been drug switches mutations may have reverted back to wild-type or intermediary forms (revertants). Therefore, a single resistance profile must be interpreted alongside previous resistance profiles and in the context of a patient's complete drug history. A knowledge of the common mutations to arise on each drug combination is also helpful to give an idea of which mutations may have occurred but have not been identified.

The mutation was identified as a revertant mutation and the patient was asked whether he was aware of being infected by a partner receiving ART. He did not know how or when he had been infected as he had multiple casual sexual partners. Hepatitis C antibody testing was negative and he was immune to hepatitis A and B. Clinical examination and routine laboratory tests were unremarkable. He was not started on antiretrovirals, in line with guidelines at the time.

> ✚ **Learning point** Transmitted resistance
>
> All patients should undergo conventional genotyping at baseline to establish if there is any resistance present. In the UK, resistance to any drug class in drug-naïve patients was identified in 13.6% of tests in 2002, declining to 9% in 2005, possibly driven overall by a fall in NRTI resistance (http://www.hpa.org.uk/hpr/archives/2007/hpr3107.pdf).
>
> Resistance at baseline can be due to presence of transmitted drug resistance (TDR), or undisclosed prior ART. Genotyping should occur as soon as the patient is diagnosed even if there is no intention of starting therapy for some time, to increase the likelihood of detecting mutations. Mutations can revert to wild-type or intermediary forms (revertants) over time without the selective pressures of drug exposure. Even if TDR is not detected at baseline, resistant mutations may still be present in the form of proviral DNA or as minority quasi-species in plasma RNA below the level of detection of conventional assays, and have the potential to impact on future therapy. See Table 7.1.
>
> **Table 7.1 Rates of reversion of resistance mutations to wild-type**
>
> | Mutation | Time to reversion |
> | --- | --- |
> | T215Y | 23% at 2 months, 45% at 4 months |
> | M184V | 40% at 2 months, 74 % at 4 months |
> | K103N | 36% at 2 months, 63% at 4 months |
>
> Source: Data from Paquet AC et al, Differences in reversion of resistance mutations to wild-type under structured treatment interruption and related increase in replication capacity, *PloS One*, Volume 6, Issue 1, e14638, Copyright © 2011 Paquet et al.
>
> (continued)

Our patient has acquired virus with the partial revertant mutation T215C, a sentinel marker of TDR. This mutation, although not directly impacting on phenotypic resistance, represents a revertant from the thymidine analogue mutation (TAM) 215Y/F and develops due to its increased fitness over the TAM in the absence of drug selective pressure. Most partial T215 revertants require only a single nucleotide mutation to revert back to the TAM. T215C is also a marker of further resistance mutations that may not have been identified by conventional resistance testing. Ultrasensitive sequencing has identified additional RT resistance mutations in 27% (6/22) of samples with 215 revertants, including M184I, as compared to 4/29 (14%) of control samples [2].

⊕ **Clinical tip** What are TAMs?

TAMs are mutations in the enzyme RT associated with resistance to the thymidine analogues, ZDV and D4T. TAMs also cause resistance to abacavir (ABC) and other NRTIs when present in groups.

TAMs emerge sequentially on ZDV- or D4T-containing regimens. Two sequences of TAMs may occur which display differing levels of resistance and cross-resistance to other NRTIs [3]. See Figure 7.1.

The mechanism by which TAMs produce drug resistance has been partially elucidated. HIV-1 RT is a heterodimer made up of a RNA-dependent DNA polymerase and a DNA-dependent DNA polymerase. The enzyme produces a DNA copy from viral RNA through incorporating and linking nucleotides. Once phosphorylated, NRTIs mimic natural nucleotides (nucleotide analogues) and compete for incorporation into viral DNA. Once an NRTI is incorporated, further nucleotides cannot be added due to the lack of a terminal 3' hydroxyl group on the NRTI, leading to chain termination. TAMs confer resistance through mutations in RT that lead to an ATP-dependent excision of the NRTI called pyrophosphorolysis. After removal of the NRTI the 3' hydroxyl group of the preceding nucleotide is free to continue chain elongation by attachment to natural nucleotides [3].

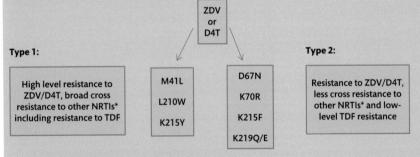

Type 1:

High level resistance to ZDV/D4T, broad cross resistance to other NRTIs* including resistance to TDF

M41L
L210W
K215Y

ZDV or D4T

D67N
K70R
K215F
K219Q/E

Type 2:

Resistance to ZDV/D4T, less cross resistance to other NRTIs* and low-level TDF resistance

* Nucleoside reverse transcriptase inhibitor (NRTI)
* For tenofovir (TDF), abacavir (ABC) and didanosine (DDI), 3 or more TAMs are usually required for high-level resistance. However, for abacavir, only 1 TAM is required if in combination with M184V. TAMs are not involved in resistance to lamivudine (3TC)/emtricitabine (FTC).

Figure 7.1 Two sequences of TAMs may occur on ZDV or D4T-containing therapy.

TAMs may also act as a marker of further UD archived resistance mutations. Therefore the decision is often made to use a PI rather than an NNRTI in the regimen because NNRTI resistance may be UD (archived) and the PI have a higher GBR. A dual NRTI combination (e.g. TDF/FTC) may still be used in the presence of TAMs in combination with a PI but this should be discussed at a resistance meeting.

❝ Expert comment

As this patient has evidence of transmitted resistance, he should be discussed at a virtual clinic or other multidisciplinary team (MDT) involving senior doctors, pharmacists, and adherence support nurses before initiation of ART. Poor initial choice of therapy can necessitate switching to second-line regimens which may be complicated by pill burden and increased toxicity.

❝ Expert comment

These are the most common mutations detectable after virological failure on Atripla.™ M184V is usually the first to be detected, followed by K103N. TDF resistance, usually associated with K65R, might subsequently occur if this combination is continued [5]. Broader NNRTI resistance may also subsequently arise which would compromise future etravirine (ETV)-containing regimens.

Two years later the patient's CD4 count had declined to 348 cells/mm^3 (16%) and VL was 110,000 copies/mL. He saw a registrar who commenced treatment as the CD4 count was now < 350 cells/mm^3, below which BHIVA guidelines recommended initiation of ART [4].

He commenced co-formulated EFV, TDF, and FTC in the form of Atripla™ 1 tablet od. After 3 months his CD4 count was 487 (20%) cells/mm^3 and VL 5,029 copies/mL. He was tolerating treatment well and adherence was thought to be good. At 6 months after starting treatment CD4 count was 500 (21%) cells/mm^3 and VL 834 copies/mL. Because his VL was not fully suppressed at 6 months, repeat genotyping was performed, which showed RT resistance mutations M184V and K103N [1].

✪ Learning Point: M184V: What is its significance and what are the clinical implications?

M184V describes an amino acid change from methionine to valine in the structure of RT at codon 184. This structural change increases the selective ability of the enzyme to incorporate the natural nucleotide over the nucleotide analogue via steric hindrance [3]. This mechanism is known as 'discrimination'. M184V is the most prevalent HIV-1 RT mutation seen in the context of non-suppressive 3TC/FTC or abacavir-containing therapy. The mutation emerges within days to weeks of non-suppressive regimens and confers high-level resistance to both 3TC and FTC and partial resistance to abacavir and didanosine. M184V also leads to resensitization to ZDV, D4T, and TDF as well as delaying development of TAMs on ZDV/D4T-containing therapy. M184V also reduces the replicative capacity of the virus, known as 'fitness'. However, the benefit of reduced fitness is usually only employed in MDR HIV that cannot be fully suppressed [4].

If M184V alone is detected on baseline genotyping, there may be other archived NRTI and/or NNRTI resistance, and a bPI-based regimen is recommended over NNRTI or INI based-therapy. Many favour replacing all NRTIs to which there is documented or likely resistance (i.e. not using 3TC or FTC) with new or active NRTIs (e.g. TDF, ZDV) or agents from other classes. However, one study showed that even in the presence of M184V, the use of a PI with a 3TC-containing backbone is usually sufficient to provide virological suppression. For example, DRV/ritonavir plus TDF and 3TC is usually sufficient [6].

✪ Learning point First- and second-generation NNRTI resistance

NNRTIs, unlike NRTIs, are non-competitive inhibitors of RT and bind to a hydrophobic pocket close to the active end of the enzyme. The presence of the NNRTI bound near to the active site blocks the nucleotides from binding (steric hindrance). Resistance occurs when amino acid changes occur in (e.g. Y181C) or near to (e.g. K103N) the binding pocket on RT so that the NNRTI cannot access the site.

Only one mutation is required for resistance to occur (low GBR) to first-generation NNRTIs like nevirapine and EFV. The pharmacokinetic properties of these drugs also favour the occurrence of resistance. They have long half-lives so that if the drugs are stopped suddenly, exposure continues at sub-therapeutic levels, leading to resistance. If these drugs are stopped for any reason the tail period should be covered with other active drugs. For these two reasons NNRTI resistance can develop rapidly. For example, after a single dose of nevirapine given intrapartum to reduce MTCT of HIV-1, 4/50 (8%) women were found to harbour CD4+ cells latently infected with K103N-mutant virus >6 months later [7].

K103N confers high-level resistance to both EFV and nevirapine. It is the most likely NNRTI resistance mutation to occur when a patient is failing treatment with EFV. Y181C is another common NNRTI

(continued)

mutation that is more likely to occur on failing treatment with nevirapine. If a patient fails one first-generation NNRTI, another first-generation NNRTI drug should not be used.

ETV, a second-generation NNRTI, has a higher GBR and has activity against viruses with single NNRTI mutations, including K103N and Y188L. This is achieved through more flexible binding of ETV to the specific NNRTI-binding pocket of RT. However, continued exposure to first-generation NNRTIs in the presence of single mutation resistance can lead to selection of further mutations which may prejudice subsequent second-generation NNRTI regimens [8].

✚ Clinical tip Barriers to resistance

Some drugs require only one mutation to confer high-level resistance. These drugs are referred to as having a low GBR. An example of a drug class with a low GBR are the first-generation NNRTIs which require only one point mutation to confer resistance, e.g. K103N. Other drugs like the PI may be referred to as having a high GBR because they require several mutations before susceptibility is reduced significantly. How likely a regimen is to fail is due not only to the GBR of the drugs but also to other features like the pharmacokinetics (PK) of the drug, how well the PKs of each drug in a regimen match, and the type of non-adherence a patient exhibits. For example, a patient taking Atripla™ (EFV/TDF/FTC) who is prone to stopping his medications for whole weeks would develop resistance to EFV very quickly due to the long half-life of EFV compared to TDF/FTC (effectively monotherapy). A regimen containing a PI with a short half-life would be better. However, a sporadic missed dose would not be such a problem with Atripla™ due to the long half-lives of the drugs.

❝ Expert comment

In switching to PI-based therapy, preferred options would be ATV or DRV, both boosted with ritonavir. Both agents can be taken as part of od regimens. These newer PIs show more favourable tolerability profiles over Kaletra™ and therefore improved adherence. In the Artemis study of treatment-naïve individuals commencing first-line PI-based therapy, fewer GI side effects were observed in the DRV/ritonavir arm compared to Kaletra™ [9]. Similar findings were seen for ATV/ritonavir over Kaletra™ in the Castle study [10].

He was switched to ritonavir-boosted LPV (Kaletra™) two tablets twice daily, RAL 400 mg twice daily, an INI, and co-formulated TDF-FTC (Truvada™) one tablet daily. However, he developed nausea and diarrhoea and subsequently admitted to taking only around half his Kaletra™ in an attempt to mitigate his symptoms.

After 4 months, CD4 count was 440 cells/mm^3 (19%) and VL 1,021 copies/mL. Genotyping showed RT mutations as above with L10F, V82A, and L90M in protease (PR), and N155H in integrase (IN). Tropism testing revealed virus that was R5 tropic, suggesting that the CCR5 antagonist MVC could be used.

✚ Clinical tip Protease and INI resistance

Protease is responsible for cleavage of the viral precursor proteins to produce mature infectious virus. PI mimic the natural substrates of protease and inhibit this enzyme by binding specifically to the active site and reducing its affinity for the natural substrate.

PI have a high GBR in that they require multiple mutations for significant resistance to occur. Our patient has two major mutations, V82A and L90M, and one minor mutation, L10F. In combination these mutations confer intermediate or high-level resistance to all PIs except DRV/ritonavir and tipranavir/ritonavir.

Integrase is responsible for transfer and integration of the viral DNA into the host chromosomal DNA in a multistep process. The first step is termed 3′ processing whereby integrase binds to the viral DNA, removes the terminal dinucleotide from the 3′ end, and along with other proteins forms the preintegration complex (PIC). The PIC enters the nucleus and the integrase enzyme nicks the chromosomal DNA, revealing hydroxyl groups, and enables covalent bonding of the viral DNA to the host DNA. The second step is known as strand transfer. Current INIs act at the strand transfer step by

(continued)

binding to the active site on integrase so that the host DNA cannot bind. First-generation INI (e.g. RAL) have a low GBR and require only one of the following primary mutations to become ineffective: Q148H, N155H, or Y143R/C. N155H emerges early but is replaced by the Q148H/G140S mutant over time due to the latter's fitness advantage. The second-generation INI DTG has a higher GBR and is likely to be active in the presence of a single primary mutation. As with NNRTIs, if second-generation INI are going to be used in the future, a failing regimen containing a first-generation INI should be stopped early to prevent further mutations occurring.

> **❝ Expert comment**
>
> PI resistance is considerably less common than NRTI, NNRTI, or first-generation INI resistance. In patients failing first-line therapy with a PI and two NRTIs at 48 weeks, less than 1% demonstrate PI mutations and 10–20% NRTI mutations, while 75% have wild-type virus. By comparison, in individuals failing first-line therapy with an NNRTI and two NRTIs, up to two-thirds have NNRTI mutations and half have NRTI mutations.

> **❝ Expert comment**
>
> DRV/ritonavir can be prescribed od as 800 mg/100 mg respectively for most patients. Twice-daily dosing is indicated in the presence of darunavir resistance-associated mutations (DRAMs).

> **❝ Expert comment**
>
> Mental health problems are common in people living with HIV. Patients should be referred promptly to specialist services. ART should be continued, if necessary with additional adherence support, as treatment interruption is associated with adverse outcomes.

> **❝ Expert comment**
>
> The previously detected M184V mutation has now been archived after removal of FTC from the current combination.

He was switched to ritonavir-boosted DRV 600 mg/100 mg twice daily, ETV 400 mg od, and MVC 150 mg twice daily. His diarrhoea improved rapidly and his VL was < 50 copies/mL after 2 months. He was maintained on this regimen for 1 year.

However, in 2011, following bereavement, he suffered an episode of severe depression. He consequently took his ART erratically for 4 months.

He also started taking St John's wort for 2 months but, as his depressive symptoms persisted, consulted a psychiatrist who stopped this medication and commenced 20 mg citalopram od. He was reviewed by his HIV physician and was found to have a CD4 count of 480 (18%) cells/mm^3 and VL of 1,900 copies/mL.

Genotyping showed:

- K103N E138K Y181C (RT)
- L10F I50V L76V V82A L90M (protease)
- X4-tropic

He was switched to ritonavir-boosted tipranavir 500 mg/200 mg twice daily, co-formulated ZDV and 3TC (Combivir™) 1 tablet twice daily, ENF 90 mg twice daily subcutaneously, and dolutegravir (DTG) 50 mg twice daily which at the time was only available within an expanded access programme. Full viral suppression was achieved by 3 months.

Discussion: A commentary on drug choices for this patient

This case highlights several challenges in the choice of effective ART for a patient who has a sentinel marker of transmitted resistance at baseline and then develops multidrug resistance due to poor choice of first-line ART by the doctor and poor subsequent adherence by the patient (Figure 7.2).

First treatment regimen
The patient commenced therapy with Atripla™, which was an inappropriate choice, given the likelihood of TDR. TDR should have been suspected because of the reversion

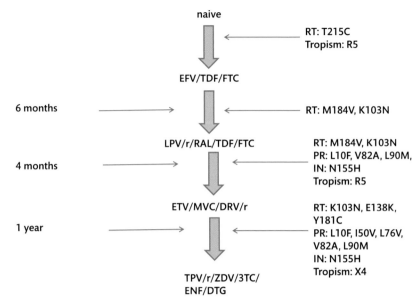

Figure 7.2 Flow diagram of antiretroviral regimens and resistance mutations over time. DTG, dolutegravir; DRV, darunavir; EFV, efavirenz; ENF, enfuvirtide; ETV, etravirine; FTC, emtricitabine; IN, integrase; LPV, lopinavir; MVC, maraviroc; P, protease; r, ritonavir boosting; RAL, raltegravir; RT, reverse transcriptase; 3TC, lamivudine; TDF, tenofovir; TPV, tipranavir; ZDV, zidovudine.

mutation T215C. The most appropriate choice of first-line therapy in a patient with TDR is usually a PI-containing regimen because of the higher GBR.

Second treatment regimen

When M184V and K103N were identified the patient was appropriately switched to therapy with a PI, RAL, and Truvada™. In patients failing first-line therapy with NNRTI plus two NRTIs with resistance, a switch to a PI-based regimen is recommended, given the higher GBR. A PI plus Truvada™ could have been an option if no other resistance mutations were suspected. However, as TAMs were likely, as indicated by the sentinel revertant mutation, two new agents were commenced. There is some evidence that a PI with RAL alone could provide complete virological suppression in individuals failing a previous regimen with a low VL and few PI-associated mutations [11]. However, there is also evidence that this dual combination does not always suppress VLs adequately. One single-arm study of ART-naïve patients found relatively frequent virological failures in those with high VLs receiving dual therapy with DRV/ritonavir and RAL alone and so TDF was continued [12]. The fourth drug, FTC, was probably excessive.

Third treatment regimen

At this stage the patient had developed PI resistance on Kaletra™, integrase resistance (N155H) on RAL, and continued to have the previous RT resistance mutations. Drug choices at this stage were very limited. After discussion he was switched to DRV/ritonavir, ETV, and MVC. DRV is a second-generation PI with substantial activity against many PI-resistant viruses. In patients with virological failure on a PI, DRV/ritonavir remains the main backbone of a new treatment regimen.

ETV was chosen, given its activity against K103N mutant virus, although it may not have been fully active in the presence of other potentially archived NNRTI mutations. Data from the DUET studies support a role for ETV with DRV/ritonavir in the context of an optimized background regimen in non-suppressed treatment-experienced patients, particularly as it may limit the emergence of darunavir-associated mutations [13].

> ✅ **Evidence base** ETV for those failing a first-line regimen with NNRT plus NRTI [8]
>
> **Study design:** This is a phase II multinational randomized controlled open-labelled trial to look at whether ETV plus two active NRTIs could be used as a second-line regimen when failure on a first-line NNRTI regimen had been documented on genotypic or phenotypic testing prior to or on trial entry. All patients were PI naïve and the comparator arm was the use of a PI plus two active NRTIs. In an unplanned interim analysis it was observed that those in the ETV group had poor virological response compared to the comparator arm and these patients were subsequently switched to a PI regimen.
>
> A total of 53 patients in each group completed the pre-switch phase. Baseline characteristics were similar (including baseline VLs and number of NNRTI-resistance-associated mutations (RAMs)) between the groups except that the median CD4 count range was lower in the ETV group (180 cells/mm^3) compared to the PI group (245 cells/mm^3) and the number of patients with at least two NRTI RAMs was higher in the ETV group (51% vs. 37%).
>
> **Results:** Up to 8 weeks of treatment, virological responses were similar between the groups, with about 30% achieving a VL <50 copies/mL. In the control group the number of responders continued to increase up to 12 weeks, but in the ETV group a plateau was reached and rebound was observed in some patients. In a multivariate analysis of baseline resistance and correlation with virological response a reduced response at 12 weeks was associated with the mutation Y181C in combination with other NNRTI mutations, increasing numbers of ETV-associated RAMs, and with increasing numbers of nucleoside analogue RAMs (e.g. TAMs, M184V, K65R). However, there was no association with the primary NNRTI resistance mutation K103N. ETV was better tolerated for GI, lipid, and liver-related side effects. It was concluded that ETV is not appropriate for use with two NRTIs in the presence of multiple NNRTI and NRTI RAMs. The DUET studies went on to look at ETV with a PI in the presence of NNRTI resistance and showed that its use improved virological response.

MVC was included in view of its novel mechanism of action and the R5 tropism result. Although there are as yet limited data for the regimen of DRV/ritonavir, ETV, and MVC from clinical trials, pharmacokinetic studies are reassuring. A meta-analysis of 10 trials between 2003 and 2010 involving patients with triple-class resistance in which new drugs were added to optimized background therapy and compared to placebo showed that the main predictive factor for efficacy was the number of fully active new drugs [14].

Fourth treatment regimen

The patient now has evidence of further resistance, with DRAMs I50V and L76V as well as development of further NNRTI resistance, E138K, and Y181C. The St John's wort he was taking is a potent inducer of cytochrome P450 cyp3A4 which increases the hepatic metabolism of ritonavir boosted PIs as well as MVC and ETV, lowering their plasma levels. Through this mechanism, as well as his poor adherence, further resistance has developed. This patient is relatively unusual, because many individuals failing treatment with DRV/ritonavir do not display DRAMs. With the two DRAMs plus the previous PI mutations the Stanford algorithm predicts intermediate or high-level resistance to all PIs except tipranavir/ritonavir. The NNRTI resistance mutations suggest that ETV would no longer be effective and the tropism result shows X4 virus, implying MVC resistance.

⊗ **Learning point** Resistance to CCR5 receptor antagonists

In order for HIV-1 to enter human cells the envelope protein gp120 must bind to the CD4 protein and to a chemokine co-receptor on host cells. The co-receptor is usually the CCR5 receptor in early infection and the CXCR4 receptor in advanced infection. CCR5 receptor antagonists inhibit virus entry by binding to the CCR5 receptor. Resistance to CCR5 antagonists arises through (i) switching co-receptor from CCR5 to CXCR4 as infection progresses or (ii) mutations in gp120 (in particular, the area known as the V3 loop which binds to CCR5). V3 loop mutations are rare in antiretroviral-naïve patients. See Figure 7.3.

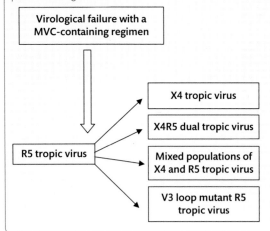

Figure 7.3 Resistance to CCR5 receptor antagonists.

The options for this patient who has resistance to four drug classes (NRTI, NNRTI, PI, INI) as well as probable resistance to CCR5 antagonists are limited. Essential to the success of any subsequent salvage regimen is adherence support.

A regimen of tipranavir/ritonavir, DTG, ENF, and Combivir™ (ZDV and 3TC) was prescribed and, fortunately, full viral suppression occurred at 3 months. This salvage regimen was selected for several reasons. Many PI-associated mutations, such as L24I, I50V, I54L, and L76V, confer hypersusceptibility to tipranavir/ritonavir. DTG, a second-generation INI, was chosen, which seems to have less cross-resistance than the first-generation INI [15]. The fusion inhibitor ENF represents an agent acting through a novel mechanism; however, it must be administered subcutaneously. There are some data for the inclusion of 3TC even in the presence of M184V-containing virus [4]. 3TC would drive M184V which reduces viral fitness and increases susceptibility to ZDV.

However, this regimen represents considerable pill burden and has the potential to incur significant toxicity including ENF-related injection site reactions, tipranavir-related hepatitis, and ZDV-related anaemia, lipoatrophy, and peripheral neuropathy. When feasible, the patient should be re-referred to the virtual clinic for consideration of treatment simplification.

⟨⟨ Expert comment

At this point, directly observed therapy should be strongly considered as well as intensive adherence counselling.

A final word from the expert

This patient develops MDR HIV after an inappropriate choice by the physician of first-line ART with NNRTI-based therapy on a background of transmitted resistance and subsequent poor patient adherence. All patients with TDR or virological failure should be referred for expert advice and discussion before treatment initiation or switch. In the context of TDR, PI-based therapy, with its higher GBR, is usually the most suitable choice. The newer PIs, ATV and DRV, are preferred over Kaletra™. In all situations of initiation and switching of therapy, the patient should be an active partner in the decision. Where patients fail therapy, a detailed discussion should take place including assessment of adherence, tolerability, toxicity, drug–drug and drug–food interactions, recreational drug use, co-morbidities, and mental health problems. Resistance testing should be performed while the patient is on failing therapy and all previous resistance tests and ART history must be evaluated. Where virological failure is confirmed, a new regimen should be constructed, if possible with three fully active agents. Tropism testing must be performed before prescribing MVC. The development of newer agents with novel mechanisms of action, such as CCR5 receptor antagonists and INI, has enabled construction of fully suppressive regimens in most patients with MDR virus. Where this is not feasible, patients should be enrolled into a pharmaceutical study to access novel investigational products.

References

1 British HIV Association. BHIVA guidelines for the routine investigation and monitoring of adult HIV-1-infected individuals 2011. *HIV Medicine* 2012; 13: 1–44.

2 Mitsuya Y, Varghese V, Wang C et al. Minority human immunodeficiency virus type 1 variants in antiretroviral-naive persons with reverse transcriptase codon 215 revertant mutations. *J Virol* 2008; 82: 10747–10755.

3 Menéndez-Arias L. Mechanisms of resistance to nucleoside analogue inhibitors of HIV-1 reverse transcriptase. *Virus Research* 2008; 134: 124–146.

4 British HIV Association. BHIVA guidelines for the treatment of HIV-1 positive adults with antiretroviral therapy 2012. Available from http://www.bhiva.org/documents/Guidelines/Treatment/2012/120430TreatmentGuidelines.pdf.

5 Miller MD. K65R, TAMs and tenofovir. *AIDS Rev* 2004; 6: 22–33.

6 Hull M, Moore D, Harris M et al. *A lamivudine (3TC)-based backbone in conjunction with a boosted protease inhibitor (PI) is sufficient to achieve virologic suppression in the presence of M184V mutations.* 49th ICAAC San Francisco. Abstract H-916, 49th ICAAC 2009, San Francisco.

7 Wind-Rotolo M, Durand C, Cranmer L et al. Identification of nevirapine-resistant HIV-1 in the latent reservoir after single-dose nevirapine to prevent mother-to-child transmission of HIV-1. *J Infect Dis* 2009; 199: 1301–1309.

8 Ruxrungtham K, Pedro RJ, Latiff GH et al. Impact of reverse transcriptase resistance on the efficacy of TMC125 (etravirine) with two nucleoside reverse transcriptase inhibitors in protease inhibitor-naive, nonnucleoside reverse transcriptase inhibitor-experienced patients: study TMC125-C227. *HIV Med* 2008; 9: 883–896.

9 Orkin C, DeJesus E, Khanlou H. Final 192-week efficacy and safety of once-daily darunavir/ritonavir compared with lopinavir/ritonavir in HIV-1-infected treatment-naïve patients in the ARTEMIS trial. *HIV Med* 2013; 14: 49–59.

10 Molina JM, Andrade-Villanueva J, Echevarria J et al. Once-daily atazanavir/ritonavir compared with twice-daily lopinavir/ritonavir, each in combination with tenofovir and emtricitabine, for management of antiretroviral-naive HIV-1-infected patients: 96-week efficacy and safety results of the CASTLE study. *J Acquir Immun Defic Syndr* 2010; 53: 323–332.

11 Burgos J, Crespo M, Falco V et al. Dual therapy based on a ritonavir-boosted protease inhibitor as a novel salvage strategy for HIV-1-infected patients on a failing antiretroviral regimen. *J Antimicrob Chemother* 2012; 67: 1453–1458.

12 Taiwo B, Zheng L, Gallien S et al. Efficacy of a nucleoside-sparing regimen of darunavir/ ritonavir plus raltegravir in treatment-naive HIV-1-infected patients (ACTG A5262). *AIDS* 2011; 25: 2113–2122.

13 Peeters M, Vingerhoets J, Tambuyzer L et al. Etravirine limits the emergence of darunavir and other protease inhibitor resistance-associated mutations in the DUET trials. *AIDS* 2010; 24: 921–924.

14 Pichenot M, Deuffic-Burban S, Cuzin L, Yazdanpanah Y. Efficacy of new antiretroviral drugs in treatment-experienced HIV-infected patients: a systematic review and meta-analysis of recent randomized controlled trials. *HIV Med* 2012; 13: 148–155.

15 Eron JJ, Clotet B, Durant J et al. Safety and efficacy of dolutegravir in treatment-experienced subjects with raltegravir-resistant HIV type 1 infection: 24-week results of the VIKING Study. *J Infect Dis* 2013; 207: 740–748.

HIV: opportunistic infections and immune reconstitution

Ellen Dwyer and Amber Arnold

ⓘ **Expert commentary** Derek Macallan

Case history

A 34-year-old Brazilian HIV-positive man presented to a GUM walk-in clinic with a 2-week history of a productive cough, fevers, and weight loss. He had been diagnosed with late-stage HIV infection at the clinic one year previously (at which time his CD4 count was 60×10^6 cells/L) but had not returned after receiving his HIV diagnosis.

On examination he was apyrexial, his chest and abdominal examination were normal, and he had no peripheral lymphadenopathy. Blood was taken for HIV VL, resistance screen, baseline virology, CD4 count, as well as routine blood samples for full blood count, urea and electrolytes, LFT, and CRP. Sputum was sent for microscopy and routine and mycobacterial culture. He had a normal chest radiograph (CXR) and he did not desaturate on exertion. A clinical diagnosis of community-acquired lower respiratory tract infection was made and he was discharged with a 5-day course of co-amoxiclav, and co-trimoxazole for PCP prophylaxis. A follow-up appointment was arranged for one week's time and an outpatient CT chest examination was requested (Table 8.1).

> ⓘ **Expert comment**
>
> Respiratory presentation is the most common presentation of OI in advanced HIV infection. A 2-week history is possibly too extended for that of an uncomplicated community-acquired pneumonic infection, especially when there are no radiographic changes. In terms of management, one might make the case that a patient with respiratory symptoms with such a low CD4 count and a normal CXR should have gone on to have a CT scan of the chest sooner rather than later. The CXR is 'normal' in about a quarter of patients with PCP, for example, and CT may reveal other pathologies such as TB.

On review the following week the patient's symptoms had improved, and it was felt that the *H. influenzae* cultured on sputum was the likely responsible respiratory pathogen. He was no longer experiencing fevers, but weight loss continued. The baseline virological serology screen revealed past infection with EBV, CMV, measles, hepatitis A, no evidence of hepatitis B or C, and a negative serum CrAg. Atripla™ (EFV, FTC, and TDF) ART was initiated and the patient was then discharged.

Fifteen days later (22 days post culture), before the outpatient CT scan had taken place, AFB were isolated on culture from the patient's sputum. When contacted he was found to have clinically deteriorated, and was feeling more generally unwell with a worsening cough. He was admitted to the local ID unit for investigation. He had a fever of 38.5°C but otherwise examination was unremarkable. Blood tests revealed a

> ⓘ **Expert comment**
>
> This patient was appropriately started on combined antiretroviral therapy (cART) promptly after diagnosis of advanced HIV infection. Although, at this stage, an OI had not been formally diagnosed, the ACTG 5164 study is relevant here. It showed that early cART resulted in decreased AIDS-associated morbidity and mortality, with no increase in adverse events or loss of virological response compared to deferred cART in patients presenting with OIs [1].

Table 8.1 Patient's results reviewed in clinic a week later

CD4	$32 \times 10^6 1/L$ (4%)	Na⁺	132 mmol/L	Platelets	121×10^9/L
VL (HIV-1 RNA)	272,000 copies/mL	K⁺	3.2 mmol/L	CRP	72 mg/L
Resistance screen	No resistance-associated mutations	Urea	8 mmol/L	ALT	32 iu/L
Sputum culture	H. influenza sensitive to amoxicillin and co-amoxiclav	Creatinine	72 µmol/L	ALP	100 iu/L
TB Sputum smear	AFB negative	Hb	9.7 g/dL		
Culture	Pending				
Blood culture	No growth	WCC	3.2×10^9/L (neutrophils 2.6, lymphocytes 0.4)		

worsening CRP of 127 mg/L, a WCC in normal range (8.9×10^9/L) but again reduced lymphocytes (0.3×10^9/L). His CXR remained unremarkable, and a high-resolution CT (HRCT) scan of the chest was carried out, which demonstrated evidence of bronchiectasis in the lingual and right middle lobe but no lymphadenopathy. A CT scan of the abdomen and pelvis was also negative for any lymphadenopathy or abnormalities. Further sputum samples and mycobacterial blood cultures were sent.

As well as investigations for the extent and differentiation of the presumed mycobacterial disease, further screening was performed to exclude other OIs. An ophthalmological examination and PCR test on blood was negative for active CMV disease. A Mantoux test was anergic and an interferon-gamma release assay (IGRA) was negative. The negative Mantoux and T spot were felt to be compatible with the patient's level of immunosuppression, and he was started on quadruple therapy for a presumed *Mycobacterium tuberculosis* (*Mtb*) infection, as well as clarithromycin to cover possible atypical mycobacterial infections such as *Mycobacterium avium* complex (MAC).

⭐ **Learning point** MAC: Clinical manifestations [2,3]

MAC consists of two species that are difficult to differentiate: *M. avium* and *M. intracellulare*. MAC is the atypical *Mycobacterium* most commonly associated with human disease and is the commonest atypical mycobacterial infection causing disease in HIV-positive individuals.

Three typical presentations of MAC infection are described:

• Pulmonary MAC infection in immunocompetent hosts
• MAC lymphadenitis in children
• Disseminated disease in those with advanced HIV (CD4 <50)

The primary features of pulmonary MAC include productive cough, fevers, and night sweats. Disseminated MAC infections tend to present more non-specifically with symptoms including night sweats, weight loss, diarrhoea, anorexia, and abdominal pain (a number of which were seen in the case described above), and these symptoms are often wrongly attributed to the underlying HIV infection, or other OIs. MAC is a common cause of PUO in those with advanced HIV disease, when no other clinical localizing signs are present.

MAC infections less commonly cause septic arthritis, osteomyelitis, and infections in the skin and soft tissue.

⊕ Clinical tip

It is important to consider both *MTb* and atypical mycobacterial infections (e.g. MAC) in patients with a CD4 count under 50 in whom an AFB has been isolated in a sputum sample. Quadruple medication for TB plus clarithromycin or azithromycin will treat both MAC and *MTb*. Treatment can be individualized once results of culture are available. If results do not fit the clinical picture it is important to send further specimens and continue treatment for both mycobacterial infections to cover dual infection.

Ten days later the patient's fevers had subsided, he was significantly clinically improved, and his CRP decreased to 41 mg/L. At this point the cultured mycobacterium was identified as MAC by the reference laboratory.

✪ Learning point Diagnosis of MAC [2,3]

Diagnosis of patients with MAC requires consideration of both clinical history and investigation findings. MAC can be a commensal organism, however it should not be thought of as such in an HIV patient with a low CD4 count. Non-specific biochemical markers include low haemoglobin (Hb), low WCC, low albumin, and raised ALP.

Chest imaging is required. CXR may be normal, though lesions are often seen on CT scanning. Typical appearances vary, but include ground-glass opacities and consolidation, and may show fibronodular bronchiectasis, especially where the lung is the primary site of infection. In disseminated disease abdominal imaging may show lymphadenopathy and hepatosplenomegaly.

In patients who may have pulmonary infection with MAC, diagnostic testing includes AFB staining and culture of sputum specimens.

In order to definitively diagnose disseminated MAC, the organism must be cultured from a sterile body site (e.g. blood or bone marrow). Although not definitive, culture from non-sterile sites including urine, stool, and sputum can be useful in deciding whether to initiate treatment in those with an indicative clinical picture. Stains of biopsy specimens from bone marrow, lymph node, or liver may demonstrate acid-fast organisms or granulomata weeks before positive blood culture results.

Blood for mycobacterial culture is a very sensitive method for diagnosing disseminated MAC. Blood cultures have been reported to be positive in 86–98% of cases in which disseminated MAC infection was confirmed on autopsy [4]. One study showed that a single blood culture identifies 91% of cases whereas two cultures will identify 98% [5].

The patient's treatment was therefore rationalized to clarithromycin, ethambutol, and rifabutin. The rifabutin dose was increased to 450 mg od from a standard dose of 300 mg od in view of the enzyme induction from the co-administration of EFV.

❝ Expert comment

Here 'rationalized' means that it was decided that cover for *Mtb* could be discontinued. Of course, *Mtb* and MAC can coexist so one would want to be fairly sure that *Mtb* really was not present before stopping the four-drug regime. It is always easier to say something is present than that it is absent. The risk here, of course, is that if co-infection with TB had been missed one might end up inadvertently treating active TB with only two drugs and so might promote the development of resistance. In this case, the clinical scenario and radiological and microbiological findings probably justify this treatment switch, but the possibility of a dual infection scenario (*Mtb* plus MAC) needs to be considered.

❝ Expert comment

'Covering the bases' in unidentified mycobacterial disease is a practice strategy that appears to safely treat both potential infections. One concern is which rifamycin to use. Most MAC guidelines suggest rifabutin [2,3]. The only published head-to-head study (which showed superiority of a rifabutin-containing regime) had different backgrounds so was not a true comparison. Interestingly, although most guidelines for MAC only mention rifabutin, the current (2012) Johns Hopkins guidelines for MAC in non-immunocompromised patients recommend rifampicin (RIF). The rifamycin is the "third agent" in MAC treatment (the macrolide and ethambutol are the most important components), so which agent is chosen is probably an academic issue only.

> ⭐ **Learning point** Treatment of MAC infection [2]
>
> The main treatment for MAC is initiation of cART in association with directed antimicrobials. These include at least two agents: a macrolide (clarithromycin 500 mg twice daily or azithromycin 500 mg once a day) and ethambutol (15 mg/kg/day), with a third agent (rifabutin 300 mg od) being added in some instances. Indications for a third agent include markedly symptomatic disease, profound immunosuppression, and the inability to construct an adequate cART regime.
>
> Treatment should continue until patients have shown a clinical improvement and an adequate immune response has emerged following cART (CD4 >100 and a virological response sustained for at least 3 months). If no such immune response occurs then treatment should be lifelong. In deciding which macrolide to use, it should be noted that studies have shown more rapid clearance of MAC from the blood with clarithromycin; however, azithromycin interacts with fewer other drugs, and also requires only od dosing, leading to greater adherence to therapy (see Table 8.2).

> ➕ **Clinical tip**: It is important to consider interactions between commonly prescribed MAC therapy and ART as these may lead to alterations in drug concentrations [2,6]
>
> See Table 8.2.

Table 8.2 Interactions between MAC therapy and standard ART

MAC treatment drug	PI with ritonavir boosting (PI/r)	Non-nucleotide reverse transcriptase inhibitors (NNRTI)
Drug effect on clarithromycin concentration	↗ by PI/r Suggest alternative agent (e.g. azithromycin)	↙ by NNRTIs. Suggest alternative agent (e.g. azithromycin)
Drug effect on rifabutin concentration	↗ by PI/r Decrease dose of rifabutin	↙ by EFV Increase dose of rifabutin ↗ by nevirapine No dose adjustment, use with caution No dose adjustment with ETV
Rifabutin effect on antiretroviral drug	Drug interactions but not significant and no need for dose adjustment of PI/r	Drug interactions with EFV and nevirapine, but no need for dose adjustment ↙ Rilpivirine with rifabutin Do not co-administer

Comment: RIF should not be used with PI due to reduction in PI drug levels >75%; ethambutol: no interactions; azithromycin: no significant interactions.

Source: Data from Panel on Antiretroviral Guidelines for Adults and Adolescents, *Guidelines for the use of antiretroviral agents in HIV-1-infected adults and adolescents*, Department of Health and Human Services, 2013, available at http://aidsinfo.nih.gov/ContentFiles/AdultandAdolescentGL.pdf and British HIV Association and British Infection Association Guidelines for the Treatment of Opportunistic Infection in HIV-seropositive Individuals 2011, *HIV Medicine*, Volume 12, Supplement 2, Copyright © 2011.

> 🕐 **Expert comment**
>
> For drug interactions an excellent resource is www.hiv-druginteractions.org.

On the day of discharge the patient complained of the emergence of new facial lesions. These were noted to be painless flesh-coloured nodules of approximately 0.5 cm in diameter. One was seen to have a central punctum, and these were diagnosed as molluscum contagiosum, to be managed conservatively, and being systemically well the patient was discharged with outpatient follow-up.

Two weeks later the patient attended clinic due to concerns regarding these lesions. They had significantly increased in size, become purple in colour, pustular, and painful, and had also begun to appear on his hands and feet. The patient also described odynophagia and subsequent weight loss. On examination ulcerating lesions were seen

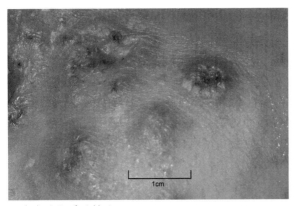

Figure 8.1 Photograph depicting facial lesions.

on both his hard and soft palate. He was admitted to hospital due to dehydration and he was treated with systemic antibiotics for presumed super-added staphylococcal infection. The diagnosis of molluscum was now in question and skin biopsy of a facial lesion was performed.

The differential diagnosis at this time included molluscum contagiosum (especially in giant or pseudocystic form), malignant lesions (e.g. KS), fungal infections (cryptococcus, coccidiocomycosis, histoplasmosis), CMV, HSV, and non-specific HIV ulceration [7] (Figures 8.1, 8.2, and 8.3).

The results of the skin biopsy demonstrated the presence of a fungal element suggestive of histoplasmosis, which was later confirmed on culture. Investigations to assess the extent of the disseminated disease were performed including an oesophagogastroduodenoscopy (OGD) examination which showed lesions in the mouth and larynx only, ophthalmic examination which was normal, and a further CT scan of the chest and abdomen which revealed new disseminated lymphadenopathy.

Treatment was commenced with intravenous liposomal amphotericin (AmBisome®) at a dose of 5 mg/kg once a day.

> **⊕ Expert comment**
>
> As part of the assessment for the extent of dissemination, ophthalmic assessment including fundoscopy is essential; LP should be considered as CNS disease is treated with higher doses and longer durations of amphotericin and may mandate use of fluconazole rather than itraconazole in the continuation phase [8].

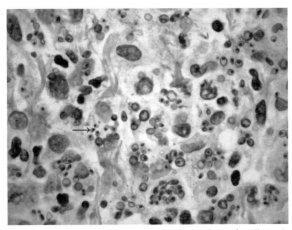

Figure 8.2 Biopsy specimen demonstrating the presence of histoplasma (small circular yeasts, marked by arrow) stained with periodic acid–Schiff diastase (PAS) stain.

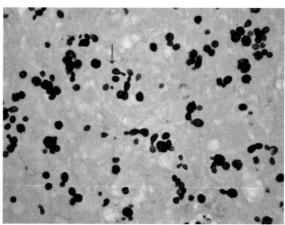

Figure 8.3 Biopsy specimen demonstrating the presence of histoplasma (black circular yeasts) stained with Grocott's methenamine silver stain. Some of the yeasts can be seen to be budding (arrow).

⭐ **Learning point** Histoplasmosis [2,3,8]

Histoplasma capsulatum is a diamorphic fungus found in soil and in bat and bird guano (especially in caves) in certain areas of the world. *Histoplasmosis capsulatum* var *capsulatum* is endemic in areas of the United States, Central and South America, and Southern and East Africa. *Histoplasmosis capsulatum* var *duboisi* is endemic in central and western Africa.

Infection is initiated when microconidia from the mould stage of the organism are inhaled.

In the immunocompetent, including patients with good CD4 counts, primary infection may be asymptomatic and often requires no treatment. Cell-mediated immunity is required to contain the infection, and relapses from previously unidentified infection can occur during a period of immunosuppression. In the immunocompromised host, infection can disseminate to multiple organs (e.g. lymphatics, adrenal glands, liver, spleen, bone marrow, and eyes). Presentation is often non-specific as PUO or can be more focal related to the area of dissemination.

Cutaneous lesions in HIV-associated histoplasmosis are commonly manifestations of more diffusely disseminated disease. These lesions can be papular, pustular, punched as ulcers, or nodules with molluscum or wart-like appearance. They can be purpuric or skin-coloured and tend to occur most often on the face, extremities, and trunk.

Definitive diagnosis is primarily made through culture of the organism from sputum, blood, bone marrow, and biopsy specimens from other sites and is positive in over 85% of HIV-infected patients with disseminated disease [3]. However, culture can take up to 6 weeks.

For a rapid diagnosis, histology of bone marrow aspirate or biopsy of an affected site such as lung, liver, or skin lesions is helpful. In tissue, *H. capsulatum* manifests as small intracellular oval-to-round shaped yeast cells (2–5 μm in greatest dimension) with single narrow-based buds. Cells often cluster in histiocytes producing a vacuolated appearance within cells. This infection may be difficult to identify on hematoxylin and eosin staining alone, but can be demonstrated with periodic acid–Schiff (PAS) and Gomori methenamine stains [9].

Serological testing has a low sensitivity in the immunosuppressed and is not recommended [2,3].

Treatment for moderate to severe disseminated disease is liposomal amphotericin B intravenously for at least 2 weeks and until a clinical response has been observed. A randomized trial showed that liposomal amphotericin 3.0 mg/kg/day was more effective than 0.7 mg/kg/day [3]. Treatment should be continued with oral itraconazole for 12 months [2,3,8]. Some evidence exists for use of other azoles including fluconazole, ketoconazole, voriconazole, and posaconazole. For mild disease an azole may be adequate for the duration of therapy [8].

After approximately 4 days of IV liposomal amphotericin therapy the patient's cutaneous lesions appeared to gradually improve, decreasing in size and appearing less swollen. He was treated for 1 month with intravenous therapy initially as an inpatient and then via an outpatient antibiotic service and was then transferred to oral itraconazole therapy for 12 months.

Due to the interactions between itraconazole and the other medications (especially the rifamycin, clarithromycin, and EFV) that this patient was receiving, it was not possible to achieve adequate itraconazole serum levels despite increases in dose.

The patient's medications were therefore altered. Due to a good response to MAC treatment, completion of 3 months of therapy, and a good virological and immunological response to cART, MAC treatment was reduced to ethambutol plus azithromycin, both of which were likely to have no or less of an effect on itraconazole levels. Good itraconazole levels were achieved without having to make any other changes to the patient's medications. He completed 12 months of treatment for MAC infection and

12 months of treatment for histoplasmosis. His viral load was UD by 5 months and his CD4 count had risen to 300 cells/mL at 1 year.

Discussion

Many challenges including those of diagnosis, treatment, and drug interactions emerged in the management of the OIs affecting this man. A further challenge was the development of histoplasmosis following several weeks of cART, and the consideration of whether this could have been prevented or identified earlier. The patient was likely to have been exposed to histoplasmosis several years earlier while he was still living in Brazil as it is not endemic in the UK. The emergence of symptoms of this previously acquired quiescent infection on cART is attributable to the phenomenon of immune reconstitution or IRIS.

IRIS describes a deregulated inflammatory response to a pre-existing microbial or host antigen that occurs on starting ART. IRIS reactions are generally subdivided into two categories described as 'unmasking IRIS' and 'paradoxical IRIS' [11].

Unmasking IRIS relates to the situation as described in this case. The lack of immune function in advanced HIV allows antigens to go 'undetected' and it is not until ART restores immune function that a response to clear the antigen is initiated. Antigens are often present at high levels and the organism is usually easily cultured.

Paradoxical IRIS describes the exacerbation or recurrence of symptoms from a disease currently being treated or previously treated. In this situation organisms are harder to culture and specimens may be sterile.

ⓘ Expert comment

Delaying cART for a few weeks after initiation of OI therapy may reduce the risk of paradoxical IRIS in some diseases (e.g. TB, cryptococcus [12]), but may also be associated with an increased risk of other HIV-related complications in patients with low CD4 counts. Delaying cART to prevent unmasking IRIS is not generally recommended; other (undiagnosed) infections may contribute to worse outcomes if cART is delayed [1]. A randomized study in non-TB IRIS showed no benefit from delaying cART [6]. TB is perhaps a special case as it may present at higher CD4 counts. If the CD4 count is <50 cells/μL, early treatment reduces overall mortality, whereas at higher CD4 counts, delaying cART (e.g. for 2 months) may be a better strategy as this reduces the risk of paradoxical IRIS.

The incidence of IRIS ranges between 15% and 25% of patients on starting cART [11]. Risk factors for IRIS include [11]:

1. Antigen-related factors: disseminated infection and higher antigen load, higher number of OIs prior to cART, shorter interval between starting treatment for OI and cART.
2. HIV-related parameters: more advanced HIV disease, i.e. low CD4 (< 50 cells/μL), high VL.
3. Treatment: cART-naïve, PI-based regimen, short OI to HIV treatment interval, and treatment response factors (rapid fall in VL, a rapid rise in CD4).
4. Host factors: younger age, black race, certain genotypic polymorphisms.

Although histoplasmosis is uncommon in the UK, in areas where the pathogen is endemic it has been reported as a common AIDS-defining condition. In French Guiana disseminated histoplasmosis is second only to TB as a common AIDS-defining condition [13]. A retrospective study performed in this area of 1,551 patients in an HIV cohort showed that disseminated histoplasmosis was more common in those patients who had been on cART for 0–2 months compared to no cART or cART for over 6 months [13].

Disseminated histoplasmosis initially diagnosed by the appearance of skin lesions has been reported to occur in unmasking IRIS on starting cART in at least 3 case reports [7]. Interestingly, during treatment two of the cases developed paradoxical IRIS at 10 months and a year into treatment, despite good initial responses to therapy.

Screening for pathogens to prevent the evolution of unmasking IRIS has been the topic of much discussion [11]. A baseline screen in those with low CD4 count should include a full history and examination plus serum testing for viral infections (e.g. CMV, EBV, hepatitis A, B, C, measles), a CXR (to look for active TB and other chest pathologies), a serum CrAg test, and ophthalmic evaluation to look for CMV retinal infection [11]. Screening for latent TB infection is advocated by the current BHIVA guidelines by way of interferon-γ release assays (IGRA) [14]. In low resource settings, Mantoux testing with subsequent prophylactic isoniazid (INH) has been shown to reduce the risk of TB by 33% [11].

This patient was screened for many infections that can unmask during treatment at his first presentation, including serum testing for CrAg, a CXR, serology for viral infections, and sputum microbiological culture. It could be argued that on first presentation the patient should have had a CT scan sooner. However, the screening that was performed established the MAC diagnosis, and excluded many other infections. When the patient was admitted he had further investigations for OIs including a retinal examination for CMV, Mantoux and IGRA testing, and a whole-body CT scan. This scan did not show any evidence of active asymptomatic histoplasmosis infection (e.g. no lymphadenopathy). Without an obvious site to biopsy, diagnosis is difficult in the UK as serology has a low sensitivity in HIV-positive patients and the urinary antigen test is not available routinely. Another option to prevent fulminant histoplasmosis could have been administration of antifungal prophylaxis based on risk factors such as the patient's demographic background, if the team were certain there was no evidence of active infection. In areas where histoplasmosis is endemic, itraconazole is recommended; in the US guidelines this applies for patients with a CD4 < 150 from endemic areas [3]. This recommendation is based on evidence that prophylaxis reduces histoplasmosis infection rates but not mortality [3].

A final word from the expert

The pivotal feature of this case is to be found in the first paragraph: this patient was a 'late-presenter' who then defaulted from care. Most, if not all, of the subsequent complications could have been prevented by earlier diagnosis and treatment with cART. If we are to advance HIV care we must achieve far higher rates of early diagnosis. PHE estimates that in the UK almost a quarter of HIV-infected people remain undiagnosed [15]. Cases such as this emphasize the importance of proactive diagnostic strategies.

This case also illustrates that multiple pathologies frequently coexist in HIV/AIDS. The traditional medical dogma to settle for one diagnosis rather than many ('Occam's razor') does not apply in HIV—indeed, the opposite is more commonly the case; 'plurality is the norm in HIV/AIDS'.

Differentiating atypical mycobacterial infections from TB is a major diagnostic issue and becomes a decision based on probabilities. Dual infection must be considered, especially as MAC infection may grow more rapidly than *Mtb*. The key is to make sure that plenty of samples have been taken and sent for culture. Newer molecular tests are becoming more useful in this regard.

Histoplasmosis can be difficult to diagnose, as illustrated by this case, and a high index of suspicion is key to diagnosis. Suspicious lesions should be biopsied, as in this case. Bone marrow aspiration may be useful in diagnosing disseminated disease.

Unmasking IRIS is well illustrated by this case and the key features are well described. This aspect of the case further reinforces the 'diagnose early' message as IRIS is less common in people who start ART at higher CD4 counts.

References

1 Zolopa AR, Andersen J, Komarow L et al. Early antiretroviral therapy reduces AIDS progression/death in individuals with acute opportunistic infections: A Multicenter Randomized Strategy Trial. *PLoS ONE* 2009; 4(5): e5575. doi:10.1371/journal.pone.0005575

2 British HIV Association and British Infection Association Guidelines for the Treatment of Opportunistic Infection in HIV-seropositive Individuals 2011, http://www.bhiva.org/documents/Guidelines/OI/hiv_v12_is2_Iss2Press_Text.pdf

3 Guidelines for Prevention and Treatment of Opportunistic Infections in HIV-Infected Adults and Adolescents. Recommendations from CDC, the National Institutes of Health, and the HIV Medicine Association of the Infectious Diseases Society of America. *MMWR Recomm Rep* 2009; 58: RR-4.

4 Wallace JM, Hannah JB. *Mycobacterium avium* complex infection in patients with the acquired immunodeficiency syndrome: A clinicopathologic study. *Chest* 1988; 93: 926–932.

5 Yagupsky P, Menegus MA. Cumulative positivity rates of multiple blood cultures for *Mycobacterium avium intracellulare* and *Cryptococcus neoformans* in patients with the acquired immunodeficiency syndrome. *Arch Pathol Lab Med* 1990; 114: 923–925.

6 Panel on Antiretroviral Guidelines for Adults and Adolescents. Guidelines for the use of antiretroviral agents in HIV-1-infected adults and adolescents. Department of Health and Human Services. Available at http://aidsinfo.nih.gov/contentfiles/lvguidelines/AdultandAdolescentGL.pdf (accessed 7 April 2013).

7 Lehloenya R, Meintjes G. Dermatologic manifestations of the immune reconstitution inflammatory syndrome. *Dermatol Clin* 2006; 24: 549–570.

8 Wheat J, Sarosi G, McKinsey D et al. Practice guidelines for the management of patients with histoplasmosis. Infectious Diseases Society of America. *Clin Infect Dis* 2000; 30: 688–695.

9 Norgan AP, Berbari EF, Roberts GD, Pritt BS. A 79-year-old man with swelling and crusted cutaneous ulceration of both hands. *Clin Infect Dis* 2010; 50: 933–934.

10 Buitrago MJ, Berenguer J, Mellado E, Rodriguez-Tudela, Cuenca-Estrella M. Detection of imported histoplasmosis in serum of HIV-infected patients using a real-time PCR-based assay. *Eur J Clin Microbiol Infect Dis* 2006; 25: 665–668.

11 Lawn SD, Meintjes G. Pathogenesis and prevention of immune reconstitution disease during antiretroviral therapy [review]. *Expert Rev Anti Infect Ther* 2011; 9: 415–430.

12 Bisson GP, Molefi M, Bellamy S et al. Early versus delayed antiretroviral therapy and CSF fungal clearance in adults with HIV and cryptococcal meningitis. *Clin Infect Dis* 2013; 56: 1165–1173.

13 Nacher M, Sarazin F, el Guedj M et al. Increased incidence of disseminated histoplasmosis following highly active antiretroviral therapy initiation. *J Acquir Immune Defic Syndr* 2006; 41: 468–470.

14 AL Pozniak, KM Coyne. British HIV Association guidelines for the treatment of TB/HIV coinfection 2011. *HIV Med* 2011; 12: 517–524.

15 HIV in the United Kingdom: 2013 Report: http://www.hpa.org.uk/Publications/ InfectiousDiseases/HIVAndSTIs/1311HIVintheUk2013report/

HIV: cryptococcal meningitis and timing of antiretroviral treatment

Angela Loyse

⊕ Expert commentary Tom Harrison

Case history

A 34-year-old female presented to her local general practitioner with recurrent head-aches for 2 months. The headaches were intermittent in nature, frequently severe, and occasionally accompanied by blurred vision. The patient had had two episodes of vomiting in the last 48 hours which had prompted her to attend her GP. She wasn't aware of any known TB contacts and was unsure as to whether she had been bacillus Calmette-Guérin (BCG) vaccinated previously.

The patient was otherwise fit and well, with no previous medical or family history of note. Seven years ago she had moved to the United Kingdom from Zimbabwe. There was no recent travel history. She was a non-smoker and did not consume alcohol.

On examination, the patient was fully orientated and complained of a severe headache. There was no meningism and a full neurological examination revealed a possible left sixth nerve palsy. In particular there was no other focal neurology or lymphadenopathy, and no positive findings on cardiovascular, respiratory, or abdominal examination.

The GP referred the patient to the local district general hospital for further assessment. On arrival in the emergency department the doctor confirmed the presence of a left sixth nerve palsy and arranged an emergency CT brain scan with contrast. Routine blood tests revealed a normocytic anaemia but were otherwise normal. The results of a postero-anterior CXR and CT of the brain were unremarkable. The patient gave consent for an HIV test.

LP revealed a clear, lymphocytic CSF (20 WCC per mm^3), borderline raised protein and glucose levels (0.50 g/L protein, 3.2mmol/L glucose, serum glucose 6.5 mg/dL), and an opening pressure of 28 cmH$_2$O. No organisms were seen.

The patient was kept under close observation as her headaches persisted. She was treated with simple analgesics and fluids and the presumptive diagnosis of viral meningitis was made. On the second day of her admission, her HIV test came back positive. The patient's CSF was subsequently examined for the presence of fungi. India ink staining and the CSF CrAg titre, at a titre of 1:264, were positive.

€€ Expert comment

This patient should not have been left overnight with the diagnosis of viral meningitis. The length of the history and the sixth nerve palsy with high CSF pressure would both be highly unusual. In a young adult from a very high HIV seroprevalence area, underlying HIV must be strongly considered. It was, but the clinical implication that her meningitis was likely cryptococcal was not urgently pursued. India ink and/or CrAg testing must be done out of hours if clinically indicated, so that treatment can be initiated without delay. The new lateral flow format for CrAg testing [1] requires less technician time than the older latex agglutination test. Testing for cryptococcal infection did not have to wait for confirmation of HIV infection.

✪ Learning point Epidemiology

CM is caused by *C. neoformans*, an ubiquitous environmental saprophyte, that is distributed worldwide. Most HIV-related cases of CM are caused by *Cryptococcus neoformans* var. *grubii* (serotype A), with var. *neoformans* (serotype D) responsible for a proportion of cases, mainly in Europe.

Despite the increasing availability of widespread, early ART, CM remains a major opportunistic disease and leading cause of mortality in much of the developing world [2]. In sub-Saharan Africa alone CM is estimated to cause 504,000 deaths annually [2]. Ten-week mortality in the most resource-poor settings in Africa ranges from 24% to 95% [3]. The incidence of CM in high-income countries has, however, decreased [4] with 10-week mortality rates in the range of 10% to 26% in this context [3]. The high mortality in LMICs reflects a combination of poor access to facilities for CM diagnosis, laboratory monitoring, supportive care, and antifungal therapy [3].

✪ Learning point Presentation and microbiological diagnosis

HIV-associated CM usually presents as a subacute meningoencephalitis in profoundly immunosuppressed patients with a CD4 cell count <100 cells/μL. Symptoms may include headache, fever, malaise, visual disturbance, and drowsiness. Signs may be absent but can include meningism, papilloedema, cranial nerve palsies, and reduced level of consciousness. The presence of sixth nerve palsies in particular may reflect the presence of raised intracranial pressure (ICP). Diagnostic tests include India ink (II) stain and CrAg testing of CSF or serum. The sensitivity of II staining is approximately 80% in HIV-associated CM. Both the sensitivity and specificity of CSF and serum CrAg are well over 90%.

The patient was started on amphotericin B (AmB) and flucytosine (5-FC). Despite receiving optimal antifungal therapy, the patient was drowsy and reported a deterioration in her vision on day 3 of her treatment for CM. On examination her visual acuity was 6/12 and 6/60 in her left and right eyes, respectively. She underwent a repeat LP the following day and the opening pressure (OP) was found to be 30 cmH$_2$O.

€€ Expert comment

The therapeutic LP should not have been delayed until symptomatic deterioration. The initial high pressure and sixth nerve palsy should have prompted, in the presence of a normal CT brain scan, careful CSF drainage, either on the day of admission, or, failing that, the following day, assuming on follow-up LP the CSF pressure was found to have remained high. Raised CSF pressure, if not managed, is associated with increased acute mortality [5]. On the other hand, if systematic therapeutic LPs are performed in patients with high CSF pressure there is no longer any association of high initial pressure and poor outcome [6].

✚ Clinical tip Amphotericin B deoxycholate (AmBd) administration

AmBd-induced nephrotoxicity is mediated by a combination of decreased renal blood flow and increased tubular membrane permeability. Renal impairment, electrolyte imbalance, and anaemia are common side effects of AmBd, particularly during the second week of therapy. Renal impairment and anaemia have been reported in up to 50% and 75% of CM patients receiving AmBd, respectively. With careful administration and close monitoring of AmBd, these common side effects are manageable and reversible on stopping therapy. See Figure 9.1.

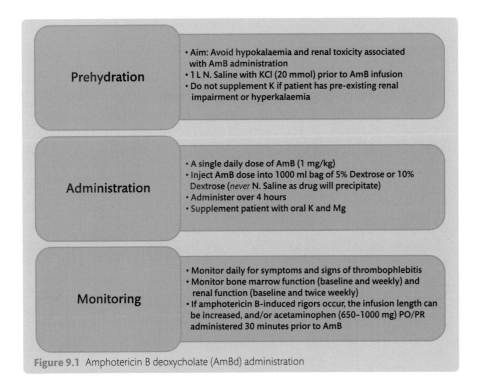

Prehydration	• Aim: Avoid hypokalaemia and renal toxicity associated with AmB administration • 1 L N. Saline with KCl (20 mmol) prior to AmB infusion • Do not supplement K if patient has pre-existing renal impairment or hyperkalaemia
Administration	• A single daily dose of AmB (1 mg/kg) • Inject AmB dose into 1000 ml bag of 5% Dextrose or 10% Dextrose (*never* N. Saline as drug will precipitate) • Administer over 4 hours • Supplement patient with oral K and Mg
Monitoring	• Monitor daily for symptoms and signs of thrombophlebitis • Monitor bone marrow function (baseline and weekly) and renal function (baseline and twice weekly) • If amphotericin B-induced rigors occur, the infusion length can be increased, and/or acetaminophen (650–1000 mg) PO/PR administered 30 minutes prior to AmB

Figure 9.1 Amphotericin B deoxycholate (AmBd) administration

A volume of 20 mL of CSF was carefully removed with good symptomatic effect. Advice was sought at this stage from a regional ID unit and the patient was transferred. At the regional unit the patient required daily LPs for 3 days before the raised ICP normalized, and her headache, visual symptoms, and intermittent drowsiness resolved. An MRI scan of the brain revealed the presence of dilated Virchow-Robin spaces and cryptococcomas (Figure 9.2).

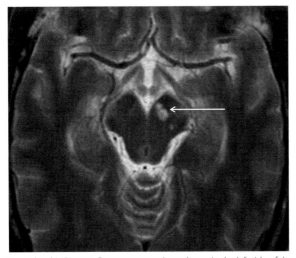

Figure 9.2 Axial T2-weighted MRI scan. Cryptococcoma/pseudocyst in the left side of the midbrain (arrow).

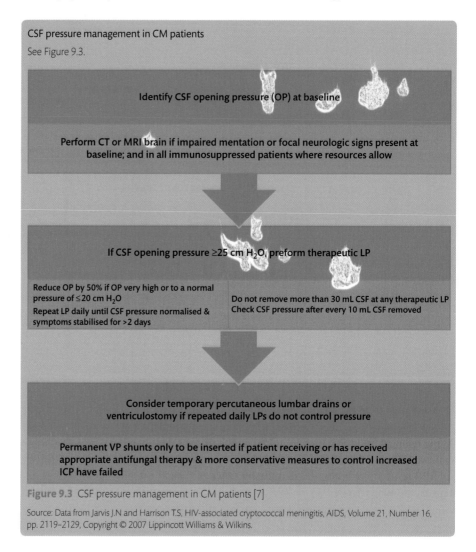

CSF pressure management in CM patients

See Figure 9.3.

Identify CSF opening pressure (OP) at baseline

Perform CT or MRI brain if impaired mentation or focal neurologic signs present at baseline; and in all immunosuppressed patients where resources allow

If CSF opening pressure ≥25 cm H_2O, preform therapeutic LP

Reduce OP by 50% if OP very high or to a normal pressure of ≤20 cm H_2O

Repeat LP daily until CSF pressure normalised & symptoms stabilised for >2 days

Do not remove more than 30 mL CSF at any therapeutic LP
Check CSF pressure after every 10 mL CSF removed

Consider temporary percutaneous lumbar drains or ventriculostomy if repeated daily LPs do not control pressure

Permanent VP shunts only to be inserted if patient receiving or has received appropriate antifungal therapy & more conservative measures to control increased ICP have failed

Figure 9.3 CSF pressure management in CM patients [7]

Source: Data from Jarvis J.N and Harrison T.S, HIV-associated cryptococcal meningitis, AIDS, Volume 21, Number 16, pp. 2119–2129, Copyright © 2007 Lippincott Williams & Wilkins.

🟢 **Learning point** Raised ICP in CM [7]

Raised ICP is an important and common contributor to the morbidity and mortality associated with CM [5], with approximately three-quarters of patients having a CSF opening pressure >25 cm in a large series [5]. In this study, higher CSF opening pressures were associated with higher frequency of headache and neurologic findings, and reduced short-term survival compared to patients with baseline pressures of <25 cmH$_2$O [5]. The pathophysiology underlying raised ICP is most likely mechanical obstruction to CSF outflow by organisms or shed polysaccharide, although an osmotic effect of fungal mannitol, and increased vascular permeability and cerebral oedema resulting from cytokine-induced inflammation, have also been proposed. The fact that CSF pressure is positively correlated with CSF CrAg titre, the proportion of patients with positive India ink smears, and cryptococcal colony forming units (CFU) in CSF, is consistent with the obstruction to CSF outflow theory. Current guidelines recommend aggressive management of raised CSF pressure through repeat LPs with careful drainage of CSF based on this hypothesis, and in view of the adverse associations of raised ICP (see Clinical Tip: Amphotericin B deoxycholate (AmBd) administration) [5,7].

The patient received 2 weeks' induction therapy and was then switched to fluconazole 800 mg daily for the consolidation phase of treatment. The baseline CD4 came back at 75 cells/μL, with a VL of 100,000 copies/mL. The patient was investigated for the presence of other OIs such as TB, and after discussion subsequently started on ART, 4 weeks following diagnosis.

Discussion

This case highlights the difficulties of treating CM patients. The main challenges outlined in the clinical case are a rapid definitive diagnosis, the choice of antifungal induction therapy, managing raised ICP, and the timing of ART. This discussion will focus on the evidence supporting current guidelines for antifungal regimens, and the current evidence underlying optimal timing of ART.

Antifungal treatment

Antifungal therapy for CM is divided into three phases. The current gold standard for induction treatment is 2 weeks of AmB (1 mg/kg/day) and 5-FC (100 mg/kg/day) [7,8]. The choice of this induction antifungal regimen is upheld by data from key RCTs. However, this rapidly fungicidal combination regimen is rarely implemented in LMICs where disease burden is greatest. Indeed, many LMICs have limited facilities to enable the safe administration and monitoring of AmB, and have no access to 5-FC, a key second drug in combination induction therapy for CM. The latest World Health Organization (WHO) and Infectious Diseases Society of America (IDSA) guidelines are therefore tailored to the patient's clinical context, notably to the presence of adequate facilities for the safe administration and monitoring of AmB, and the availability of 5-FC [7,8].

> **🟢 Expert comment**
>
> MRI is a much more sensitive imaging modality than CT for the detection of cryptococcal-related lesions. Cryptococcal-related lesions include: dilated Virchow-Robin spaces, cryptococcccomas/pseudocysts, radiological meningitis, intracerebral nodules/masses, and infarcts. Large intracerebral cryptococcomas, hydrocephalus, and cerebral oedema are more common in non-HIV-related CM. Virchow-Robin spaces are perivascular spaces surrounding vessels as they course from the subarachnoid space through the brain parenchyma. Many of these abnormalities reflect the fact that the infection is an encephalomyelitis with organisms seen throughout the brain parenchyma in histopathology studies.

> **✪ Learning point** Treatment of CM
>
> CM antifungal treatment schema [7,8] (see Figure 9.4).
>
> The latest 2011 BHIVA CM guidelines advocate the use of liposomal formulations of AmB as first line, over standard deoxycholate formulations (AmBd). The recommendations are based on the nephrotoxicity associated with AmBd and the finding, in a small RCT of 28 patients, that liposomal AmB sterilized CSF faster than AmBd [9]. However, a subsequent larger RCT comparing AmBd 0.7 mg/kg/day to AmBisome® at 3 or 6 mg/kg/day found no difference in CSF clearance between the regimens, although AmBisome® caused less nephrotoxicity [10]. For many clinical settings, liposomal formulations of AmB are unaffordable. Furthermore, manageable and reversible renal impairment and electrolyte imbalance has been demonstrated in cohorts of HIV-infected patients treated with AmBd 0.7–1 mg/kg/day with careful prehydration and electrolyte monitoring and supplementation [11]. In view of the huge cost differential, and as per the latest 2011 WHO and 2010 IDSA guidelines, careful administration and monitoring of deoxycholate formulations of AmB as first line would seem most appropriate for HIV-associated CM patients with normal baseline renal function.
>
> **Alternative induction regimens**
>
> For resource-poor clinical settings where AmBd cannot be monitored safely, and/or 5-FC is unavailable, alternative treatment regimens may be considered [7,8]. See Figure 9.5.
>
> (continued)

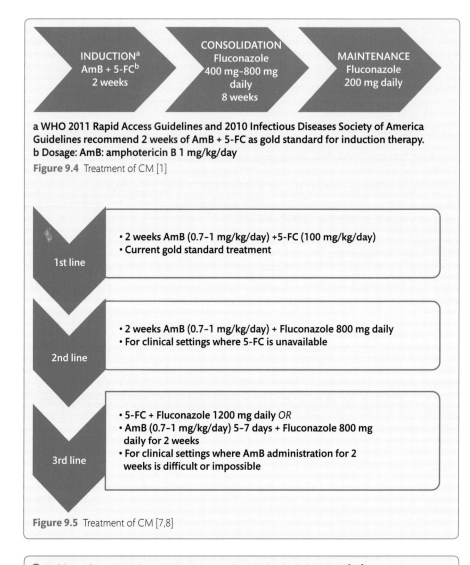

a WHO 2011 Rapid Access Guidelines and 2010 Infectious Diseases Society of America
Guidelines recommend 2 weeks of AmB + 5-FC as gold standard for induction therapy.
b Dosage: AmB: amphotericin B 1 mg/kg/day

Figure 9.4 Treatment of CM [1]

1st line
- 2 weeks AmB (0.7–1 mg/kg/day) +5-FC (100 mg/kg/day)
- Current gold standard treatment

2nd line
- 2 weeks AmB (0.7–1 mg/kg/day) + Fluconazole 800 mg daily
- For clinical settings where 5-FC is unavailable

3rd line
- 5-FC + Fluconazole 1200 mg daily *OR*
- AmB (0.7–1 mg/kg/day) 5–7 days + Fluconazole 800 mg daily for 2 weeks
- For clinical settings where AmB administration for 2 weeks is difficult or impossible

Figure 9.5 Treatment of CM [7,8]

✓ **Evidence base** Low dose AmB versus Low dose AmB + high dose 5-FC [12]

- Double-blind multicentre phase III trial
- 381 patients with first episode of HIV-associated CM randomized to:
  o AmB (0.7 mg/kg/day)
  o AmB (0.7 mg/kg/day) + 5-FC (100 mg/kg/day)
- Trial endpoint: mycological and clinical outcome at 2 and 10 weeks
- Trend towards increased CSF sterilization at 2 weeks was noted with combination therapy (60% vs. 51% for AmB alone, p = 0·06)
- In a multivariate model, the addition of 5-FC was independently associated with 2-week CSF sterilization (OR 1.92, 95%CI 1.15–3.22, p = 0.01). Not receiving 5-FC during the initial 2 weeks of induction treatment was the factor most strongly associated with CM relapse at a time when no highly active antiretrovirals were available (RR 5.9; p = 0·004).
- Note that patients who were comatose, or had moderate-severe hepatic, renal, or haematological dysfunction were ineligible for initial study inclusion. Also at 2 weeks, only patients who were stable or improved were re-randomized to alternative consolidation therapy with either fluconazole or itraconazole for the following 8 weeks. In effect, the sickest patients were excluded from study inclusion and this may explain in part the relatively low 2-week and 10-week mortality rate.

> ✓ **Evidence base** Mortality benefit of AmB + 5-FC over AmB monotherapy [13]
>
> - Phase III RCT
> - 298 patients with a first episode of CM were randomized to three induction treatment arms:
>   a) 4 weeks of AmB (1 mg/kg/day) alone
>   b) AmB + 5-FC (100 mg/kg/day) for 2 weeks
>   c) AmB + fluconazole (FLU) 400 mg twice daily for 2 weeks
> - For the first time, a mortality benefit was identified with addition of 5-FC compared to AmB monotherapy (HR 0.7 (0.30, 1.08), p = 0.08 at 2 weeks; HR 0.61 (0.39, 0.97), p = 0.04 at 10 weeks)
> - Note that this study was conducted prior to the widespread availability of ART
> - The rate of clearance of AmB + 5-FC was significantly greater than for AmB monotherapy or AmB +fluconazole 800 mg
> - Although a secondary adjusted analysis identified a mortality benefit at 6 months in the AmB + 5-FC arm compared to the AmB + high dose FLU, there was no statistical difference in mortality between these two arms at the co-primary 2-week and 10-week study endpoints.
>
> In view of the widespread lack of accessibility of 5-FC, whether more readily available high-dose fluconazole represents an equally effective second drug in combination with AmB remains an important question for resource-limited settings where the greatest disease burden lies. A phase III trial addressing this question, and evaluating short-course AmB, and oral combination therapy with high-dose fluconazole and 5-FC, against the current standard of 2 weeks of AmB and 5-FC is currently ongoing in Africa (ACTA trial ISRCTN45035509).

Fluconazole (FLU) is a cornerstone of both consolidation and maintenance phases of CM treatment [7,8]. It is also used in the pre-emptive treatment of patients with asymptomatic antigenaemia [7,8]. The dose of FLU for the 8 weeks of consolidation therapy is 400–800 mg daily followed by fluconazole 200 mg daily as maintenance therapy.

> ⊕ **Clinical tip** Prevention of cryptococcal disease [8]
>
> Early ART initiation is the most important and cost-effective preventive strategy to reduce the incidence and high mortality linked to HIV-associated CM. Patients should ideally initiate ART at a CD4 count of 350 cells/mm^3 [8].
>
> Primary prophlaxis in CrAg-negative (or where CrAg status is not known) HIV-associated CM patients with a CD4 count <100 cells/mm^3 is not recommended prior to ART initiation, unless a prolonged delay in ART initiation is likely [8]. While five RCTs showed a reduction in the incidence of cryptococcal disease with azole primary prophylaxis, there was no clear impact on survival.
>
> Routine serum or plasma CrAg screening in ART-naïve adults, followed by pre-emptive antifungal therapy if CrAg-positive, may be considered prior to ART initiation in populations with high prevalence of CrAg in patients with a CD4 count <100 cells/mm^3 [8]. A serum or plasma CrAg assay (latex antigen or lateral flow assay) is recommended for screening.
>
> In the context of a positive serum CrAg, it remains unclear whether all asymptomatic patients require a diagnostic LP to determine whether there is active neurological involvement and raised ICP. IDSA guidelines recommend that all CrAg positive patients receive a diagnostic LP. If the LP precludes a diagnosis of CM, the optimal antifungal regimen has yet to be determined; however, the latest WHO and IDSA guidelines recommend treatment with fluconazole [7,8]. For asymptomatic CrAg, WHO suggests fluconazole 800 mg daily for 2 weeks followed by a further 8 weeks of fluconazole 400 mg daily [8].

Timing of ART

The optimal timing for ART remains uncertain. To date two published trials have sought to identify the optimal timing of ART in the context of CM.

In a multicentre AIDS Clinical Trials Group (ACTG) phase IV strategy study, 282 patients with acute AIDS-related OIs or serious BIs were randomized to either early or deferred ART [14]. Patients in the early arm of the study started ART at a median of 12 days, and patients in the deferred arm commenced ART at a median of 45 days after initiation of OI treatment. A total of 35/282 (12%) patients had CM as their entry OI, although *Pneumocystis jirovecii* pneumonia accounted for the majority (63%) of OIs [14]. There was no statistically significant difference in the ordered three-category primary endpoint at 48 weeks: alive without AIDS progression and with HIV VL < 50 copies/mL; alive without AIDS progression and with detectable HIV VL; and AIDS progression or death at any time. IRIS occurred in 5.6% in the early arm versus 8.5% in the deferred ART arm [14]. A difference in clinical outcomes between study arms was detected in a secondary analysis that evaluated AIDS progression or death. Early ART appeared to be associated with less clinical progression, compared to deferred ART, and this difference was statistically different for study patients overall, fungal infections (including cryptococcosis and histoplasmosis), and for patients with baseline CD4 counts of less than 50 cells/mm^3. Although the trial was not powered to examine the impact of ART timing in specific OIs, a non-significant trend favoured earlier ART in patients with CM who were treated with AmB. It is important to stress that this statistically significant difference in a secondary outcome is based on a small numbers of patients, with death or AIDS progression, when broken down by OI study entry category.

The question of early versus delayed initiation of ART for CM was examined further in a recent Zimbabwean study [15]. A total of 54 patients were randomized to receive early ART, within 72 hours of diagnosis of CM, or delayed ART, following 10 weeks of fluconazole monotherapy [15]. The primary study endpoint was all-cause mortality. The median duration of survival was 28 and 637 days in the early and delayed ART arms, respectively (p = 0.031, by log-rank test), with a three times greater mortality risk in the early ART group (adjusted hazard ratio (AHR) 2.85; 95% CI 1.1–7.23). Excessive mortality in the early ART arm prompted early termination of the study by the data safety monitoring committee (DSMC). Overall 3-year mortality was 73%. IRIS cases were not routinely identified or reported for logistical reasons, although the authors claim 'early initiation of ART most likely resulted in increased rates of cryptococcal IRIS'. High residual CSF fungal burden following fluconazole monotherapy may have predisposed patients to the development of CM IRIS. All study patients received suboptimal induction therapy with fluconazole 800 mg daily and this will have undoubtedly contributed to the high early mortality, with most deaths occurring in the first 2 weeks following study enrolment.

Lastly, a National Institutes of Health (NIH)-funded RCT of early versus deferred ART in Uganda and South Africa randomized patients presenting with a first episode of HIV-associated CM receiving AmB to early ART (at median 8 days) or ART at ≥4 weeks after study entry [16]. Induction therapy consisted of AmB and fluconazole 800 mg daily. 'A substantial excess 6-month mortality rate in the early ART compared with the delayed ART arm' (hazard ratio (HR) for death for early ART = 1.71 [95% CI 1.03, 2.87] vs. delayed ART) prompted the trial DSMC to terminate the trial early (NIAID Press Release, 30 May 2012); 15% patients are currently accruing follow-up (September 2012). Initial analyses indicate that early ART was linked to poor outcomes particularly in patients with altered mental status (HR ~3 for early ART) and paucity of CSF inflammation (CSF WBC ~5 cells/mL) (HR ~6.6 for early ART) [17]. The number of IRIS cases in either arm has yet to be reported.

In conclusion, although the exact timing of ART in the context of CM remains unclear, there is no evidence currently to support starting ART during the induction phase of CM therapy. On the contrary, the available data suggest that ART within the first 2 weeks may be harmful, particularly in patients with altered mental status and/or paucity of CSF inflammation. Additional data from the prematurely terminated COAT trial will further inform the debate on timing of ART in CM. The latest WHO guidelines recommend that, in recently diagnosed HIV-associated CM patients, ART initiation should be deferred until there is evidence of a sustained clinical response to antifungal therapy after 2–4 weeks of induction and consolidation treatment with amphotericin B-based combination regimens, or after 4–6 weeks of induction and consolidation treatment with a high-dose oral fluconazole regimen [8]. The long-term benefit of ART must be balanced against the risk of life-threatening intracranial IRIS, especially in the context of suboptimal induction therapy such as fluconazole monotherapy.

A final word from the expert

The case underlines the importance of thinking of and recognizing OIs in patients without a prior diagnosis of HIV infection. As in all cases, in this case there were usual and unusual features of cryptococcal infection. Typical were the subacute onset, lack of meningism, the low CSF WCC, high CSF pressure (with no hydrocephalus), and false localizing sixth nerve palsy. On the other hand, a barely raised CSF protein is rare, and double rather than blurred vision would be the more frequent initial visual symptom.

Rapid diagnosis and treatment are essential and require good liaison between clinician and laboratory. The tests are rapid and simple and should not be delayed for patients presenting out of hours.

In terms of antifungal therapy, amphotericin B and 5-FC can be safely given to this patient group for 2 weeks provided pre-emptive fluid and electrolyte replacement is given, and blood test results monitored and acted upon promptly [8]. Patients are very frequently dehydrated and the Normal saline supplement should be in addition to normal fluid replacement. Proteinuria should be checked to identify patients with underlying HIV-related nephropathy who will need even closer monitoring. The consolidation dose of fluconazole was 400 mg/day in the van der Horst study [12]. A dose of 800 mg/day is sensible if a less rapidly fungicidal induction regimen is used, or induction is for less than the full 2 weeks. Of note, fluconazole should probably be reduced to 400 mg/day if nevirapine is used for ART, due to an increase in nevirapine levels with concomitant fluconazole and lack of safety data with this combination with doses of fluconazole above 400 mg/day.

Daily therapeutic LPs are effective in controlling raised pressure in the great majority of cases. Of note, pressure often increases and becomes a clinical problem during the second and third weeks of therapy and despite successful sterilization of the CSF. Thus, if patients deteriorate on therapy, a repeat LP should be done to measure pressure. Lumbar drains are highly effective in the small number of patients in whom therapeutic LPs do not control pressure [18]. Patients need careful instruction and should be nursed on a neurosurgery ward if possible with staff familiar with such drains. The drain may be clamped after some days, and removed if CSF pressure does not subsequently rise.

Successive trials have narrowed the time interval during which ART should be introduced to between 2 and 6 weeks. In our experience, treating over 500 patients with HIV-associated CM in prospective clinical studies, following gold standard induction with amphotericin B plus 5-FC for 2 weeks, ART can be safely initiated at a median of 23 days [19]. In this recent trial, the survival curve appeared to flatten a little earlier, suggesting ART at this time point may have prevented some later non-cryptococcal, HIV-related deaths. It is probably wise to wait until 4 weeks if less rapidly active induction therapy is used.

Between 10% and 20% of patients may develop cryptococcal immune reconstitution inflammatory syndrome (CM-IRIS), at a median of around 1 month after ART initiation. Risk factors are low initial CD4 cell count and rapid rise in count on ART, low initial markers of inflammation, and a high organism load (CrAg titre or CFU count) at baseline and at time of ART initiation. The prognosis of CM-IRIS may be better now than in earlier papers, due to earlier recognition and appropriate management—with CSF pressure control, continued antifungal and ART, and selective use of dexamethasone in patients whose condition deteriorates. It is vital, given that this is a diagnosis of exclusion, that other possible diagnoses are urgently and actively investigated.

References

1 Jarvis JN, Percival A, Bauman S et al. Evaluation of a novel point of care cryptococcal antigen (CRAG) test on serum, plasma and urine from patients with HIV-associated cryptococcal meningitis. *Clin Infect Dis* 2011; 53: 1019–1023.
2 Park BJ, Wannemuehler KA, Marston BJ et al. Estimation of the global burden of cryptococcal meningitis among persons living with HIV/AIDS. *AIDS* 2009; 23: 525–530.
3 Jarvis JN, Bicanic T, Harrison TS. Management of cryptococcal meningoencephalitis in both developed and developing countries. In: *Cryptococcus, from human pathogen to model yeast.* Eds Heitman J, Kozel TR, Kwon-Chung KJ, Perfect JR, Casadevall A. Washington DC: ASM Press.
4 Mirza SA, Phelan M, Rimland D et al. The changing epidemiology of cryptococcosis: an update from population-based active surveillance in 2 large metropolitan areas, 1992–2000. *Clin Infect Dis* 2003; 15; 36: 789–794.
5 Graybill JR, Sobel J, Saag M et al. Diagnosis and management of increased intracranial pressure in patients with AIDS and cryptococcal meningitis. The NIAID Mycoses Study Group and AIDS Cooperative Treatment Groups. *Clin Infect Dis* 2000; 30: 47–54.
6 Bicanic T, Brouwer A, Meintjes G et al. Relationship of raised CSF opening pressure, fungal burden and outcome in HIV-associated cryptococcal meningitis patients managed with serial lumbar punctures. *AIDS* 2009, 23: 701–706.
7 Perfect JR, Dismukes WE, Dromer F et al. Clinical Practice Guidelines for the Management of Cryptococcal Disease: 2010 Update by the Infectious Diseases Society of America. *Clin Infect Dis* 2010; 50: 291–322.
8 World Health Organization. *Rapid advice: Diagnosis, prevention and management of cryptococcal disease in HIV-infected adults, adolescents and children.* Geneva: WHO, December 2011.
9 Leenders ACAP, Reiss P, Portegies P et al. Liposomal amphotericin B(AmBisome) compared with amphotericin B both followed by oral fluconazole in the treatment of AIDS-associated cryptococcal meningitis. *AIDS* 1997; 11: 1463–1471.
10 Hamill, RJ, Sobel JD, El-Sadr, W et al. Comparison of 2 doses of liposomal amphotericin B and conventional amphotericin B deoxycholate fortreatment of AIDS-associated acute

cryptococcal meningitis: a randomized, double-blind clinical trial of efficacy and safety. *Clin Infect Dis* 2010; 51: 225–232.

11 Bicanic T, Wood R, Meintjes G et al. High-dose amphotericin B with flucytosine for the treatment of cryptococcal meningitis in HIV-infected patients: a randomized trial. *Clin Infect Dis* 2008; 47: 123–130.

12 Van der Horst CM, Saag MS, Cloud G et al. Treatment of cryptococcal meningitis associated with the acquired immunodeficiency syndrome. *N Engl J Med* 1997; 337: 15–21.

13 Day JN, Chau TT, Wolbers M et al. Combination antifungal therapy for cryptococcal meningitis. *N Engl J Med* 2013; 368: 1291–1302.

14 Zolopa AR, Andersen J, Komarow et al. Early antiretroviral therapy reduces AIDS progression/death in indivisuals with acute opportunistic infections: a multicentre randomized strategy trial. *Plos One* 2009; 4(5): e5575. Doi: 10.1371/journal.pone.0005575.

15 Makadzange AT, Ndhlovu CE, Takarinda K et al. Early versus delayed initiation of antiretroviral therapy for concurrent HIV infection and cryptococcal meningitis in Sub-Saharan Africa. *Clin Infect Dis* 2010; 50: 1532–1538.

16 Cryptococcal Optimal ART Timing (COAT) *Trial Clinicaltrials.gov NCT01075152.*

17 Boulware D. *Oral presentation, Interscience Conference on Antimicrobial Agents and Chemotherapy (ICAAC)*, San Francisco, US, September 2012.

18 Macsween K, Bicanic T, Brouwer AE, Marsh H, Macallan DC, Harrison TS. Lumbar drainage in control of cerebrospinal fluid pressure in cryptococcal meningitis: Case report and review. *J Infect* 2005; 51: 221–224.

19 Jarvis JN, Meintjes G, Rebe K et al. Adjunctive interferon-γ immunotherapy for the treatment of HIV-associated cryptococcal meningitis: a randomized controlled trial. *AIDS* 2012; 26: 1105–1113.

10 Candida infection in the intensive care unit

Luke Moore

ⓘ **Expert commentary** Silke Schelenz

Case history

A 56-year-old man with a past medical history of dyslipidaemia was admitted to the intensive care unit (ICU) after a right hemicolectomy and end-to-end anastomosis for an obstructing caecal tumour. Postoperatively there were persistent inotropic and oxygen requirements. Formal central venous access was sited and he was commenced on total parental nutrition (TPN). Admission screening cultures were sent to bacteriology. His meticillin-resistant *Staphylococcus aureus* (MRSA) screen was reported as negative, and his rectal screen was reported as growing a yeast. The persisting inotropic requirement in the context of abdominal surgery prompted empiric antimicrobial treatment with piperacillin-tazobactam. Over the following 6 days the inotropic support was weaned and he was extubated.

However, on day 7 of his ICU admission he developed a fever, a leucocytosis of 16×10^9/L, and a CRP rise to 189 mg/L. Further abdominal cross-sectional imaging was reported as showing fluid in the right paracolic gutter but there were no obvious large collections to drain. Blood cultures and repeat screening swabs were sent. The piperacillin-tazobactam was empirically converted to meropenem.

On day 9 of his ICU admission his blood cultures remained negative but his rectal swab grew a germ tube negative yeast as did his abdominal wound swab. He remained pyrexial and his CRP continued to climb. Fluconazole was added to the meropenem and his central line was changed over a guide-wire.

ⓘ **Expert comment** Routine screening of Candida colonization in ICU

Routine screening of patients for *Candida* colonization is debatable unless an intensive care unit deals with a large number of very high-risk patients. Although routine screening has in some studies shown to have a good NPV, the positive predictive value is low (66%) and would need to involve quantitative culture in order to increase its sensitivity, which is very costly [1]. It is recommended that all yeast isolates from high-risk patients (i.e. those in ICU) should be routinely identified to species level as this will guide the empirical treatment of suspected or confirmed cases of invasive candidiasis [2]. This recommendation would also be applicable to the yeast isolated from this patient's rectal swab. If it were to be identified as *C. glabrata* it could have led to starting a more appropriate antifungal agent such as an echinocandin rather than fluconazole.

On day 11 of ICU admission his temperature remained at 38.2°C and his inflammatory markers were persistently raised. He developed a mild hepatitis with an alanine transaminase of 150 iu/L but also a marked rise in CK to 3600 iu/L. His central line tip grew *Candida glabrata*, with a fluconazole minimum inhibitory concentration (MIC_{90}) of 8 microgram/mL and a caspofungin MIC_{90} of 0.07 microgram/mL. The fluconazole was changed to caspofungin and by day 13 of his ICU admission his fever and inflammatory markers were beginning to normalize. With this slow improvement he was discharged from ICU to the surgical high dependency unit (HDU), still continuing TPN.

Five days into his caspofungin treatment he complained of blurring of vision in his right eye.

> **⚙ Expert comment** Ocular candidiasis
>
> Chorioretinitis is the most common site of dissemination following candidaemia and if untreated can progress into vitritis (cotton ball appearance in the vitreous visible on fundoscopy), also known as endogenous endophthalmitis. It is important to know that some antifungal agents such as echinocandins and amphotericin B have a large molecular weight and penetrate the blood–ocular barrier poorly, leaving ocular candidiasis inadequately treated if given as a single agent. In contrast fluconazole, voriconazole, and 5-FC penetrate the blood–ocular barrier well and can be detected in sufficient concentration in the vitreous fluid.

That evening he developed a flaccid right-sided paralysis and despite re-admission to ICU and further inotropic support he died the following day. Three days after death, a blood culture taken during the terminal deterioration grew a yeast (Figure 10.1) further identified as *Candida glabrata*. Post-mortem examination revealed a right chorioretinitis and a left hemisphere cerebral abscess.

Discussion

This patient presents with a history and findings typical of the complications that can follow a candidaemia. The absence of an ante-mortem positive blood culture does not refute the diagnosis and, as is commonly the case, pre-emptive antifungal therapy must often be commenced on the basis of supportive evidence. This supportive evidence is often in the form of risk factors for invasive candidiasis (in this case, surgery and

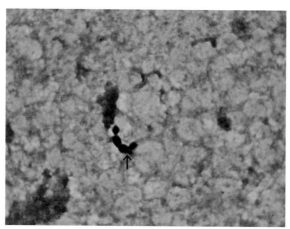

Figure 10.1 Gram stain of blood culture showing a budding yeast (arrow) identified as *Candida glabrata*. Image courtesy of Luke Moore.

presence of an indwelling central line being used for TPN), evidence of colonization (in this case two non-contiguous sites growing yeast), and indirect evidence of intra-vascular candida (in this case a line tip growing a yeast).

> ⊗ **Learning point** Candidaemia epidemiology
>
> A recent prospective observational study by Das et al. [3] looked at 107 episodes of candidaemia between 2005 and 2008 in a UK university hospital. They found an incidence of 10.9 episodes/100,000 bed-days. The most common predisposing factors were found to be:
>
> - Preceding use of broad-spectrum antibiotics (92%)
> - Presence of an intravascular device (82%)
> - Intensive care unit admission (51%)
> - Recent surgery (50%)
>
> *C. albicans* accounted for 43% of episodes, *C. glabrata* 31%, and *C. parapsilosis* 20%. Overall *C. tropicalis*, *C. krusei*, *C. norvegensis*, and *C. lusitaniae* caused 7% of episodes. The relative prevalence of *Candida* species must be considered at a local level, however, when constructing antimicrobial policies as significant variation in fluconazole-susceptible vs. non-fluconazole-susceptible species can exist.
>
> The crude 30-day mortality rate in the study by Das et al. [3] approximated 37% with advanced age (p = 0.003) and the presence of septic shock (p = 0.038) associated with increased mortality. Factors affecting mortality was also looked at in a 9-year retrospective study by Fortún et al. [4] in a large university hospital in Spain. This group looked at factors affecting mortality in 419 patients with candidaemia. They also found a 30-day mortality of 37% that did not significantly change between the periods 2000–2004 and 2005–2009. According to a multivariate analysis, the independent factors associated with higher mortality were:
>
> - Shock
> - Age >50 years
> - Elevated comorbidity score (Charlson index >6)
> - Source of candidaemia other than intravenous catheter

Intense debate historically took place regarding the possibility that candidaemia could be an insignificant finding, with early reports suggesting that candidaemia was often a trivial process that could simply be ignored or would resolve solely with removal of the intravascular device. This idea was gradually reversed by reports showing that candidaemia was associated with significant morbidity and mortality (see Learning point: Candidaemia epidemiology). The importance of candidaemia in critically ill patients is now indisputable but the species epidemiology continues to develop, with the ratio of *C. albicans* to non-albicans candida markedly variable. The cause of these changes is likely to be multifactorial. In immunosuppressed patients the use of fluconazole as a prophylactic agent has been strongly associated with the changes towards non-albicans candida causing candidaemia in this population. However, other causes must also play a role as trends towards non-albicans candidaemia have occurred in populations not exposed to this agent. Postulated alternatives focus on the prescription of antifungal therapy for non-invasive cutaneous and muco-cutaneous infections in the general populace exerting an ecological pressure on species prevalence.

The aetiology of the candidaemia in this case potentially included intra-abdominal sources (breakdown of the end-to-end anastomosis) or the central line. Bodey, Anaissie, and Edwards [5] describe four forms of invasive candidiasis, which may manifest with overt candidaemia: (1) catheter-related candidaemia; (2) acute disseminated candidiasis; (3) deep organ candidiasis; and (4) chronic disseminated candidiasis.

Catheter-related candidaemia

Intravascular devices are perhaps the most frequent attributable cause of invasive candidiasis. Introduction through the line, particularly those used for total parenteral nutrition (TPN) and development of an infected fibrin clot at the catheter tip, can lead to candidaemia and seeding. Removal of the line is key, along with appropriate antifungal therapy for a sufficient period of time to cover any distant seeding. In this case the line was changed, but railroading is not appropriate for a potentially infected line.

> ⊕ **Clinical tip** Fundoscopy in candidaemia
>
> Ophthalmic complications of candidaemia are common. In a recent study by Oude Lashof et al. [6] of 370 non-neutropenic candidaemia patients, 49 had findings consistent with the diagnosis of ocular candidiasis at baseline, and an additional 11 patients developed abnormalities during treatment, culminating in 60 patients, or 16%, with eye involvement. Prospective studies performed during the 1980s reported variable incidence of candidal endophthalmitis (range 5–78%, median 29%). The spectrum of disease is variable—in the study by Oude Lashof et al. [6] only 6 patients had endophthalmitis with 54 having chorioretinitis.
>
> The duration of candidaemia was significantly longer in patients with ocular complications (median 4 days; range 1–18 days) compared with patients without ocular involvement (median 3 days; range 1–26 days).
>
> The IDSA guidelines [7] on candidaemia management suggest that at least one careful ophthalmological examination should be performed, preferably at a time when the candidaemia appears controlled and new spread to the eye is unlikely. A proviso to this is made for neutropenic candidaemia patients in whom there may not be manifestation of visible endophthalmitis until recovery from neutropenia, and ophthalmological examination should therefore be performed after recovery of the neutrophil count.

Acute disseminated candidiasis

The source may well be related to an intravascular device, but the resulting candidaemia rapidly disseminates to the parenchyma of distant organs, most frequently resulting in ophthalmic complications (as in this case; see Clinical tip: Fundoscopy in candidaemia), endocarditis (predominantly onto prosthetic valves, with native valve endocarditis being less commonly affected), cerebral emboli (also seen in this case), renal tract abscesses, and pulmonary seeding.

Deep organ candidiasis

Candidaemia, while part of the pathogenesis of this form of invasive candidiasis, is not evident clinically at the time of diagnosis. What is evident is dissemination to distal organs which includes those noted above, as well as less frequently affected sites such as bones, joints, and pancreatic tissue. Deep organ candidiasis can occur in any patient who has endured a period at risk for candidaemia.

Chronic disseminated candidiasis

Also known as hepatosplenic candidiasis, this is a particular form of deep organ candidiasis. It specifically occurs in those patients who experience prolonged periods of neutropenia, most frequently being seen in the haematological population rather than the solid-organ tumour cohort. Frank candidaemia is rarely detected in this form, instead it is characterized by micro-abscesses of liver, spleen, and on occasion kidney.

The decision to instigate pre-emptive antifungal therapy for the patient in this case on day 9 of his ICU stay is consistent with published data. Preceding *Candida* species colonization is widely recognized as being the strongest predictor of subsequent invasive disease, and is therefore accepted as an indication for early antifungal treatment in at-risk patients. Historically fluconazole has been the pre-emptive antifungal of choice with previously accepted practice being initiation on isolation of *Candida* from at least two non-contiguous skin and mucosal sites in high-risk patients. However, there is some evidence that fluconazole pre-emptive therapy based upon colonization of at least two sites may be inadequate. In an 8-year study by Troughton et al. [8] looking at invasive candidiasis in a university hospital in Northern Ireland, 43% of candidaemic patients had no evidence of prior colonization, 67% of whom had candidaemia due to *C. glabrata*. Many institutes have therefore instead developed local policies based on the large multicentre observational trials that have looked at other risk factors for invasive candidiasis in addition to two-site colonization in non-neutropenic critically ill patients.

> **✔ Evidence base** Invasive candida scoring systems
>
> The EPCAN (Estudio de Prevalencia de CANdidiasis; Candidiasis Prevalence Study) study group has looked at serial admissions to intensive care units across Spain. The EPCAN study group have published several landmark trials refining scoring systems for identifying non-neutropenic critically ill patients who would benefit from early antifungal administration.
>
> The trial published in 2006 [9] identified 1,765 patients across 70 intensive care units. Using a logistic regression model to identify relevant risk factors, a receiver operating curve was constructed to delineate a score that provided the optimal sensitivity and specificity for those at risk of invasive candidiasis.
>
> The score incorporates:
>
> - TPN = 1
> - Surgery on ICU admission = 1
> - Multifocal *Candida* species colonization = 1
> - Severe sepsis = 2
>
> A cut-off of 2.5 generates a sensitivity of 81% and a specificity of 74% for risk of invasive candidiasis. This corresponds to a risk ratio of 7.75 for proven invasive candidiasis (95% CI 4.74–12.66) in patients with a score >2.5 compared with a score of <2.5.

The decision on day 9 in this case to use fluconazole as the pre-emptive therapy agent could be questioned, however. As noted above, this patient does warrant pre-emptive therapy, but the delineation of the yeasts as being germ tube negative equates to a decreased confidence in the effectiveness of fluconazole in this case.

> **✪ Learning point** Clinical impact of germ tube
>
> A germ tube positive yeast can be presumptively identified as *C. albicans* pending further identification methods. As such this isolate should be susceptible to fluconazole and, where there is a clinical indication for an antifungal therapy, this agent is advocated. The Global Antifungal Surveillance Programme tracked the susceptibility of *Candida* bloodstream infection isolates from 1992 to 2004, and among 7,725 *C. albicans* found a mean MIC_{90} of <0.5 microgram/mL [10].
>
> Germ tube negative isolates, of which the most commonly identified in the Global Antifungal Surveillance Programme were in descending order *C. glabrata*, *C. parapsilosis*, *C. tropicalis*, and *C. krusei*, had a variable fluconazole MIC_{90}. The mean values were 32, 2, 2, and >64 microgram/mL, respectively. Therefore, in treating germ tube negative yeast invasive infections, alternative agents to fluconazole may be indicated. Depending upon local guidelines these may include amphotericin (predominantly
>
> (continued)

liposomal derivatives) or echinocandins. Three echinocandins are currently licensed in the UK and the USA: caspofungin, micafungin, and anidulafungin. These agents are similar with respect to *in vitro* activity against *Candida* species, with micafungin and anidulafungin having similar MIC_{90} that are generally lower than the MIC_{90} of caspofungin. The MIC_{90} of the echinocandins is highest against *Candida parapsilosis*; however, the impact of this in clinical practice has not been quantified. Micafungin and anidulafungin generally have a lower frequency of adverse reactions compared with caspofungin. The most common adverse events are phlebitis (up to 25% of patients) and elevated liver enzyme levels (up to 15%) with caspofungin, with micafungin and anidulafungin having half the adverse events rates.

The concern that the germ tube negative yeast may not be sensitive to fluconazole is borne out in this case when the central line tip is confirmed as growing *C. glabrata* with a fluconazole MIC_{90} of 8 microgram/mL, against which the fluconazole will not have had a high level of activity (see Learning point: Clinical impact of germ tube). Delineation of germ tube positivity in the laboratory provides a quick and cheap method to guide use of antifungal agents in the clinical setting.

⊕ Clinical tip   Laboratory germ tube

Speciation of *Candida* isolates can take 24–48 hours after growth is detected, but bench-top laboratory information can allude to presumptive identifications and hence fast, appropriate antifungal prescription in the clinical setting. The germ tube test provides a simple, reliable, and economical procedure for the presumptive identification of *Candida albicans* with 95% of isolates producing a germ tube in 3 hours. The only non-albicans candida which can be misidentified through this method is *C. dubliniensis* which is thought to account for 1.2–2% of germ tube positive clinical isolates.

The germ tube technique:

1. Using a Pasteur pipette, dispense 3 drops of fresh pooled human serum into tube
2. Lightly touch a yeast colony and suspend the yeast in the serum
3. Incubate the tube at 35°C for 2.5–3 hours
4. Place a drop of the suspension on a clean microscope slide and cover. Use ×10–×40 objective lens to confirm the presence (see Figure 10.2) or absence of germ tubes (see Figure 10.3).

❝ Expert comment   Germ tube test and Candida speciation

The germ tube test provides an inexpensive and timely result for the identification of *C. albicans/C. dubliniensis* but the interpretation of the microscopy appearance of true germ tube formation depends very much on the experience of the person performing the test. While this test is easy to be performed by an experienced mycologist, most biomedical scientists in UK laboratories no longer have the necessary experience to interpret such tests. Many laboratories also no longer stock serum for the germ tube test, and yeast identification has largely been replaced by other technologies needing less expertise and hands-on time such as chromogenic agar, automated biochemical tests (Vitek), or mass spectrometry (MS) (MALDI-TOF).

E-test MIC quantification can be used for yeasts but interpreting zone sizes does require experience. Care must be taken to look for the zone of reduced growth rather than the zone of complete inhibition, as a trailing effect can be seen with some strains. As a result *Candida* species MICs do have the potential to be misreported as higher than expected, making use of control strains in susceptibility testing particularly important. Broth microdilution, most easily and practically achieved through microtitre plates, is a preferred method of susceptibility testing.

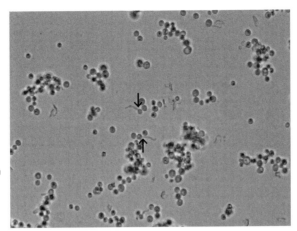

Figure 10.2 A germ tube positive (arrows) yeast after colony incubation in human serum for 3 hours seen under light microscopy at ×40 objective.
Image courtesy of Luke Moore.

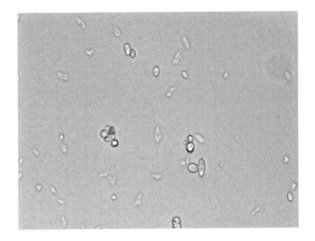

Figure 10.3 A germ tube negative yeast after colony incubation in human serum for 3 hours seen under light microscopy at ×40 objective.
Image courtesy of Luke Moore.

At 48 hours after the pre-emptive fluconazole was commenced in this patient two biochemical dyscrasias were noted. While the transaminitis was mild, a marked rise in the CK was found and this does have the potential to contribute to acute kidney injury and onwards to exacerbating metabolic dysfunction. The use of fluconazole in this patient who is on long-term atorvastatin may well have been the cause of these biochemical abnormalities.

⊗ **Learning point** Drug interactions

Up to 5% of those treated with fluconazole develop an asymptomatic mild to moderate transaminitis that frequently resolves during the course of the therapy and clears fully following discontinuation. Hepatotoxicity to a degree that is clinically relevant is rare. In addition to hepatotoxicity, rarely drug hypersensitivity can occur manifesting as fever, rash, and eosinophilia.

Fluconazole has over 80 documented severe drug interactions, of which two are worth particular mention. The first relates to the potential for fluconazole to cause QT interval prolongation. Of itself this effect rarely causes clinical sequelae but co-administration with other agents that also cause QT prolongation is not advisable—one such antimicrobial is moxifloxacin. The second interaction of particular note relates to the potent inhibition of CYP450 3A4 by azole antifungal agents. Administration of fluconazole at doses of >200 mg/day may therefore significantly increase the plasma concentrations of substrates of this isoenzyme such as statins (HMG-CoA reductase inhibitors). This can potentiate the
(continued)

adverse effects of statins, particularly the increased risk of musculoskeletal toxicity. Clinically this may manifest as myopathy, myalgia, and elevated CK, as in this case. Significant rhabdomyolysis may lead to acute renal impairment.

The decision to switch treatment to an echinocandin in this case did result in a clinical improvement and, as noted, echinocandin treatment is a valid strategy. If events had not overtaken this patient, further blood cultures should be serially taken and the minimum treatment duration should be 14 days from the first negative blood culture.

> ✔ **Evidence base** Echinocandin versus fluconazole
>
> The clinical efficacy of the three echinocandins has been investigated in multicentre randomized double-blind trials primarily involving adult non-neutropenic patients with candidaemia. Non-inferiority has been shown between caspofungin and conventional amphotericin B, micafungin and liposomal amphotericin B, and micafungin and caspofungin. Previous work has established the non-inferiority of amphotericin B against fluconazole. However, the first candidaemia trial to establish a significant favourable outcome from an echinocandin compared with fluconazole was the landmark trial by Reboli et al. [11]. This RCT looked at 245 predominantly non-neutropenic patients, 89% of whom had candidaemia only and in whom the species ratio was *Candida albicans* 62% to non-albicans candida 38%. They found at the end of intravenous therapy that treatment was successful in 75.6% of patients treated with anidulafungin, compared with 60.2% of those treated with fluconazole (15.4% difference; 95% CI 3.9–27.0). In addition to this end-of-treatment outcome, anidulafungin had significantly higher success rates at 2 weeks post-therapy. It is thought the faster clearance of the pathogens from the intravascular compartment accounts for the higher global efficacy of anidulafungin—the study found sterilization for *C. albicans* after a median of 2 days in patients receiving anidulafungin and 5 days in the arm receiving fluconazole. Failure in terms of persistent *Candida* infection at the end of the intravenous regime was observed in 6.3% of anidulofungin patients against 14.4% of patients receiving fluconazole. In subgroup analysis of cohorts with recognized risk factors for poor outcomes anidulofungin achieved higher success rates. These included intensive care patients, patients with retained central venous catheters, patients with organ failure/severe sepsis, and older age groups. In conclusion, this study showed anidulafungin to be non-inferior to, and possibly more efficacious than, fluconazole for the primary treatment of the candidaemic form of invasive candidiasis, and with a safety profile similar to that of fluconazole. However, it should be noted that the study was supported by a research grant from Vicuron (now merged with Pfizer), the pharmaceutical company holding the anidulofungin patent.

When culture-based techniques fail to provide definitive evidence of invasive candidiasis other modalities of microbiological diagnosis are needed. Non-invasive diagnostics, particularly tests aimed at detecting components of the fungal cell wall, have been developed of which two are becoming more commonly used—galactomannan (GM) (useful in invasive aspergillosis) and beta-D-glucan (BDG) as a panfungal diagnostic test (the test cannot differentiate between yeasts and moulds). BDG is included in the EORTC/MSG 2008 [12] mycological criteria for probable invasive fungal infection caused by fungi other than zygomycetes and *Cryptococcus* species and has been validated in non-neutropenic critically ill patients. The great strength of the BDG test is its consistently high NPV; however, the ubiquitous nature of BDG in the environment makes the assay somewhat prone to false-positive results. A meta-analysis by Karageorgopoulos et al. [13] looked at 2,979 patients (594 with proven or probable invasive fungal infections) included in 16 studies. The pooled sensitivity of BDG was 76.8% (95% CI 67.1–84.3%) and the specificity was 85.3% (95% CI 79.6–89.7%).

One potentially useful diagnostic tool that may become more widely used in the future is polymerase chain reaction (PCR) nucleic acid amplification. The use of PCR

> ⊕ **Clinical tip** BDG
>
> Experience with the BDG assay is not as comprehensive as the GM assay and as such its utility data is not as highly validated. It is likely however that its true utility will be in serial testing, as with GM, and that 2–3 times per week testing should be used during the period of high risk to detect early invasive fungal disease (IFD) and monitor response.

to diagnose invasive fungal infections has been advocated due to the theoretical high sensitivity of the test compared with the myriad of limitations associated with current serological assays [14]. Unfortunately, thus far the potential of PCR has not been translated into clinical practice, and it is not included as a diagnostic criterion in the EORTC/MSG guidelines. Until the problems associated with false-positive results from fungal PCR, predominantly due to environmental contamination, are managed, this modality will struggle to obtain widespread uptake.

A final word from the expert

The case illustrates a classic example of candidaemia occurring in the intensive care setting. The combination of abdominal surgery, central venous line, TPN, and broad-spectrum antibiotics are all classic risk factors for the development of *Candida* bloodstream infection, and dissemination of the yeast to other sites is not unusual. Involvement of the eye is one of the most common infection-related complications, followed by endocarditis and bone/joint infection. However, cerebral abscesses are rare event in adults.

There are a number of important points to bear in mind when managing invasive candidiasis in the intensive care unit:

- The isolation of *Candida* from a vascular line tip is rarely a contaminant and treatment should always be considered, as in this case. A vascular line is a common source of candidaemia and it is therefore advisable to perform a surveillance blood culture prior to starting antifungal treatment. Other non-culture-based diagnostic approaches such as the detection of fungal (1,3)-BDG, mannan, or anti-mannan antibodies in serum samples have been investigated for the diagnosis of invasive candidiasis but are currently not recommended for routine use in the UK due to their relatively poor sensitivity and specificity.

- The detection of yeasts in a blood culture always warrants antifungal treatment even in the absence of clinical signs of infection such as fever. The recently published guidelines of the European Society of Clinical Microbiology and Infectious Diseases (ESCMID) no longer recommend the use of fluconazole as the first-line empirical treatment [15]. Echinocandins are now considered to be superior over fluconazole. Second-line agents are liposomal amphotericin B or voriconazole depending on local epidemiology and organ involvement.

- TOE and eye fundoscopy are recommended following candidaemia to detect dissemination of the infection. These investigations may also be warranted following a positive *Candida* culture from a vascular line tip in a high-risk patient. The dissemination of *Candida* to other organs also has a considerable impact on the length of treatment as well as choice of antifungal agent due to differences in tissue penetration, e.g. some drugs poorly cross the blood–ocular or –brain barrier. In some cases where endophthalmitis, endocarditis, or bone involvement is present, antifungal treatment would have to be combined with surgery (vitrectomy, valve replacement, or debridement of necrotic tissue).

- The duration of treatment for an uncomplicated candidaemia (without dissemination) is on average 14 days from the last negative surveillance blood culture. A step down to oral therapy may be considered after 5–10 days of intravenous therapy [7,15].

All in all, it is advisable that hospitals have an antifungal stewardship programme in place which normally includes an antifungal policy for the management of invasive fungal infections, the monitoring of appropriate antifungal prescribing, and the regular surveillance of antifungal susceptibility and incidence of candidaemia and their species distribution.

References

1 Pittet D, Monod M, Suter PM et al. *Candida* colonization and subsequent infections in critically ill surgical patients. *Ann of Surgery* 1994; 220: 751–758.

2 Denning DW, Kibbler CC, Barnes RA. British Society for Medical Mycology proposed standards of care for patients with invasive fungal infections. *Lancet Infect Dis* 2003; 3: 230–240.

3 Das I, Nightingale P, Patel M, Jumaa P. Epidemiology, clinical characteristics, and outcome of candidemia: experience in a tertiary referral centre in the UK. *Int J Infect Dis* 2011; 15: e759–763.

4 Fortún J, Martín-Dávila P, Gómez-García de la Pedrosa E et al. Emerging trends in candidemia: A higher incidence but a similar outcome. *J Hosp Infect* 2012; 65: 64–70.

5 Bodey GP, Anaissie EJ, Edwards JE. Definitions of Candida infections, pp. 407–408. In: Bodey GP (ed.), *Candidiasis: Pathogenesis, Diagnosis, and Treatment.* 1993; New York: Raven Press Ltd.

6 Oude Lashof AM, Rothova A, Sobel JD et al. Ocular manifestations of candidemia. *Clin Infect Dis* 2011; 53: 262–268.

7 Pappas PG, Kauffman CA, Andes D, et al. Clinical Practice Guidelines for the Management of Candidiasis: 2009 Update by the Infectious Diseases Society of America. *Clin Infect Dis* 2009; 48: 503–35.

8 Troughton JA, Browne G, McAuley DF, Walker MJ, Patterson CC, McMullan R. Prior colonisation with *Candida* species fails to guide empirical therapy for candidaemia in critically ill adults. *J Infect* 2010; 61: 403–409.

9 León C, Ruiz-Santana S, Saavedra P et al.; EPCAN Study Group. A bedside scoring system ('Candida score') for early antifungal treatment in nonneutropenic critically ill patients with *Candida* colonization. *Crit Care Med* 2006; 34: 730–737.

10 Pfaller MA, Diekema DJ, Sheehan DJ. Interpretive breakpoints for fluconazole and *Candida* revisited: a blueprint for the future of antifungal susceptibility testing. *Clin Microbiol Rev* 2006; 19: 435–447.

11 Reboli AC, Rotstein C, Pappas PG et al.: Anidulafungin Study Group. Anidulafungin versus fluconazole for invasive candidiasis. *N Engl J Med* 2007; 356: 2472–2482.

12 De Pauw B, Walsh TJ, Donnelly JP et al.; European Organization for Research and Treatment of Cancer/Invasive Fungal Infections Cooperative Group; National Institute of Allergy and Infectious Diseases Mycoses Study Group (EORTC/MSG) Consensus Group. Revised definitions of invasive fungal disease from the European Organization for Research and treatment of Cancer/Invasive fungal infections Cooperative group and the National Institute of Allergy and infectious diseases mycoses study group (EORTC/MSG) consensus group. *Clin Infect Dis* 2008; 46: 1813e21.

13 Karageorgopoulos DE, Vouloumanou EK, Ntziora F, Michalopoulos A, Rafailidis PI, Falagas ME. β-D-glucan assay for the diagnosis of invasive fungal infections: a meta-analysis. *Clin Infect Dis* 2011; 52: 750–770.

14 Klingspor L, Jalal S. Molecular detection and identification of *Candida* and *Aspergillus* spp. from clinical samples using real-time PCR. *Clin Microbiol Infect* 2006; 12: 745–753.

15 Cornely OA, Bassetti M, Calandra T et al.; ESCMID Fungal Infection Study Group. ESCMID guideline for the diagnosis and management of *Candida* diseases 2012: non-neutropenic adult patients. *Clin Microbiol Infect* 2012; 18(Suppl. 7): 19–37.

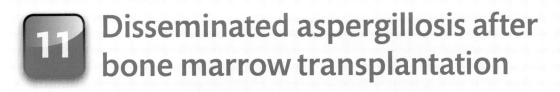

Disseminated aspergillosis after bone marrow transplantation

Jonathan Lambourne

ℭ **Expert commentary** Carolyn Hemsley

Case history

A 64-year-old patient was referred for cardiothoracic assessment of a mass in her left ventricular outflow tract (LVOT), identified incidentally on CT scanning.

The patient had a history of chronic lymphocytic leukaemia (CLL), diagnosed 6 years previously, which had been refractory to marrow-ablative chemotherapy (alemtuzumab, fludarabine, and cyclophosphamide) and necessitated an allogeneic haematopoietic cell transplant (HCT) from a matched unrelated donor, 11 months ago. A number of complications occurred post-HCT. The first was delayed engraftment leading to prolonged neutropenia (> 6 weeks). While she was neutropenic she had suffered from prolonged high fevers which had not settled until the neutropenia resolved. She was investigated for fungal infection during this period but there was no microbiological or radiological evidence and she did not receive treatment-dose antifungals.

✓ Evidence base Empiric vs. pre-emptive antifungal therapy

Growing confidence in diagnostic tools has led to a paradigm shift in the management of fever in immunocompromised patients. Standard practice had been to commence empiric antifungal therapy in all neutropenic patients with an antibiotic-unresponsive fever lasting >3–4 days [1]. A number of studies, including one by Maertens et al. [2], challenged this view by investigating the impact of restricting antifungal therapy to only those patients with prolonged fever and serological, radiological, or culture results suggestive of invasive fungal infection. This approach was termed 'pre-emptive' therapy.

Design
- 138 treatment episodes for patients 'at risk' of IFD
- No mould-active antifungal prophylaxis prescribed
- Daily GM assays (positive = two consecutive samples with optical density ≥0.5)
- Febrile episodes treated initially with broad-spectrum antibiotics, no antifungals
- Antifungal therapy commenced only if positive GM or combination of fever, suggestive CT findings, and positive fungal culture
- Antifungal used compared to what would have been used if current IDSA guidelines observed [1]

Results
- 78% reduction in rate of antifungal use for febrile neutropenia (from 35% down to 7.7%)
- No missed cases of aspergillosis, 1 missed case of zygomycosis
- Initiation of antifungal therapy prior to development of clinical symptoms in 10 cases
- 12-week survival for invasive aspergillosis = 63%

Following this and other studies, updated IDSA guidance now recommends pre-emptive management as an acceptable alternative to empirical antifungal therapy [3].

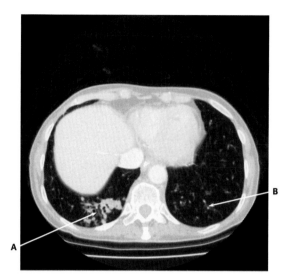

Figure 11.1 CT scan of the thorax showing nodular lesions in the lung parenchyma (A+B).

Another complication post-HCT was the development of GI graft versus host disease (GvHD) 6 months post-transplant, requiring treatment with high-dose methylprednisolone and mycophenolate mofetil. Due to escalation in immunosuppression antimicrobial prophylaxis was recommenced, including cotrimoxazole, acyclovir, and thrice-weekly intravenous liposomal amphotericin B.

Ten months after the transplant and 6 weeks prior to her cardiothoracic referral, she had developed a cough, breathlessness, and pleuritic pain. A CT scan demonstrated nodular lesions in the lung parenchyma (Figure 11.1).

Clinical tip

Radiographic features of IA are variable and depend upon the host and the timing in the disease process. No radiological feature is pathognomonic of IA. Plain radiographs can demonstrate an array of abnormalities including nodular pulmonary infiltrates, wedge-shaped opacities, and cavitatory lesions. Early CT findings include single or multiple nodules, representing focal areas of infection. Next, the 'halo' sign appears characterized by nodules with surrounding ground-glass infiltrates, the infiltrates representing focal areas of haemorrhage. Finally, the 'air-crescent' sign appears. This is due to coalescence and cavitation of nodules and most typically occurs during immune recovery. Infections with other angio-invasive pathogens, such as the *Zygomycetes*, *Fusarium* sp., *Scedosporium* sp., *Pseudomonas aeruginosa* (PSA), and *Nocardia* spp and other conditions affecting the pulmonary vasculature such as GVHD, KS, and Wegener's granulomatosis may also cause nodules, the halo sign, and the air-crescent sign.

Broad-spectrum antibiotics were commenced. Cultures of sputum and blood were negative for bacterial and fungal pathogens, no viral pathogens were identified, and fungal antigen testing was not performed.

Learning point Antigen testing as part of diagnosis

Definitive diagnosis as in this case requires isolation of the organism. However, obtaining tissue for culture is often too invasive for many patients where *Aspergillus* infection is suspected. Antigen detection can be useful in suspected disease to add weight to a possible diagnosis.

(continued)

Antigen detection: GM

GM is a cell wall polysaccharide present in most *Aspergillus* and *Penicillium* species. Circulating GM levels are associated with the fungal load in tissue. Two GM assays have United States Food and Drug Administration (FDA) approval, using serum and BAL fluid. They may also be useful when performed on CSF. False-positive results have been reported due to: use of medicines that contain GM including piperacillin-tazobactam; infection with other fungi whose cell wall GM is similar including *Fusarium, Histoplasma, Penicillium*, and *Blastomyces*; and patients with severe mucositis or GI GvHD. The performance of the GM assay varies depending on the cut-off used, the use of mould-active antifungal prophylaxis, and the prevalence of *Aspergillus* infection in patients under investigation. A meta-analysis of 27 studies by Pfeiffer and colleagues reported an overall sensitivity of 0.71, specificity of 0.89, and an NPV of >95% for proven invasive aspergillosis [4]. Sustained high levels of GM during antifungal therapy are associated with treatment failure, and serial GM levels can be used to monitor treatment response.

Antigen detection: PCR

A number of techniques based on amplification of *Aspergillus* genetic material have been described. A meta-analysis of these for IA diagnosis reported a sensitivity of 88% and specificity of 75% [5]. Significant inter-assay differences in DNA extraction and PCR target(s) prevented the EORTC from including PCR in their list of supportive mycological evidence. One approach is to perform wide-ranging fungal PCR (e.g. 18s rRNA) on tissue samples in which fungal hyphae have been seen, for which fungal culture remains negative.

ⓕ Expert comment

These assays can certainly be of value in clinical practice in high-risk patients but care must be taken when interpreting a result. The prevalence of fungal disease is crucial when translating sensitivity and specificity into predictive value. In a setting where *Aspergillus* infection occurs at low prevalence (even in a high-risk group such as HSCT recipients, with an incidence of approximately 15%) a test with 80% sensitivity and 80% specificity equates to a positive predictive value of only 31% and an NPV of 97%. When prior probability of disease is increased because of the presence of clinical features then these predictive values will also change. Tests detecting *Aspergillus* antigens should perhaps not necessarily be considered diagnostic but more as providing information regarding the probability of disease occurring, given each patient's clinical scenario. A second sample to confirm a positive result is recommended.

Histological examination and microbiological culture of transbronchial biopsy tissue demonstrated *Aspergillus fumigatus*.

⊕ Clinical tip Histopathology

Invasive aspergillosis is characterized histopathologically by invasion across tissue planes, angioinvasion, infarction, and tissue necrosis. On histological microscopy *Aspergillus* sp. appear as 3–6 μm wide, acute angle (45°) branching, septate hyphae, in contrast to the Mucorales which appear as non-septate broad hyphae with branching at 90°. Hyphae of *Scedosporium* sp., *Penicillium* sp., and *Fusarium* sp. have similar appearances histologically to *Aspergillus*, which is why definitive speciation requires microscopic examination of spore-bearing structures that only arise during laboratory culture, and is essential for choosing the most appropriate antifungal therapy.

ⓕ Expert comment

Even with improving molecular diagnostics, diagnosis still relies heavily on standard microscopy and culture of specimens (blood, respiratory tract secretions, fluid from sterile sites including CSF, urine and tissue), but there are known problems with sensitivity and/or specificity. Visualization

(continued)

of fungal elements within the affected tissue is required to be absolutely confident that a patient has invasive local or disseminated fungal infection. However, there are problems with reliance on histological diagnosis. Histology lacks sensitivity due to sampling error. The presence of fungal elements within tissue denotes infection but it may not be possible to define the species or the species may be misidentified. Tissue sampling itself is often precluded in this group of patients because of thrombocytopenia and the risk of bleeding. BAL fluid is often easier to obtain than tissue and should be attempted. Although BAL cultures have a sensitivity of only 50%, in immunosuppressed individuals with focal pulmonary lesions, isolation of *Aspergillus* sp. from respiratory tract specimens is highly predictive of invasive disease. Microscopy of BAL specimens is more sensitive than culture and should be performed on all BAL samples.

⭐ **Learning point** Diagnosis of *Aspergillus*

Timely diagnosis and initiation of effective antifungal therapy is associated with improved survival. However, diagnosing *Aspergillus* remains a major challenge. The definitive diagnosis of invasive *Aspergillus* infection requires microbiological culture. However, obtaining tissue culture via surgery, aspiration, or biopsy is often difficult (too invasive) for patients at risk. Therefore a decision on whether to treat is usually based on an assessment of risk factors, suggestive clinical features, radiology, and other indirect mycological tests (GM and 1,3-BDG). Although created for research purposes, clinically it can be useful to think about a case according to the European Organisation for Research and Treatment of Cancer (EORTC) definitions of fungal disease and make a decision about treatment based on degree of diagnostic certainty [6]. British Society for Medical Mycology (BSMM) guidelines describe how the various investigations should be performed [7].

The EORTC definitions of IFD [6]

Degrees of diagnostic certainty
- 'Proven': Fungus detected, by culture or histological analysis, in tissue taken from a site of disease.
- 'Probable': Requires host risk factor(s), suggestive clinical features, radiographic features and supporting mycological evidence.
- 'Possible': Requires host risk factor(s), suggestive clinical and radiological features but no requirement for mycological evidence.

Host factors
- Recent history of neutropenia: $<0.5 \times 10^9$ neutrophils/L (or <500 neutrophils/mm^3) for >10 days
- Receipt of an allogeneic HCT
- Prolonged use of corticosteroids: mean min. dose 0.3 mg/kg/day of prednisone or equivalent for >3 weeks
- Treatment with recognized T-cell immunosuppressants during the past 90 days
- Inherited severe immunodeficiency (e.g. CGD or severe combined immune deficiency (SCID))
- Mannan-binding protein deficiency

Radiological criteria (site-specific)
- Respiratory infection: nodules (with or without a halo), air-crescent sign or cavity
- Sino-nasal infection: sinusitis plus with extension of disease across bony barriers, e.g. into the orbit
- CNS infection: focal lesions or meningeal enhancement

Mycological criteria
- Direct tests: detection of *Aspergillus* sp. by microscopy or culture
- Indirect tests: detection of GM or 1,3-BDG

Source: data from Ben De Pauw et al, *Clinical Infectious Diseases*, Volume 46, Issue 12, pp. 1813–1821, Copyright © 2008 by the Infectious Diseases Society of America.

Voriconazole was commenced as treatment for acute invasive pulmonary aspergillosis. The follow-up CT scan that prompted her cardiothoracic referral showed an improvement in the pulmonary lesions but also a new LVOT mass.

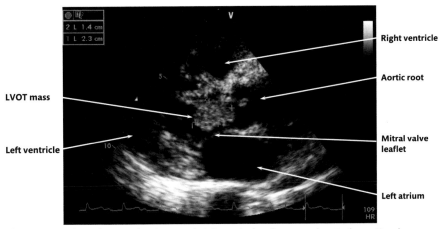

Figure 11.2 Echocardiogram showing mass in left ventrical outflow tract close to the aortic valve. Image courtesy of Professor John Chambers, Cardiovascular Services, Guy's and St Thomas' NHS Trust. Annotation thanks to Dr Rani Robson.

Echocardiography confirmed the presence of a large, pedunculated, intracardiac mass measuring 2.5 × 1.7 cm attached to the left ventricular septum (Figure 11.2).

Shortly after transfer, the patient complained of pain and diminished visual acuity in her left eye. Ophthalmic examination was suggestive of endophthalmitis, a vitreous aspiration was performed, and intra-vitreal ceftazidime, vancomycin, and amphotericin were administered. An MRI scan of the brain revealed multiple lesions in both hemispheres, suggestive of cerebral emboli. Medical treatment was intensified by the addition of caspofungin to voriconazole.

> ⊕ **Clinical tip** Treatment failure
>
> Progression of CT appearances within the first 10 days of antifungal treatment does not necessarily imply treatment failure. Repeat CT imaging is useful for assessing treatment response but the number and size of lesions may initially increase in individuals in whom treatment is ultimately successful. This may reflect immune reconstitution. Serial GM levels may help differentiate between these possibilities. If failure is suspected the following should be considered:
>
> 1. Is the diagnosis correct, or could there be another pathogen or co-infection?
> 2. Is antifungal therapy being administered at the appropriate dose, via the most appropriate route? Consider monitoring drug levels.
> 3. Although uncommon, the possibility of antifungal resistance should be considered.
> 4. Management of a failing regimen includes the use of surgery, change in antifungal therapy, and consideration of immunomodulatory adjunctive therapies.

Given the size of the endocardial lesion and evidence of embolic phenomena, cardiothoracic surgery was performed. At surgery, the intracardiac mass was removed; however, there was evidence of infiltration into the intraventricular septum and abnormal deposits were seen on the epicardial surface. *A. fumigatus* was grown from both the excised mass and from vitreous fluid, and histology of the cardiac mass demonstrated hyphae suggestive of *Aspergillus* (Figure 11.3). Despite dual antifungal therapy the patient died several weeks later, following an intracerebral haemorrhage.

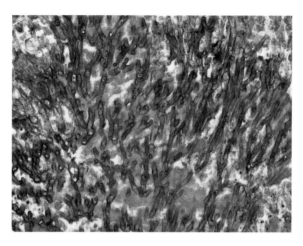

Figure 11.3 Periodic acid–Schiff (PAS) stain of histological specimen from ventricular mass showing septate branching hyphae.

ⓕ Expert comment

Therapeutic drug monitoring is essential when treating proven or probable invasive fungal infection with voriconazole. Voriconazole has a complex pharmacokinetic profile. The oral formulation sometimes has limited bioavailability and metabolism of drug in the liver is variable according to individual genetic configuration of the host cytochrome P450. Voriconazole can also interact with many hepatically metabolized drugs. It has a narrow therapeutic index. Toxicity is common and is related to high drug levels and can be cumulative over time. There is also evidence that inadequate serum levels (<1.0 mg/L) are associated with treatment failure.

It is not clear if this patient has progressed through adequate voriconazole dosing and levels or failed simply as a result of low drug levels. Not knowing which of these has happened is an indication to confirm susceptibility pattern of the *Aspergillus* isolated from the heart valve and treat with an alternative antifungal agent at least initially or, as in this case, consider combination therapy.

Discussion

This case illustrates the all-too-familiar scenario of invasive aspergillosis in the setting of profound immunosuppression and the capacity of *Aspergillus* species, ubiquitous environmental organisms, to cause devastating human infection. Unlike many cases of *Aspergillus* infection, diagnosis in this case was not a problem because the patient was well enough to undergo bronchoscopy and biopsy in the early stages of the illness. However, despite the correct diagnosis and timely intervention, the patient died. Two challenges posed by this case, and central to many others, are: could *Aspergillus* infection have been prevented and, once infection had been diagnosed, could alternative management have resulted in an improved outcome?

Given that invasive mould infections have become one of the leading causes of infection-related mortality in HCT recipients, with rates of *Aspergillus* infection as high as 20% in the first year following HLA mismatched transplants, preventing IFD is clearly a priority (Box 11.1).

However, the benefits of prophylaxis in preventing infection must be balanced against antifungal toxicity and cost. The risk of IFD is not the same for all immunocompromised patients; for example, the rate of invasive aspergillosis following autologous HCT is <2%. Some transplant centres advocate using anti-mould prophylaxis

> **Box 11.1** Infection control
>
> Exposure to *Aspergillus* is universal. Conidia 2–5 μm in diameter are easily dispersed into the air and remain airborne for prolonged periods. In an average day, hundreds of conidia are inhaled and deposited into the peripheral airways and sinus cavities. However, the high mortality of invasive aspergillosis leads to a desire to reduce exposure in those at risk of infection.
>
> The poor outcome of invasive aspergillosis emphasizes the importance of preventing infection in at-risk patients, by both physical and pharmacological means. Guidelines published by the American Society of Blood and Marrow Transplantation [8] and endorsed by IDSA [1] give recommendations for the design and maintenance of accommodation for HCT recipients, including ventilation of patients' rooms using positive pressure ventilation, with >12 air changes/hour and high-efficiency particulate air (HEPA) filtration. In addition, patients' rooms should be correctly sealed, especially during construction work. Despite meticulous attention, control of the physical environment is not 100% effective. In addition, these measures only protect patients in hospital, usually in the immediate post-transplant period. However, as previously discussed, invasive aspergillosis is increasingly occurring in those who have been discharged from hospital but who have their immunosuppression escalated to treat GvHD, which is why chemoprophylaxis is also required.

in patients with a predicted risk of IFD of >6% per year. Pre-transplant, transplant, and post-transplant factors influence each individual's risk for IFD. For example, in this case, extensive pre-transplant chemotherapy, the use of an unrelated donor, and the development of GvHD are all significant risk factors. The major determinants of IFD risk are the duration of neutropenia and T-cell suppression as both are essential in the normal immune response to *Aspergillus*. Neutrophils phagocytose conidia and effect extracellular killing of hyphae, and an intact Th1 response is required to sustain phagocytic recruitment and activity [9]. There is growing evidence supporting the 'second-hit' hypothesis; that additional defects in the immune response to *Aspergillus*, such as mutations in genes coding for pattern-recognition receptors (PRRs) such as MBL, TLR2 and dectin-1, influence an individual's risk of developing IA. These mutations, in and of themselves, do not cause an immunodeficiency sufficient to cause IA but significantly increase the risk of IA in those with coexistent impaired neutrophil and/or T-cell function [10].

> ⊕ **Learning point** Immune defects associated with susceptibility to *Aspergillus* infection
>
> **Impaired mucociliary clearance**
>
> Respiratory epithelial cells act as a physical barrier and the mucociliary system effects early clearance of conidia and hyphae. Patients with abnormal pulmonary architecture but a healthy immune response can limit fungal invasion but mechanical clearance is impaired. The result is saprophytic forms of aspergillosis such as aspergillomas and chronic necrotizing, cavitatory or fibrosing pulmonary aspergillosis.
>
> **Impaired phagocyte number and/or function**
>
> Alveolar macrophages, PBMCs, and neutrophils phagocytose conidia. Hyphae, however, are too big to be phagocytosed and neutrophil-mediated extracellular killing is required. Neutrophils release substances that damage hyphae, e.g. reactive oxygen species (ROS), and that starve growing fungi of essential nutrients, e.g. lactoferrin. Patients with impaired phagocyte number and/or function are at significantly increased risk of developing invasive aspergillosis (IA).
>
> Causes of prolonged neutropenia include aplastic anaemia, acute myeloid leukaemia (AML), myelodysplastic syndromes (MDS), HCT, and chemotherapy. Causes of impaired phagocyte function include chronic granulomatous disease (CGD), SCID, and prolonged corticosteroid use.
>
> (continued)

Impaired Th1 immune response

The balance between Th1 and Th2 responses is critical in determining the outcome of IFD. Th1 cells produce proinflammatory cytokines, e.g. IFN-γ, TNFα, IL-1, and IL-6 that recruit and activate phagocytes promoting *Aspergillus* eradication. In contrast, CD4+ Th2 cells release IL-4 and IL-10, which induce an antibody-mediated response and downregulate the Th1 response.

An impaired Th1 immune response is associated with a significantly increased risk of developing IA and is usually a consequence of immunomodulatory therapy given to solid organ transplant (SOT) recipients, to prevent rejection, or to HCT recipients with GvHD. Among SOT recipients, IA is most commonly seen following lung transplantation.

Mannose-binding lectin (MBL) deficiency

MBL is a non-specific opsonin and part of the innate immune system. In a study of neutropenic patients suffering from invasive aspergillosis, MBL deficiency was common [10]. MBL has been cloned and expressed in sufficient quantities for therapeutic trials and may be useful both in prophylaxis and treatment of immunocompromised patients with infection. Clinical trials are in progress.

✚ Clinical tip Risk periods for infection after bone marrow transplantation (BMT)

Infection with *Aspergillus* is related both to duration and degree of neutropenia and to the degree of Th1-cell dysfunction. There are two main periods when *Aspergillus* infection is most common: first, during the neutropenic period and second, during prolonged immunosuppression, as occurs with GvHD. Figure 11.4 shows the periods when different types of infection are most likely to occur post-transplant (Figure 11.4).

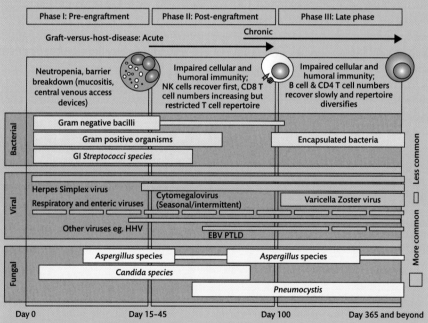

Figure 11.4 Phases of OIs among allogeneic HCT recipients. EBV, Epstein–Barr virus; HHV6, human herpes virus 6; PTLD, post-transplant lymphoproliferative disease.
Reproduced from *Biology of Blood and Marrow Transplantation*, Volume 15, Issue 10, Marcie Tomblyn et al, Guidelines for Preventing Infectious Complications among Hematopoietic Cell Transplantation Recipients: A Global Perspective. Figure 2, p. 1152, Copyright © 2009 American Society for Blood and Marrow Transplantation with permission from Elsevier, http://www.sciencedirect.com/science/journal/10838791

The epidemiology of IFD is changing. It is becoming less frequent in the early post-transplant period, as newer transplant regimens reduce the duration of neutropenia. However, incidence of IFD post-engraftment is increasing, due to the increasing use of mismatched transplants and consequent increased incidence of GvHD. In GvHD, donor-derived T-cells recognize tissues in the transplant recipient as foreign and cause immune-mediated tissue damage. GvHD occurs in 30–50% of patients receiving transplants from HLA-matched, related donors and 50–70% of patients receiving mismatched, unrelated donors. Current therapeutic approaches for the prevention and treatment of GvHD target T cells and include anti-T-cell agents including corticosteroids, anti-thymocyte globulin (ATG), cyclosporin, tacrolimus, mAbs (e.g. alemtuzumab), and purine analogue chemotherapy (fludarabine). Given the necessity of T cells in the immune response against *Aspergillus*, the relationship between GvHD and invasive aspergillosis is clear. This case demonstrates how an individual's risk for IFD is not static and may increase if transplant complications, such as GvHD, necessitate re-escalation of immunosuppression. Measures to prevent IFD in the immediate post-transplantation period are common to all transplant protocols and include the use of positive pressure isolation rooms and antifungal prophylaxis. However, once engraftment has occurred and the neutrophil count has returned to normal, these precautions are, understandably, lifted. Escalation of immunosuppression following engraftment may not always be accompanied by re-initiation of antifungal prophylaxis and, in contrast to an easily noticeable low neutrophil count, there are as yet no reliable indicators of T-cell immune function. In this case, antifungal prophylaxis was restarted, using thrice-weekly intravenous liposomal amphotericin, chosen due to the patient's intolerance of other antifungals and a favourable interaction profile between this and concurrent medication. Any antifungal agent with activity against *Aspergillus* can theoretically be used for prophylaxis. Evidence supports the use of itraconazole, posaconazole, voriconazole, micafungin, and nebulized amphotericin. The optimal agent depends on multiple factors including interactions with co-prescribed medications, reliability of absorption, and the presence of renal and/or hepatic impairment. Use of azole prophylaxis theoretically increases the possibility of breakthrough infection with azole-resistant organisms. However, azole resistance is rare and, on balance, 'breakthrough' infection is more likely to have occurred due to ineffective drug levels from poor adherence or absorption and drug interactions. Therefore, voriconazole is still appropriate first-line treatment for IA arising on a background of azole prophylaxis.

Despite receiving prophylaxis this patient went on to develop pulmonary aspergillosis complicated by endocarditis, and died, despite seemingly appropriate antifungal therapy. Without antifungals, invasive aspergillosis is almost invariably fatal. Even with antifungal therapy and intensive care support, invasive aspergillosis has an attributable mortality of 30–40%. Cardiac aspergillosis carries a particularly poor prognosis with mortality typically >90%, due to the catastrophic complications of both dissemination and local invasion through endocardial tissue. Even in individuals who survive surgery and in whom the disease appears to be cured, the rates of relapse are so high that lifelong antifungal therapy is recommended. A major determinant of survival of aspergillosis is immune recovery, either as a result of curtailing immunosuppressive therapy or successful engraftment following HCT. Voriconazole and amphotericin B dexoycholate (D-AMB) are the only two compounds licensed for primary treatment of invasive aspergillosis.

> **✅ Evidence base** Voriconazole vs. amphotericin B for primary therapy of invasive aspergillosis [12]
>
> **Design**
> - 277 patients with definite or probable IA
> - 144 randomized to voriconazole, 133 to AmBd
>
> **Results**
> Voriconazole associated with:
> - Greater likelihood of treatment success at week 12 (53% vs. 32%)
> - Improved survival at 12 weeks (71% vs. 58%)
> - Fewer severe adverse reactions
> - More frequent transient visual disturbances (45%)
>
> **Issues**
> - The trial compared voriconazole vs. D-AMB, not the newer lipid formulations which have improved side-effect profiles [12].
>
> Voriconazole is considered the treatment of choice for invasive aspergillosis. Subsequent studies have shown high rates of cure of CNS and osteoarticular aspergillosis with voriconazole. Due to inter-individual variation in serum voriconazole levels and the association between levels and treatment success and adverse effects, IDSA recommends checking a trough concentration after one week of therapy (target range >1 microgram/mL and <5.5 microgram/mL).

Other agents, such as the echinocandins or other mould-active azoles, are licensed for 'salvage therapy', for patients either failing or intolerant of voriconazole and amphotericin. Voriconazole is considered first-line therapy for invasive aspergillosis [13]. However, in cases of IFD in which the causative pathogen has not been unequivocally demonstrated, the use of amphotericin is advised, as voriconazole has no activity against the *Mucorales*.

The reasons for treatment failure in this case are not clear. One possibility could be that voriconazole drug levels were not checked and were low. Another possible reason for treatment failure is resistance to antifungals. In contrast to most bacterial pathogens, routine susceptibility testing of *Aspergillus* isolates is not recommended as methods and breakpoints have not been well established. It should be considered in infection with species associated with high levels of azole resistance, e.g. *A. ustus* and *A. lentulus*, and in patients with progressive disease during antifungal therapy. Isolates from this case were submitted to the UK Mycology Reference Laboratory and found to be susceptible to voriconazole, amphotericin, and the echinocandins.

Following cardiac surgery the patient was treated with dual antifungals, in recognition of the poor prognosis. Debate continues whether two antifungals are better than one. *In vitro* evidence suggests that some combinations are synergistic while others are antagonistic. Clinical trial data has yet to convincingly show a benefit in dual over monotherapy.

> **❛❛ Expert comment**
>
> There has been much interest and debate for years around the role of dual antifungal therapy in treatment of invasive aspergillosis (IA). There is currently no recommendation for dual therapy in the treatment of IA. *In vitro* studies of fungal growth have shown dual therapy to have a synergistic, additive, antagonistic, or no effect compared to monotherapy. Some animal models of IA provide evidence in support of the combination of a triazole and echinocandin. Results from the first prospective, randomized, double-blind clinical trial of combination therapy for IA comparing voriconazole with anidulafungin to voriconazole
>
> (continued)

monotherapy in patients with proven or probable IA were available in 2012 (277 patients included in primary analysis [14]., NCT00531479). Unfortunately the results were not as clear-cut as many would have hoped, although there was a trend towards improved overall survival in those treated with dual therapy as compared to monotherapy, but this was not significant. The jury is still out.

Investigation continues into the role of immunomodulatory therapies for invasive fungal infection. The British Committee for Standards in Haematology (BCSH) does not recommend the use of colony-stimulating factors in aspergillosis but IDSA guidelines suggest neutropenic patients may benefit from G-CSF. Granulocyte transfusions have been associated with stabilization of invasive pulmonary aspergillosis in some patients with infection refractory to standard treatment. Interferon-γ augments the phagocytosis by macrophages and neutrophils of a variety of fungal pathogens and there is limited data supporting its use in treatment of invasive aspergillosis. However, one concern is its potential to worsen GvHD in allograft HCT recipients. Following the discovery of MBL deficiency as an independent risk factor for IA, recombinant-human MBL is being investigated as an adjunctive therapy in IA [10].

A final word from the expert

There is a growing number of severely immunocompromised patients that are at risk of developing invasive fungal infection and the incidence of disease is likewise increasing. This trend will continue as the population begins to age and more patients undergo treatment for haematological malignancies and receive solid organ and stem cell transplantation. Yet the diagnosis and management of invasive fungal infection and particularly invasive mould infection continues to be taxing. There are management uncertainties at every step of the way from appropriate use of diagnostics to choice of antifungal agent and use of adjunctive therapy. There are some points to highlight:

1. Knowledge of the expected pattern of disease in the patient population in question is essential to interpreting the likelihood of disease and translating this into appropriate use of novel diagnostics. Without this knowledge, assessment of the predictive value of any serological test is impossible.

2. There is evidence that integrated care pathways involving structured multidisciplinary input and the use of nationally and locally agreed standards of practice lead to improved patient care. Such pathways require active participation from transplant consultants, haematologists, infection specialists, radiologists, and respiratory physicians. Each has a key role to play when ensuring the best possible patient care.

3. Although mortality remains high there has been a trend towards improved outcome from treatment for invasive aspergillosis in the last decade.

References

1 Hughes WT, Armstrong D, Bodey GP et al. 2002 guidelines for the use of antimicrobial agents in neutropenic patients with cancer. *Clin Infect Dis* 2002; 34: 730–751.
2 Maertens J, Theunissen K, Verhoef G et al. Galactomannan and computed tomography-based preemptive antifungal therapy in neutropenic patients at high risk for invasive fungal infection: a prospective feasibility study. *Clin Infect Dis* 2005; 41: 1242–1250.

3 Freifeld AG, Bow EJ, Sepkowitz KA et al. Clinical practice guideline for the use of antimicrobial agents in neutropenic patients with cancer: 2010 Update by the Infectious Diseases Society of America. *Clin Infect Dis* 2011; 52: 427–431.

4 Pfeiffer CD, Fine JP, Safdar N. Diagnosis of invasive aspergillosis using a galactomannan assay: a meta-analysis. *Clin Infect Dis* 2006; 42: 1417–1427.

5 Mengoli C, Cruciani M, Barnes RA, Loeffler J, Donnelly JP. Use of PCR for diagnosis of invasive aspergillosis: systematic review and meta-analysis. *Lancet Infect Dis* 2009; 9: 89–96.

6 De Pauw B, Walsh TJ, Donnelly JP et al. Revised definitions of invasive fungal disease from the European Organization for Research and Treatment of Cancer/Invasive Fungal Infections Cooperative Group and the National Institute of Allergy and Infectious Diseases Mycoses Study Group (EORTC/MSG) Consensus Group. *Clin Infect Dis* 2008; 46: 1813–1821.

7 Denning DW, Kibbler CC, Barnes RA. British Society for Medical Mycology proposed standards of care for patients with invasive fungal infections. *Lancet Infect Dis* 2003; 3: 230–240.

8 Guidelines for preventing opportunistic infections among hematopoietic stem cell transplant recipients. *Biol Blood Marrow Transplant* 2000; 6: 659–713, 715, 717–727, quiz 729–733.

9 Park SJ, Mehrad B. Innate immunity to *Aspergillus* species. *Clin Microbiol Rev* 2009; 22: 535–551.

10 Lambourne J, Agranoff D, Herbrecht R et al. Association of mannose-binding lectin deficiency with acute invasive aspergillosis in immunocompromised patients. *Clin Infect Dis* 2009; 49: 1486–1491.

11 Tomblyn M, Chiller T, Einsele H et al. Guidelines for preventing infectious complications among hematopoietic cell transplantation recipients: a global perspective. *Biol Blood Marrow Transplant* 2009; 15: 1143–1238.

12 Herbrecht R, Denning DW, Patterson TF et al. Voriconazole versus amphotericin B for primary therapy of invasive aspergillosis. *N Engl J Med* 2002; 347: 408–415.

13 Walsh TJ, Anaissie EJ, Denning DW et al. Treatment of aspergillosis: clinical practice guidelines of the Infectious Diseases Society of America. *Clin Infect Dis* 2008; 46: 327–360.

14 Marr KA, Schlamm H, Rottinghaus ST. *A randomised, double-blind study of combination antifungal therapy with voriconazole and anidulafungin versus voriconazole monotherapy for primary treatment of invasive aspergillosis. Poster presented at the 22nd European Congress of Clinical Microbiology and Infectious Diseases (ECCMID)*, London, 31 March–3 April 2012.

Hepatitis B reactivation

Gayatri Chakrabarty

ⓘ **Expert commentary** Daniel Forton

Case history

A 59-year-old male was referred to the viral hepatitis clinic for assessment and management of hepatitis B virus (HBV) infection by his general practitioner. His GP had
tested for hepatitis B when the patient registered with the practice. He was found to be
HBV surface antigen (HBsAg) positive. His past medical history included diffuse large
B-cell lymphoma, diagnosed 12 months previously. At that time he had presented with
a cough and shortness of breath. A lung biopsy in another hospital revealed intravascular diffuse large B-cell lymphoma. It was not clear whether he had been screened for
blood-borne infections at this time but his baseline LFTs were normal.

⊗ **Learning point** HBV screening: who should be screened for hepatitis B infection?

Chronic hepatitis B (CHB) can lead to cirrhosis, liver failure, and hepatocellular cancer. The United
Kingdom has a low prevalence of CHB of about 0.3% [1]. However, the prevalence is higher among
people from countries with high or intermediate prevalence and people with high-risk behaviours [2].
There is no universal screening programme, except for pregnant women, and best practice is to screen
individuals at increased risk [3]:

- Persons born in high or intermediate endemic areas and their children
- Persons with chronically elevated liver enzymes
- Individuals needing immunosuppressive therapy, including chemotherapy. The European Association
  for the Study of the Liver (EASL) recommends screening ALL patients before chemotherapy [4]
- MSM
- Persons with multiple sexual partners or history of sexually transmitted disease
- Prisoners
- Persons who have ever used injecting drugs
- Patients on haemodialysis
- Persons who have HIV or HCV infection
- Family and household members and sexual contacts of HBV-infected individuals

---

He had received eight cycles of chemotherapy with rituximab and CHOP (cyclophosphamide, doxorubicin, vincristine, and prednisolone) leading to complete remission. He subsequently underwent autologous bone marrow stem cell transplantation
which occurred 4 months prior to his family doctor's referral to the hepatitis clinic.
The full details of his treatment were not available at the time of his first consultation
in the hepatitis clinic but the patient did not recall a previous diagnosis of or treatment
for hepatitis B infection.

There was no other significant past medical history and he was currently asymptomatic. He was born in Korea and had emigrated to the United Kingdom 30 years

Table 12.1 Initial blood results

Haematology		Biochemistry		Viral serology			
Hb	14.4 g/dL	Bilirubin	10 IU/mL	HBsAg	Positive	HBV DNA	7000 IU/mL
WCC	7.2×10^9/L	ALT	28 IU/mL	HBeAg	Negative	HCV-ab	Negative
Platelet	300×10^9/L	ALP	120 IU/mL	HBeAb	Positive	HIV-ab	Negative
INR	1.1	GGT	50 IU/mL	HBcAb IgM	Negative		
		Albumin	40 g/L	HBcAb	Positive		

previously. He was not aware of a family history of hepatitis B infection. He had no risk factors for transmission of blood-borne viruses. He was married with two children. He did not smoke and his alcohol consumption was minimal (2–4 units per week).

His general physical examination was unremarkable with no evidence of jaundice, chronic liver disease, or pedal oedema. His pulse was 76 per minute with a blood pressure of 118/58 mmHg. He weighed 78 kg with a body mass index of 24.1. The cardiorespiratory examination was unremarkable and the abdominal examination was normal with no organomegaly or ascites. His initial blood results performed by the GP are shown in Table 12.1.

The GP had arranged an ultrasound of the abdomen which showed normal liver echo-texture and outline. No focal parenchymal lesions were seen. The biliary tree looked normal and the spleen size was normal. There was no evidence of hepatocellular carcinoma.

Expert comment

HBV infection is endemic in parts of Asia including China and Korea and is frequently transmitted from mother to infant. This man's country of birth is in itself a risk factor for HBV infection and serological testing should definitely have been performed prior to immunosuppressive treatment. Positive HBsAg serology indicates chronic HBV infection and antiviral prophylaxis is required during profound immunosuppression to prevent hepatitis flares. Negative HBsAg serology together with a positive anti-HBcAb (hepatitis B core antibody) indicates prior infection and natural immunity but there still remains a risk of viral reactivation during chemotherapy and BMT.

Clinical tip Assessment of liver disease

The initial assessment of the severity of liver disease due to chronic HBV infection should include LFTs including ALT, AST, ALP, GGT, bilirubin, serum albumin, full blood count (FBC), prothrombin time, alpha-fetoprotein, and a liver ultrasound. A low or progressive decline in serum albumin concentrations and/or prolongation of the prothrombin time, often accompanied by a low platelet count, suggests cirrhosis. However, advanced fibrosis and cirrhosis can occur when these tests are normal. Thus assessment by a specialist with the ability to order liver biopsy or non-invasive markers of liver fibrosis such as Fibroscan is suggested. Fibroscan is a non-invasive ultrasound technique which allows quantitative analysis of fibrosis based on elastography. Patients with serological evidence of chronic HBV infection should be followed longitudinally with serial measurements of LFTs, serology, and HBV VL to determine the current phase of their infection. This affects the likelihood of liver disease and the need for repeat fibrosis assessment and treatment.

Repeat blood tests were ordered from clinic and subsequently showed an increasing viral HBV DNA at 150,000 IU/mL and a rise in ALT to 159 IU/mL. His serum bilirubin was 15 IU/mL, ALP 92 IU/mL, AST 151 IU/mL, GGT 54 IU/mL, albumin 41 g/L, and the INR was 1.1. A Fibroscan of the liver was performed which showed a reading of 8.8 kPa (interquartile range 1.3 kPa).

The patient was booked to return to clinic in the next days to commence treatment with oral antiviral therapy.

Learning point Aims of treatment in CHB

CHB infection is a dynamic process and its natural history is divided into four phases [4]: (1) 'immune tolerant' phase; (2) 'immune reactive hepatitis B e-antigen (HBeAg) positive' phase; (3) 'immune control inactive HBV carrier' state; and (4) 'HBeAg negative CHB'. HbsAg is positive in all four phases and is a marker of ongoing infection. These phases are distinguishable by the HBeAg status, HBV DNA level, and evidence of liver necroinflammation (see Figure 12.1).

(continued)

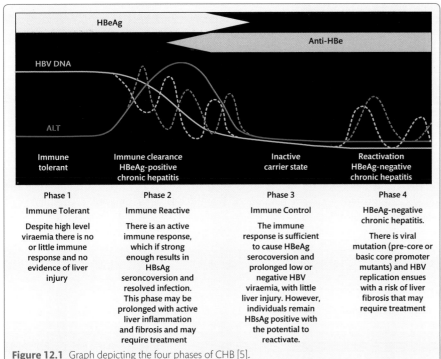

Figure 12.1 Graph depicting the four phases of CHB [5].
Adapted from Hyung Joon Yim and Anna Suk-Fong Lok, Natural history of CHB virus infection: What we knew in 1981 and what we know in 2005, *Hepatology*, Volume 43, Issue S1, pp.S173–S181, Copyright © 2006 American Association for the Study of Liver Diseases, with permission from John Wiley & Sons, Inc. All Rights Reserved.

One of the main goals of treatment of CHB is to move patients into an inactive phase where there is no detectable viral replication. An absence of replication reduces the level of liver injury and the risk of cirrhosis and hepatocellular carcinoma. There are two approaches to treatment: immunomodulatory treatment with α-interferon or viral suppression with antivirals which include the nucleoside entecavir and nucleotide TDF. Both approaches may result in HBeAg seroconversion if used in phase 2 or HBsAg seroconversion if used in phase 4, although in practice the latter is unusual (<10%). Alpha-interferon is generally used in phase 2 to achieve HBeAg serocoversion and transition to phase 3 and is a therapy of finite duration (usually 12 months). Both oral antivirals have high efficacy and a low barrier to resistance and are most commonly used as long-term viral suppressive therapies in phases 2 and 4.

The patient missed his appointment and was reviewed in the clinic 2 weeks later. At that time he complained of nausea and poor appetite. He had dark-coloured urine but normal stool. He did not give any history of recent travel. His current medication was omeprazole 40 mg per day which was started by his family doctor for dyspepsia 10 days previously. He was not taking any other prescribed drugs, over-the-counter remedies, or herbal medications.

On examination he looked tired with jaundice but no asterixis, ascites, or pedal edema. His temperature was 37.1°C, pulse rate 90 bpm with a blood pressure of 108/56 mmHg. The cardiorespiratory and remaining abdominal examinations were normal. His repeat blood tests are shown in Table 12.2.

Table 12.2 Repeat blood results

Haematology		Biochemistry				Viral serology	
Hb	12.4 g/dL	Bilirubin	249 IU/mL	Urea	7	Hep A total	Positive
WCC	5.2 × 10⁹/L	ALT	861 IU/mL	Creatinine	98	Hep A IgM	Negative
Platelet	279 × 10⁹/L	ALP	300 IU/mL	Na	138	CMV IgM	Negative
INR	1.5	GGT	301 IU/mL	K	3.8	CMV IgG	Positive
CRP	20 mg/L	AST	1412 IU/mL			HDV IgG	Negative
		Albumin	32			HBV VL	3.2×10^6 IU/mL

A repeat ultrasound of the abdomen showed coarse echo texture of the liver parenchyma suggesting diffuse parenchymal disease with possible fibrosis and no biliary dilatation.

The rapid deterioration in the LFTs with markedly elevated transaminases and jaundice indicated viral reactivation of hepatitis B as a delayed consequence of immunosuppression.

> **Clinical tip** Deterioration of LFTs in patients with CHB infection
>
> A sudden or gradual increase in liver enzymes, particularly the ALT/AST, and a rise in bilirubin in patients with CHB may be due to a flare in chronic HBV infection. This may be caused by viral reactivation or may be part of the natural history of the infection. However, other causes need to be considered when assessing a patient. The following causes need to be excluded:
>
> - Alcohol abuse
> - Prescribed or over-the-counter drugs or herbal remedies
> - Other acute viral hepatitides (hepatitis A, C, D, E, CMV, EBV)
> - Autoimmune hepatitis
> - Biliary pathology or hepatoma

> **Learning point**
>
> HBV reactivation is defined as loss of HBV immune control (due to HIV, steroid use, chemotherapy, or organ transplantation, etc.) in an individual with inactive (phase 3, HBsAg +ve, anti-HBeAb +ve, low VL) or resolved HBV infection (HBsAg -ve, UD HBV DNA). Reactivation can be clinically silent but can cause severe hepatitis with liver failure. A flare is defined as an acute exacerbation of hepatitis, which may occur as a result of reactivation but may also be part of the natural history of the infection, heralding a HBeAg seroconversion, for example. Reactivation may resolve spontaneously, but if there is prolonged immunosuppression chronic hepatitis ensues and can lead to fibrosis and cirrhosis. The most aggressive form of reactivation can lead to fulminant hepatitis and death. Reactivation of HBV infection is suggested by the reappearance or an increase in the viral replication with liver damage occurring during and/or following immune reconstitution [6].
>
> Clinically, reactivation is suggested by:
>
> 1. Rise or reappearance of serum HBV DNA and or return of HBeAg and/or HBsAg
> 2. ALT increase (mild to very high)
>
> A proportion of patients during reactivation can have a simultaneous rise in ALT and HBV DNA, but others may have low or UD HBV DNA at the time of ALT rise. Serial ALT and HBV DNA monitoring of patients on chemotherapy showed that the rise of HBV DNA precedes the ALT rise by a median of 2-3 weeks, and by the time the patient shows biochemical signs of hepatitis the HBV DNA may have decreased to an UD level [7], leading to misdiagnosis, delayed recognition of reactivation, and delayed initiation of treatment. There may also be potential poor cancer-related outcomes due to interruption of chemotherapy. HBV reactivation is not limited to patients receiving chemotherapy. Other causes of HBV reactivation include [6]:
>
> (continued)

- Spontaneous
- Immunodeficiency (HIV Infection)
- Withdrawal of antiviral therapy
- Immunosuppression for autoimmune diseases
- SOT (breast, kidney, heart, lung)
- Liver transplantation (reactivation in graft)
- BMT

❝ Expert comment

The initial serology from the GP showed that the patient was HBeAg negative with a positive anti-HBeAb. In the context of CHB infection this would be consistent with phase 3 or 4 infection. At this point there was no definite evidence of viral reactivation. The Fibroscan operates using transient elastography and gives a non-invasive measure of liver stiffness, which correlates with liver fibrosis. Cut-offs have been defined and a value of 8.8 kPa is above the threshold that excludes liver fibrosis (<7 kPa). The interquartile range value of 1.3 kPa indicates a valid set of recordings as the spread of the recorded values is low. The interquartile range should be <20% of the liver stiffness value. It is important to remember that the Fibroscan reading only gives information about liver stiffness and may be affected by ALT flares, resulting in spuriously high readings. Furthermore, unlike a liver biopsy, the Fibroscan does not give any diagnostic information. It was appropriate to repeat the LFTs and VL measurements in the clinic to look for viral reactivation, and this is exactly what was seen with the VL climbing to 150,000 IU/mL and a worsening biochemical hepatitis. Given the preceding immunosuppression, the diagnosis of a delayed reactivation was considered and the decision to institute viral suppressive therapy was correct. However, there was a delay due to a missed appointment and, when the patient returned to clinic, the LFTs showed a significant flare with evidence of impaired liver synthetic function (reduced albumin, prolonged INR) and jaundice. The repeat ultrasound in the specialist clinic indicated the possibility of fibrosis. Underlying liver fibrosis reduces the hepatic reserve and capacity to tolerate an acute hepatitic flare; treatment should have been started as soon as possible at this stage.

He was admitted to hospital the same day. He was started on TDF 245 mg per day, which he tolerated well. He was observed closely and there was no clinical evidence of hepatic encephalopathy or the development of ascites. His transminases and bilirubin fell gradually and, with a decrease in the HBV VL of 2 $\log_{10}$ IU/mL, he was discharged home after 2 weeks.

He was seen in the outpatient clinic 4 weeks later. He was feeling much better and did not report any further nausea or vomiting. His appetite had improved and he was gaining weight. There was a steady improvement in his liver function test with a reducing HBV DNA level. Repeat blood test results are shown in Table 12.3.

Table 12.3 Blood results 4 weeks after discharge

Haematology		Biochemistry			
Hb	13.5 g/dL	Bilirubin	56 IU/mL	Urea	4
WCC	5.2 × 10⁹/L	ALT	62 IU/mL	Creatinine	95
Platelet	279 × 10⁹/L	ALP	110 IU/mL	Na	141
INR	1.1	GGT	60 IU/mL	K	3.7
		AST	46 IU/mL	HBV DNA	38 IU/mL
		Albumin	38		

> **ⓘ Expert comment**
>
> The patient responded well to antiviral therapy with TDF. However, rescue therapy for viral reactivation in this setting is more often unsuccessful, and prophylactic therapy should have been instituted before immunosuppression to prevent the risk of serious hepatitis and death. In this case it is likely that he will require long-term treatment as both the hospital ultrasound scan and Fibroscan indicate that there is underlying liver fibrosis. This could be confirmed and staged accurately with a liver biopsy. Chemotherapy and BMT put the patient at particularly high risk for HBV reactivation. Immunosuppressive therapy impairs T-cell function and reduces immune-mediated virus clearance from infected hepatocytes. Corticosteroids may activate the glucocorticoid responsive element in the HBV genome and thus enhance HBV replication and gene expression. Either one or the combined effect of the two may contribute to an increase in HBV-infected cells during immunosuppression. After successful BMT and withdrawal of immunosuppression, there is immune reconstitution, often accompanied by a vigorous antiviral immune response. This 'second hit' may result in HBV DNA clearance or a severe and sometimes fatal hepatitis. Multiple RCTs have shown that reactivation of hepatitis B can be prevented by antiviral prophylaxis. Routine prophylaxis is therefore recommended for persons with HBsAg undergoing cancer chemotherapy or transplantation [6]. Reactivation can also occur in patients with resolved infection who are HBsAg negative, particularly with some regimes including rituximab, although the place of antiviral prophylaxis is still debated in this situation.

Discussion

The case illustrates the importance of screening for blood-borne viruses before immunosuppression. It is not known whether this patient was screened for HBV infection prior to chemotherapy and BMT. However, the opportunity was not taken to provide antiviral prophylaxis to prevent the severe hepatitic flare as a consequence of viral reactivation. It is highly unlikely that this was an acute *de novo* infection as the patient was HBeAg negative when first tested (stage 3 or 4). If the haematologist had screened the patient for HBV infection, the serological pattern would have allowed an assessment of the risk of reactivation, which depends on the stage of the hepatitis B and the level of planned immunosuppression.

In patients who are HBsAg positive, the rate of reactivation is in the range 20–50%. In a prospective study of 41 patients with breast cancer who were HBsAg positive and were followed during chemotherapy, 17 (41%) patients developed HBV reactivation. The study also found that there was premature termination of chemotherapy or a delay in treatment in 71% of the patients who developed viral reactivation, compared with 33% who did not develop the condition [8]. In another study of 626 consecutive cancer patients who received chemotherapy and were followed up to identify the risk factors for reactivation, 72 (12%) were HBsAg positive and among them 34 (44%) had a raised ALT during their treatment. Out of the 34 patients, 15 cases of hepatitis were attributed to HBV reactivation (44%). Male sex, younger age, HBeAg-positive patients, and patients with lymphoma were at higher risk of reactivation [9].

Several anticancer immunosuppressive agents have been associated with a greater risk of HBV reactivation [7], including corticosteroids, antitumour antibiotics (actinomycin D, bleomycin, daunorubicin, doxorubicin, epirubicin, mitomycin-C), plant alkaloids (vinblastine, vincristine), alkylating agents (carboplatin, chlorambucil, cisplatin, cyclophosphamide), antimetabolites (azuridine, citarabine, fluorouracil, gemcitabine, mercaptopurine, methotrexate, thioguanine), and mAbs (alemtuzumab, rituximab). With regard those with past hepatitis B infection (HBSAg -ve, HBcAb +ve), rates of reactivation during chemotherapy are much lower. However, rituximab has been shown to lead to high rates of reactivation even in this group **(see Evidence base: Hepatitis B virus reactivation).**

✅ **Evidence base** Hepatitis B virus reactivation in lymphoma patients with prior resolved hepatitis B undergoing anticancer therapy with or without rituximab [10]

Rituximab is a chimeric mouse human mAb against CD20+ expressed on B lymphocytes. Incorporation of rituximab into standard chemotherapy for lymphoid malignancies has improved clinical outcome. However, use of rituximab alone or in combination chemotherapy has been associated with HBV reactivation.

- This study determined the HBV reactivation rate in HBsAg-negative/anti-HBcAb-positive lymphoma patients treated with rituximab-containing chemotherapy and compared to patients not treated with rituximab.
- 80 HBsAg-negative patients were treated with either CHOP alone or rituximab plus CHOP (R-CHOP). All patients were observed for HBV reactivation defined as detectable HBV DNA with a rise in ALT during and for 6 months after chemotherapy.
- Out of the 80, 46 patients (44.2%) were HBsAg negative/anti-HBc positive; 25 of these patients were treated with CHOP, and none had HBV reactivation.
- Of 21 patients who were treated with R-CHOP, five developed HBV reactivation, including one patient who died of hepatic failure (p = 0.0148). Further analysis identified male sex, absence of anti-HBs, and the use of rituximab to be predictive of HBV reactivation.
- In conclusion, the authors noted that 25% of HBsAg-negative/HBcAb-positive lymphoma patient treated with R-CHOP developed HBV reactivation and that close observation and consideration of antiviral prophylaxis is necessary.

Source: Data from Yeo W et al, Hepatitis B virus reactivation in lymphoma patients with prior resolved hepatitis B undergoing anticancer therapy with or without rituximab, *Journal of Clinical Oncology*, Volume 27, Number 4, pp. 605–611, Copyright © 2009 by American Society of Clinical Oncology.

If the haematologist had identified this patient's major risk factors for reactivation (BMT and rituximab) prophylactic chemotherapy should have been given. Prophylaxis with 3TC, a nucleoside analogue that inhibits the HBV polymerase, has been shown to reduce reactivation rates by 80–100% in those who are HBsAg positive.

✅ **Evidence base** Use of pre-emptive 3TC reduces risk of HBV-related hepatitis

Study design: In this study the authors compared the efficacy of early and deferred pre-emptive therapy with 3TC during chemotherapy for lymphoma in 30 patients who were HBsAg positive [11].

- 30 consecutive HBSAg-positive patients having intensive chemotherapy were selected.
- They were randomized 1:1 to two groups. Group 1 received 3TC 100 mg daily for 1 week before starting the chemotherapy and then continued for 6 weeks after completion of the last course of chemotherapy. Group 2 had their treatment deferred until there was evidence of HBV reactivation based on 2-weekly serum HBV monitoring.

Results
- 8 patients (53%) in group 2 and none in group 1had hepatitis B viral reactivation after chemotherapy (p = 0.002); 7 patients in group 2 developed hepatitis (5 non-icteric, 1 icteric, 1 hepatic failure).
- Survival (free from hepatitis due to HBV reactivation) was significantly longer in group 1 than in group 2.
- The median onset of HBV reactivation in group 2 was 16 weeks (range 4–36 weeks).

(continued)

The use of pre-emptive therapy with antivirals may also reduce the risk of reactivation in HBsAg-negative, anti-HBcAb-positive individuals and, given the significant risk in some regimes, e.g. rituximab containing, prophylaxis seems a sensible approach in selected cases.

Prolonged treatment with 3TC has been associated with increased likelihood of treatment-resistant HBV mutations. The emergence of the resistant virus is usually associated with increased ALT and HBV DNA. In a follow-up study by Lok et al. [12] it was noted that the proportion of patients with a documented 3TC-resistant mutation increased from 23% in year 1 to 65% in year 5. In cirrhotic patients 3TC resistance-related flares can result in liver failure and death. Thus most experts would recommend use of a more potent HBV polymerase inhibitor with a high barrier to resistance, such as entecavir or TDF, in patients with a high HBV DNA level, liver fibrosis, or those who require prolonged or repeated courses of immunosuppression.

According to the EASL guidelines [4] and more recent UK National Institute for Health and Care Excellence (NICE) guidelines [13], this patient should have been offered prophylaxis, whether or not he was initially found to be HBsAg positive or had previously cleared infection (HBsAg-negative, anti-HBcAb-positive). The guidelines recommend that HBsAg-positive patients should be tested for HBV DNA levels and be given pre-emptive antiviral therapy during treatment (regardless of HBV DNA levels) and for 12 months after cessation of treatment. If the DNA level is under 2000 IU/mL and the patient is receiving a finite course of chemotherapy, 3TC is recommended. However, patients with high HBV DNA levels who are receiving lengthy and repeated cycles of immunosuppression should be given antivirals with high potency and high barrier to resistance, e.g. entecavir or TDF.

HBsAg-negative, anti-HBc-positive patients receiving chemotherapy should be monitored for HBV reactivation with serum ALT and HBV DNA level every 1–3 months depending on type of immunosuppression and co-morbidities. If the DNA level is detectable, antiviral therapy should be commenced. The exception is when this type of patient is offered a solid organ or stem cell transplant (as with this patient). In this setting, the patient should be treated as a HBsAg-positive patient and receive routine prophylaxis. Some also recommend that if rituximab is used (as in this patient) routine prophylaxis should also be used, regardless of HBsAg status [14]. In summary, this patient had a number of reasons to be offered antiviral prophylaxis, which were not identified. Fortunately in this case, the administration of reactive as opposed to pre-emptive therapy was sufficient to prevent a fatal hepatitis. However, this preventable eventuality is still seen, all too often, in cancer units around the world.

⊕ **Clinical tip** Risk factors for reactivation and hepatic flares

HBsAg positive

- Chemotherapy
- Glucocorticoids
- HBeAg+ve, High DNA VL (>10^5 copies/mL)
- Haematological malignancy (up to 58% of Hodgkin's lymphoma patients can reactivate)
- Male > female

HBcAb+, HBsAg–

- Rituximab
- BMT

A final word from the expert

This was a preventable case of delayed, symptomatic HBV reactivation that occurred several months after chemotherapy and BMT. The time course is not atypical and current guidelines for antiviral prophylaxis recommend that treatment continues for one year after the end of immunosuppressive therapy [4]. In cases where there is evidence of underlying liver disease, as in this case, treatment should be long term. The detection of underlying liver fibrosis is not always easy, without recourse to liver biopsy or a non-invasive test of fibrosis. An understanding of the natural history of HBV infection is important and, in this case of likely maternal-infant infection 59 years previously, the treating physician should be aware of the substantial risk of fibrosis and cirrhosis.

On infection, HBV viral DNA is incorporated into the hepatocyte nucleus as covalently closed circular DNA (cccDNA). It serves as the template for viral RNA transcription by host RNA polymerases and is rarely cleared from the hepatocyte, even when there has been an HBsAg seroconversion. If the balance between immune control and viral replication is altered, this archived viral DNA can be the source for replicating virions that infect increasing numbers of hepatocytes, leading to viral reactivation. A biochemical hepatitis ensues when the reconstituted immune system, often some time after the end of chemotherapy, leads to recognition of infection hepatocytes and cell death.

HBV screening and antiviral prophylaxis in the context of immunosuppressive therapy is recommended by the hepatological community and is included in treatment guidelines including NICE guidance [13]. There is less consensus in oncological circles and routine screening has not been recommended by the American Society of Clinical Oncology [15]. Rather, it is suggested that physicians can consider screening patients belonging to groups at heightened risk for chronic HBV infection or if highly immunosuppressive therapy is planned. It is likely that such a policy would miss patients who go on to reactivate because there is no failsafe way to determine who is at risk of this infection. Having treated a number of patients with HBV reactivation, who did not have as favourable an outcome as this man, it is this author's strong belief that all patients undergoing chemotherapy should be screened for HBV infection.

References

1 Department of Health. *Immunisation against infectious disease: the green book*, Chapter 18 Hepatitis B (pp. 161–184), 2012. Available at: http://immunisation.dh.gov.uk/green-book-chapters/.
2 Lavanchy D. Hepatitis B virus epidemiology, disease burden, treatment, and current and emerging prevention and control measures. *J Viral Hepat* 2004; 11: 97–107.
3 Lok ASF, McMahon BJ. Chronic hepatitis B: Update 2009. *Hepatology* 2009; 50: 661–662.
4 European Association for the Study of the Liver. EASL clinical practice guidelines: Management of chronic hepatitis B virus infection. *J Hepatol* 2012; 57: 167–185.
5 Yim HJ, Lok AS. Natural history of chronic hepatitis B virus infection: What we knew in 1981 and what we know in 2005. *Hepatology* 2006; 43: S173–S181.
6 Hoofnagle JH. Reactivation of hepatitis B. *Hepatology* 2009; 49: S156–S165.
7 Yeo W, Johnson PJ. Diagnosis, prevention and management of hepatitis B virus reactivation during anticancer therapy. *Hepatology* 2006; 43: 209–220.
8 Yeo W, Chan PK, Hui P et al. Hepatitis B virus reactivation in breast cancer patients receiving cytotoxic chemotherapy: a prospective study. *J Med Virol* 2003; 70: 553–561.

9 Yeo W, Chan PKS, Zhong S et al. Frequency of hepatitis B virus reactivation in cancer patients undergoing cytotoxic chemotherapy: A prospective study of 626 patients with identification of risk factors. *J Med Virol* 2000; 62: 299–307.

10 Yeo W, Chan TC, Leung NWY et al. Hepatitis B virus reactivation in lymphoma patients with prior resolved hepatitis B undergoing anticancer therapy with or without rituximab. *J Clin Oncol* 2009; 27: 605–611.

11 Lau GKK, Yiu HHY, Fong DYT et al. Early is superior to deferred preemptive lamivudine therapy for hepatitis B patients undergoing chemotherapy. *Gastroenterology* 2003; 125: 1742–1749.

12 Lok AS, Lai CL, Leung N et al. Long-term safety of lamivudine treatment in patients with chronic hepatitis B. *Gastroenterology* 2003; 125: 1714–1722.

13 National Clinical Guideline Centre. *Diagnosis and Management of Chronic Hepatitis B in Children, Young People and Adults.* www.http://guidance.nice.org.uk/CG165

14 Vigano M, Vener C, Lampertico P et al. Risk of hepatitis B surface antigen seroreversion after allogeneic hematopoietic SCT. *Bone Marrow Transplant* 2011; 46: 125–131.

15 Artz AS, Somerfield MR, Feld JJ et al. American Society of Clinical Oncology Provisional Clinical Opinion: Chronic hepatitis B virus infection screening in patients receiving cytotoxic chemotherapy for treatment of malignant diseases. *J Clin Oncol* 2010; 28: 3199–3202.

13 Developments in the treatment of hepatitis C virus infection

Tomas Doyle

ⓘ Expert commentary Daniel Webster

Case history

A 42-year-old white male returned to his routine hepatology appointment for management of chronic hepatitis C infection which had been diagnosed 8 years previously. He was keen to discuss possibilities for treating his infection. He had previously used intravenous drugs, which was the likely source of his infection. He had no other risk factors for infection and had recently had a negative HIV test result. There was no significant other medical history, no known drug allergies, and he was not taking any medications. He had a history of mild depression in the past and had no history of self-harm. He was a smoker with a 10 pack-year history but had never used alcohol heavily.

✪ Learning point Hepatitis C background

Hepatitis C virus (HCV) is a single-stranded positive-sense RNA virus of approximately 9.4 kilobases in length and is a member of the Flaviridae family. Between 130 and 170 million people are infected worldwide [1]. In Western countries, HCV is a major cause of chronic liver disease leading to cirrhosis, liver failure, and hepatocellular carcinoma. HCV is blood-borne and is primarily transmitted by contaminated blood products and intravenous drug use. Perinatal infection occurs at a rate of approximately 1–4% and sex between men is an increasingly recognized route of transmission although this is thought to be likely in the context of particularly high-risk practices. There are at least six HCV genotypes (1–6) with somewhat different geographical distribution which is of considerable importance as viral subtype is a major determinant of response to interferon-based therapy. A significant proportion of HIV-infected patients are also infected with HCV; since the introduction of ART the contribution of HCV-related liver disease to morbidity and mortality in this group has become increasingly important. Extrahepatic disease associations of HCV infection include mixed cryoglobulinaemia, non-Hodgkin's lymphoma, arthritis, diabetes, depression, and cognitive disturbance.

✪ Learning point Public health

Recent years have seen outbreaks of HCV infection in MSM in large cities in the USA, Europe, and Australia, particularly affecting those who are HIV-positive. This has been associated with high-risk sexual practices such as unprotected anal sex, particularly where increased trauma to the ano-rectal mucosa is involved. This trend may partly be due to inconsistent condom use in HIV-positive men with suppressed HIV VLs. Clinicians should be aware of the risk of HCV infection in MSM, particularly HIV-positive MSM, and provide adequate risk counselling. As HIV infection has a negative impact on the outcome of HCV infection, a rising incidence of co-infection could have important implications and appropriate targeted prevention strategies are desirable. Studies are ongoing to ascertain the most cost-effective screening strategy, but many centres perform yearly HCV serological screens in HIV-positive patients. Although the majority of acute HCV infections are asymptomatic, HCV RNA

(continued)

testing should be performed in MSM presenting with transaminitis where the history suggests possible risk of HCV acquisition. Approximately 25% of patients will clear the acute infection spontaneously. Identification of acute infection is important for the remainder as early treatment of HCV infection (within 12 weeks of infection) with pegIFN/RBV has much higher success rates (>80%) than in chronic infection.

He was infected with HCV genotype 1b. Three years previously he had undergone a 48-week course of pegylated interferon and ribavirin (pegIFN/RBV) therapy. His HCV VL had reduced by $> 2 \log_{10}$ copies/mL at week 12, and was UD at week 24 and at the end of treatment.

> ✪ **Learning point** Past standard of care (SOC)
>
> Before the approval of the new PIs, SOC for HCV infection consisted of a 24–48-week course of pegylated interferon alpha (2a or 2b) and ribavirin. A sustained virological response (SVR), defined as persistently negative HCV RNA in serum using a sensitive assay, is considered a successful treatment outcome as this indicates clearance of HCV infection. The viral subtype is a major determinant of response to interferon-based therapy with rates of SVR to pegIFN/RBV according to the common genotypes as follows: genotype 1 40–50% (subtype 1a having a slightly poorer response than subtype 1b), genotype 2 80–90%, and genotype 4 50%. Generally genotypes 1 and 4 are treated with 48 weeks of pegIFN/RBV and genotypes 2 and 3 with a 24-week course.

The patient subsequently relapsed with a detectable VL. During the treatment course he had experienced fatigue. In addition, his haemoglobin had dropped to 8.5 g/dL at week 6 of therapy, which was managed by ribavirin dose reduction and erythropoietin injection.

Relevant blood investigations were performed to re-evaluate his disease status and are listed in Table 13.1.

> ✪ **Learning point** Virological monitoring of HCV on treatment and virological response definitions
>
> Before and throughout treatment HCV RNA should be measured on the same assay platform at the same centre using a sensitive assay with a lower limit of detection of 10–50 IU/mL. On-treatment virological responses strongly predict SVR, are important in the management of pegIFN/RBV therapy, and remain so for triple therapy. Patients experiencing rapid virological response (RVR), defined as UD HCV RNA at week 4, have high rates of subsequent SVR (see Figure 13.1). In the absence of other poor-response indicators at baseline they are eligible to reduce the treatment duration of pegIFN/RBV for genotype 1 infection from 48 to 24 weeks without jeopardizing their rate of SVR. Early virological response (EVR) is defined as a reduction in HCV RNA by $>2 \log_{10}$ IU/mL at week 12 of pegIFN/RBV. Non-achievement of EVR is an indication to discontinue pegIFN/RBV therapy. Patients who fail to achieve EVR are termed null responders. Patients who achieve EVR but with virus still detectable at week 12 and subsequently UD at week 24 may benefit from an extended treatment course to 72 weeks for genotype 1 infection. Patients who achieve EVR but fail to subsequently achieve undetectability are termed partial responders (PR). Patients who are UD at the end of treatment and whose HCV VL subsequently becomes detectable again are termed relapsers. Extended RVR (eRVR) is a term which will be applied to triple therapy and is defined as a UD HCV RNA at week 4 and week 12 on telaprevir-based therapy, and UD HCV RNA at weeks 8 and 24 on boceprevir-based therapy (see Figure 13.1).

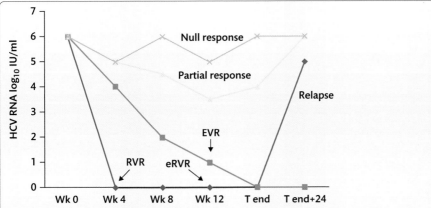

Figure 13.1 On treatment virological response definitions. Important time-points at which virological responses to treatment are clinically assessed are indicated. The significance of responses at these time-points is explained in the learning point: Virological monitoring of HCV on treatment and virological response definitions.

EVR, early virological response; RVR, rapid virological response; eRVR, extended rapid virological response.

Table 13.1 Baseline blood investigations

Hb	15 g/dL	Creatinine	70 μmol/L	HCV RNA	120,000 IU/mL
WCC	6.2×10^9/L	ALP	78 U/L	HCV genotype	1b
Platelets	120×10^9/L	ALT	64 U/L	IL28B genotype (860)	CC
INR	1.1	AST	44 U/L	HIV antibody	Negative
Alfafetoprotein	3 kU/L	Albumin	49 g/L	HBsAg	Negative

⭕ **Learning point** Baseline predictors of SVR

Although the currently approved PIs are only effective against genotype 1, the majority of patients in the UK and USA are infected with this genotype, thus their introduction has greatly improved the overall outlook for treatment. Other baseline predictors of response to pegIFN/RBV are also important in patient counselling and treatment management. These retain importance for triple therapy and are outlined below:

- Age
- Sex
- Race
- Body mass index
- Baseline HCV RNA level
- Viral genotype and subtype
- IL28B polymorphisms
- LDL-co-receptor polymorphisms
- Presence of fibrosis and cirrhosis
- Previous treatment response

IL28B polymorphisms: In 2009 a series of genome-wide association studies identified an association between SVR to pegIFN/RBV therapy and some common polymorphisms in IL28B (or IFN λ3) [2,3,4]. Single nucleotide polymorphisms rs12979860 and rs8099917 were found to be associated with SVR by different groups. IL28B is a lambda IFN in the type 3 interferon group, which have somewhat different characteristics to type 1 IFNs (containing IFNα). The mechanistic explanation for the association is unclear at present. The interferon lambda receptor complex is found primarily on epithelial cells and signalling through the receptor upregulates many of the genes upregulated by interferon-alpha. Interferon-alpha administration may induce increased production of lambda

(continued)

interferon during therapy as these cytokines work in complex cyclical cascades. Many centres are now determining patient IL28B '860' genotype to aid in predicting responses to treatment. Homozygosity for the CC allele is associated with high likelihood of response. CT and TT genotypes are associated with intermediate and low likelihood of response, respectively. The association between IL28B and SVR accounts for much of the long-recognized association between race and SVR to pegIFN/RBV treatment.

✪ Learning point Side effects of HCV treatment and management

- Pegylated interferon: flu-like symptoms, fatigue, fever, myalgia, neutropenia, thrombocytopenia, anorexia, nausea, depression, sleep disturbance, anxiety, alopecia, and exacerbation of underlying liver, cardiovascular, and autoimmune disease.
- Ribavirin: cough, shortness of breath, haemolytic anaemia, teratogenicity, rash, anorexia and weight loss
- Telaprevir: rash, anaemia, pruritus, anorectal discomfort
- Boceprevir: anaemia, neutropenia, dysgeusia (taste disturbance)

Prior to initiating pegylated interferon-based therapy it is important to take a full medical history and perform appropriate investigations to exclude the presence of underlying medical conditions which could be exacerbated by treatment. Routine blood investigations should include thyroid function tests and a tissue autoantibody screen. Any symptoms suggesting underlying cardiovascular or respiratory disease should be investigated to avoid on-treatment decompensation and a careful risk assessment should be performed in patients at risk of decompensation of their liver disease. Patients should be adequately counselled concerning the teratogenicity of ribavirin. Anaemia is a significant treatment-related adverse effect due to ribavirin therapy and this is now exacerbated by the concomitant administration of boceprevir and telaprevir. Ribavirin dose reduction is the initial management. Erythropoeitin is commonly used for moderate to severe anaemia and transfusion may be effective. Telaprevir causes an eczematous rash in a significant number of patients, usually within the first 4 weeks of initiation of therapy. When localized, recommended treatment is with oral antihistamines, topical steroids, and referral to a local dermatologist if feasible. More serious rashes may occur such as drug rash with eosinophilia and systemic symptoms (DRESS) and Steven-Johnson syndrome (SJS). Patients must therefore be warned to report rash and all therapy should be discontinued where any features suggesting the above conditions are suspected. Anecdotally, anal discomfort with telaprevir tends to resolve when patients increase their fat intake, suggesting that this side effect of the drug was the result of inadequate absorption.

An ultrasound scan of the liver was unremarkable and liver biopsy performed one year ago showed evidence of moderate fibrosis (F2). With transient elastography, the median stiffness was 8.2 kPa (interquartile range 1, success rate 100%).

⊕ Clinical tip METAVIR

The METAVIR score is a histological score which was developed specifically for use in HCV infection. It is widely used both in clinical trials and in routine clinical practice. The score has two components: a grade and a stage. A specimen is graded from 0 to 4 according to the extent of necroinflammation present. The stage relates to the amount of fibrosis present and is scored as follows: 0, no fibrosis; 1, portal fibrosis only; 2, presence of few septa; 3, presence of numerous septa but no cirrhosis; 4, cirrhosis. The accuracy of scoring is dependent on the adequacy of the specimen taken and is subject to variability between observers. Careful review by an experienced pathologist is therefore desirable where the score will affect a treatment decision.

He initiated treatment with pegIFN/RBV and telaprevir. Telaprevir was chosen because of the previous history of anaemia on therapy. HCV RNA level was measured by PCR at week 4 and 12, as results at these time-points determine whether treatment should be continued and the duration of therapy. He achieved an extended rapid virological response (eRVR). He again required ribavirin dose reduction due to a drop in his haemoglobin levels. Telaprevir and pegIFN/RBV were given for a total of 12 weeks and pegIFN/RBV treatment extended for a further 12 weeks. He remained UD at the end of treatment and 24 weeks post-treatment.

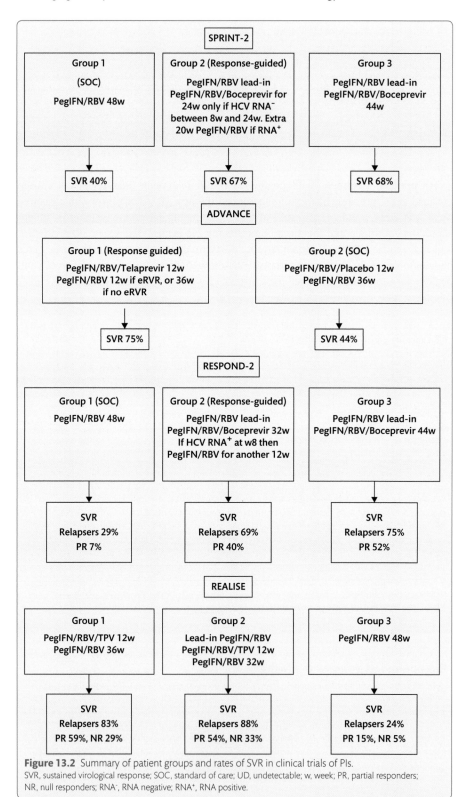

Figure 13.2 Summary of patient groups and rates of SVR in clinical trials of PIs.

SVR, sustained virological response; SOC, standard of care; UD, undetectable; w, week; PR, partial responders; NR, null responders; RNA⁻, RNA negative; RNA⁺, RNA positive.

ADVANCE was a randomized, double-blind placebo-controlled trial comparing pegIFN/RBV and telaprevir with pegIFN/RBV (SOC) in treatment-naïve patients infected with genotype 1 [7]. Rates of SVR for groups of interest are shown. Anaemia, GI disturbances, and rash occurred more commonly in the telaprevir-containing arms. Both SPRINT-2 and ADVANCE showed impressive increases in the rates of SVR in treatment-naïve patients receiving a PI-containing regimen over rates of SVR in patients receiving pegIFN/RBV alone. Rates of SVR were highest in those patients achieving eRVR. Recommendations for the use of triple therapy in treatment-naïve patients have followed thereafter [8]. For boceprevir, the use of a 4-week lead-in is recommended by the manufacturer. The US FDA and European Medicines Agency (EMA) guidance recommends that treatment-naïve patients who are non-cirrhotic should receive response-guided therapy with boceprevir (either 28 or 48 weeks of total therapy depending on response). For telaprevir, the FDA and EMA recommend that treatment-naïve patients should begin with a 12-week course of pegIFN/RBV/telaprevir followed by response-guided therapy (depending on whether eRVR is achieved) to 24 or 48 weeks. It is recommended that cirrhotic patients should receive the full 48 weeks of a telaprevir- or boceprevir-containing regimen.

⊘ Evidence base PIs in treatment-experienced patients

PegIFN/RBV treatment results in poor response rates in patients who have previously been treated with these agents and failed to achieve SVR. Rates of SVR are different in those who were prior relapsers, prior PRs, and prior null responders, with prior relapsers having the best and prior null responders having the poorest response to retreatment. RESPOND 2 was a randomized trial comparing pegIFN/RBV and boceprevir to pegIFN/RBV (SOC) in prior relapsers and prior PRs [9]. The groups were similar to SPRINT-2, as summarized in Figure 13.2, and rates of SVR for prior relapsers and PRs are shown. Null responders were not included. Anaemia occurred more commonly in the boceprevir-treated groups. Another randomized trial, REALISE, compared telaprevir with pegIFN/RBV to pegIFN/RBV in prior relapsers, PRs, and null responders [10]. Groups and rates of SVR are summarized in Figure 13.2. The telaprevir-containing arms had more grade 3 adverse events (primarily anaemia, leukopenia, and neutropenia). Both PIs, when used in combination with pegIFN/RBV, greatly increased the rates of SVR over SOC in previously treated patients. However, rates of SVR are clearly still suboptimal in this population and further improvements are greatly needed. Recommendations from the FDA and EMA for the use of triple therapy in treatment-experienced patients resulting from these trials are as follows [8]: a 48-week fixed-duration course of either a boceprevir or telaprevir-containing regimen is recommended in previous null responders. The FDA recommends that prior relapsers and PRs treated with boceprevir use response-guided therapy (albeit continuing the three-medication regimen to 36 as opposed to 28 weeks) whereas the EMA recommends a 4-week lead-in, triple therapy to week 36, and pegIFN/RBV for 12 weeks. For telaprevir the FDA and EMA recommend that previous relapsers should have telaprevir with pegIFN/RBV for 12 weeks followed by response-guided therapy with pegIFN/RBV and that PRs have a fixed-duration regimen of triple therapy for 12 weeks followed by 36 weeks of pegIFN/RBV.

✦ Learning point On treatment futility rules and resistance

As with HIV infection, high rates of mutation in the HCV genome during replication of the virus due to the low fidelity RNA polymerase means that viruses present within any given individual exhibit considerable variation and thus the virus exists as a quasi-species within individual hosts. Monotherapy with a PI leads to the rapid selection of resistant viruses present as minority variants within the quasi-species. On-treatment failure with boceprevir and telaprevir in the context of triple therapy is partly explained by the emergence of characteristic substitutions in the NS3 gene, e.g. V36M (valine to methionine at the amino acid position 36), T45A/S, and R155K seen in clinical specimens from patients failing these regimens. Studies are under way using ultra-deep sequencing technologies to determine what baseline level of these variants confers increased risk of virological failure on triple therapy. The consequences of the development of resistance to the PIs for future therapeutic options are currently unclear for HCV. At the quasi-species level, resistant variants seem to disappear sometime after treatment is withdrawn and there is not thought to be a reservoir in which to lay down these variants as

(continued)

there is for HIV. Stopping rules or treatment futility rules have been established for triple therapy partly with the aim of lessening the impact of any resistance for future therapy in addition to sparing patients the side effects of difficult and futile regimens. For telaprevir, the presence of HCV RNA >1,000 IU/mL at week 4 or week 12 is an indication for discontinuing all medication. In addition, if the HCV RNA is not detectable by week 24, pegIFN/RBV should be discontinued. For boceprevir, the presence of HCV RNA ≥100 IU/mL at week 12 is an indication to stop all medications. Treatment should also be discontinued if HCV RNA is detectable at week 24.

Discussion

This patient was a good candidate for treatment with first-generation PIs, given his previous response to interferon-based therapy and the baseline assessment of his disease status. Over the next few years it is expected that we will see the introduction of a number of directly acting antiviral drugs that will make additional dramatic improvements to HCV treatment in relation to efficacy, toxicity, and ease of administration. Thus understanding the baseline predictors of response has become increasingly important in clinic as in some patients with poorer chances of response (those with cirrhosis and previous null response to therapy, for example) or in those who are less suitable for interferon-based therapy due to co-morbidities, it may be advisable to await the introduction of new regimens. In addition to the next generation of PIs, directly acting antivirals targeting the viral NS5A protein and the NS5B polymerase are currently being tested in clinical trials. Both nucleoside and non-nucleoside inhibitors of NS5B are in development. Importantly, many of these agents have the promise of pangenotypic activity, i.e. will be active against all viral genotypes. Other classes of agent include cyclophilin inhibitors, which target host cyclophilins necessary for viral replication. There is continued interest in the development of different interferon classes and modified interferons with more favourable side-effect profiles for treatment of HCV (and other viral infections). Recently interferon lambda has shown promising results in early clinical trials [11]. Proof-of-concept studies have now demonstrated the possibility of clearing HCV infection with a combination of directly acting antiviral drugs in the absence of interferon. This is an important milestone and holds the promise of HCV treatment for the patient group who are most in need of clearing HCV infection, namely, those with advanced cirrhosis and decompensated liver disease.

A final word from the expert

This case describes a 42-year-old man with genotype 1b hepatitis C infection. He was non-cirrhotic, had a previous relapse on interferon-based treatment, and had favourable predictors of response to interferon-based therapy at baseline. He was successfully treated with a DAA-containing regimen. This case is reflective of the progress that has been made in recent years regarding the treatment of genotype 1 HCV infection with the first-generation PIs. The burden of HCV-related diseases, in terms of mortality and cost, will remain considerable over the next decade and HCV will remain a potential cause of morbidity, mortality, and need for liver transplantation in the future. Due to shared routes of transmission, HIV/HCV co-infection is also a significant problem. Existing treatments are fraught with side effects and, prior to the introduction of new drugs, have poor success rates. There is no currently licensed vaccine. For many years, patients with chronic HCV have been promised that new, more effective drugs are 'just around the corner'. Now, advances in drug discovery means that there is a pipeline of candidate drugs in development and many at the stage of clinical testing with encouraging results. A goal of therapy is now interferon-free regimens with high treatment success rates and triple oral drug therapy has shown that this is, in principle, possible. If the aim is to treat millions of patients, however, with drugs that are of very high cost, the question will be how this can be afforded, particularly in developing countries. It is hoped that lessons can be learned from the treatment of HIV (where combination therapy is more effective and less prone to resistance development) and the treatment of hepatitis B (where sequential monotherapy with drugs that have a low barrier to resistance leads to the rapid acquisition of drug resistance and treatment failure). There is also a pressing need to overcome the barriers to diagnosis, referral, care, management, and treatment of hepatitis C at this critical juncture. Although treatment success rates are likely to continue to improve, there remains an urgent need for a prophylactic vaccine to prevent infections.

References

1 Szabo E, Lotz G, Paska C et al. Viral hepatitis: new data on hepatitis C infection. *Pathol Oncol Res* 2003; 9: 215–221.
2 Ge D, Fellay J, Thompson AJ et al. Genetic variation in IL28B predicts hepatitis C treatment-induced viral clearance. *Nature* 2009; 461: 399–401.
3 Suppiah V, Moldovan M, Ahlenstiel G et al. IL28B is associated with response to chronic hepatitis C interferon-alpha and ribavirin therapy. *Nat Genet* 2009; 41:1100–1104.
4 Tanaka Y, Nishida N, Sugiyama M et al. Genome-wide association of IL28B with response to pegylated interferon-alpha and ribavirin therapy for chronic hepatitis C. *Nat Genet* 2009; 41: 1105–1109.
5 Degos F, Perez P, Roche B et al. Diagnostic accuracy of FibroScan and comparison to liver fibrosis biomarkers in chronic viral hepatitis: a multicenter prospective study (the FIBROSTIC study). *J Hepatol* 2010; 53: 1013–1021.
6 Poordad F, McCone J, Jr., Bacon BR et al. Boceprevir for untreated chronic HCV genotype 1 infection. *N Engl J Med* 2011; 364: 1195–1206.
7 Jacobson IM, McHutchison JG, Dusheiko G et al. Telaprevir for previously untreated chronic hepatitis C virus infection. *N Engl J Med* 2011; 364: 2405–2416.
8 Bacon BR, Gordon SC, Lawitz E et al. Boceprevir for previously treated chronic HCV genotype 1 infection. *N Engl J Med* 2011; 364: 1207–1217.
9 Zeuzem S, Andreone P, Pol S et al. Telaprevir for retreatment of HCV infection. *N Engl J Med* 2011; 364: 2417–2428.
10 Jacobson IM, Pawlotsky JM, Afdhal NH et al. A practical guide for the use of boceprevir and telaprevir for the treatment of hepatitis C. *J Viral Hepat* 2012; 19 Suppl 2: 1–26.
11 Muir AJ, Shiffman ML, Zaman A et al. Phase 1b study of pegylated interferon lambda 1 with or without ribavirin in patients with chronic genotype 1 hepatitis C virus infection. *Hepatology* 2010; 52: 822–832.

14 Management of viral haemorrhagic fevers in the UK

Jonathan Lambourne

Expert commentary Tim Brooks

Case history

A 62-year-old Nigerian man, resident in the United Kingdom for over 25 years, returned to Nigeria to visit friends and relatives. The patient stayed for 6 weeks, in urban Abuja for the majority of the time, spending 10 days in a semirural setting in Taraba state. The patient was well while away and did not report any illness in their travelling companions or hosts. The patient denied any direct contact with animals and did not enter any caves or mines. The patient did not take any antimalarial prophylaxis. The background medical history included diet-controlled diabetes mellitus and hypertension.

The patient began to feel feverish and shivery on the flight back to the UK. He remained at home for the first week of illness, being cared for by his spouse and children. Due to persistent fevers and mounting myalgia and fatigue the patient presented to his local hospital. On examination the patient was febrile, but there were no localizing signs and the patient denied any other symptoms.

> **Expert comment** Clinical features of viral haemorrhagic fevers
>
> It is a common misconception that viral haemorrhagic fever (VHF) always presents with haemorrhage and cardiovascular collapse, but this is not necessarily the case. In Lassa infection, clotting abnormalities and haemorrhage are rarely seen and up to 80% of infections are asymptomatic. In those who develop symptoms, the incubation period is in the range of 5–16 days and infection typically presents with an 'undifferentiated fever', i.e. fever accompanied by non-specific symptoms such as headache, myalgia, and malaise. Sore throat is reported in 10–20% of individuals and may be accompanied by tonsillar exudates and vesicular lesions. Other symptoms reported include cough, headache, retrosternal chest pain, abdominal pain, and vomiting. Examination may reveal pleural effusions, ascites, facial oedema, and lymphadenopathy [1]. Blood tests may be surprisingly normal, but a mild thrombocytopenia and transaminitis are common. High creatinine kinase and transaminase enzymes are associated with a poor prognosis.

> **Learning point** VHFs are not all the same
>
> At least 32 viruses, from four families, have been documented to cause viral haemorrhagic fever (VHF), a severe febrile illness complicated by vascular damage, increased vascular permeability, and haemorrhage. VHFs are of particular concern due to their high case fatality, their potential for person-to-person spread, and the lack of effective therapy for most VHF pathogens. The viruses causing VHFs vary significantly with respect to their reservoir, mode of transmission, geographic distribution, pathophysiology, clinical features, capacity for transmission, and responsiveness to antiviral therapy. Key features of the most significant VHFs are compared in Tables 14.1 and 14.2. The pathology of some VHFs is pathogen mediated, in others it is immune mediated. For example, disease due to Lassa virus is caused through uncontrolled viral replication; in Marburg and Ebola both viral cytopathic effect and an overly robust immune response cause disease; and in dengue, Hanta, and yellow fever virus infection, haemorrhagic complications are immune mediated.
>
> (continued)

Table 14.1 Viral haemorrhagic fevers

Virus	Reservoir	Vector	Transmission	Nosocomial spread	Geographic distribution	Incubation (days)	Case:infection ratio	Case fatality	Haemorrhage	DIC
FILOVIRIDAE										
Marburg	fruit bat, ?primates	nil	droplet (caves & mines),? ingestion (bushmeat)	yes	DRC, Kenya, Uganda, Angola, S. Africa	3–16	>75%	25–90%	25–50%	yes
Ebola	bats & primates	nil	droplet, ?ingestion	yes	DRC, Gabon, Sudan, Uganda, Ivory Coast	3–16	>75%	25–90%	25–50%	yes
FLAVIVRIDAE										
Yellow fever	primate & mosquito	Aedes mosquito	mosquito bite	no	S. America, tropical Africa	3–6	30–50% (5% of prior flavivirus exposure)	20–50%	20% of non-fatal, >70% of fatal cases	not described
Dengue	human	Aedes mosquito	mosquiton bite	no	widespread, tropics & sub-tropics	3–15	<0.1% non-immune (1% if prior DV)	10–15% (<1% with supportive Rx)	usually only in children during 'critical' phase of disease	not described
Omsk	muskrats & voles	tick	tick bite, droplet	not described	Western Siberia	3–8	not clear	1–5%	20%	not described
Kyasanur	mammals esp. rodents & bats	tick	tick bite	unknown	rural Karnatka state (India)	3–8	not clear	1–10%	20%	not described
Alkhumra	livestock	?tick ?mosquito	livestock, ?mosquito, ?tick	not described	Arabia	3–8	not clear	1–10%	25%	not described

	ARENAVIRIDAE / BUNYAVIRIDAE				Geography	Incubation (days)				Vaccine
					ARENAVIRIDAE					
Junin (*similar for other SAmerican HFs)	Calomys sp. (rodent)	nil	droplet	yes	Argentina (pampas)	7–14	>50%	15–30%	10–25%	not described
Lassa	Mastomys sp. (rodent)		droplet, sexual	yes (rare)	West Africa	5–16	<1%	2–15%	<10%	not described
					BUNYAVIRIDAE					
CCHF	mammals (incl. livestock)	ticks (Hyalomma sp.)	tick bite, butchery	yes (significant)	Middle East, SE Europe, W. China, Balkans, Africa	3–12	20–80%	15–30%	10–25%	yes
Rift Valley	domestic ruminants, Aedes mosquito	Aedes & Culex mosquito	mosquito bite, animal contact	not described	Sub-Saharan Africa, Arabian Peninsula	2–5	<1%	<1%	<10%	yes
HFRS	rodent species	nil	aerosol (urine, faeces), rodent bite	not described	Worldwide, species depends on rodent	9–35	depends on virus Hantaan 75%, Puumala 5%	Hantaan 5–15%, Puumala <1%	10–25%	yes
SFTS	unknown	?tick	?tick bite	unknown	China	not clear	not clear	15%	<10%	yes

Table 14.2 Viral haemorrhagic fevers

Virus	Virology	Cell tropism	Pathophysiology	Suggestive clinical features	Specific therapy
			FILOVIRIDAE		
Marburg	negative-sense, single-stranded, non-segmented RNA	circulating & tissue-resident mononuclear phagocytes (macrophages, Kupfer cells etc)	direct viral CPE (esp. endothelium & liver), proinflammatory cytokines, apoptosis (lymphocyte, splenic & hepatic), DIC	large effusions	no specific antiviral therapy. Passive antibody transfer of some benefit in animal studies
Ebola	negative-sense, single-stranded, non-segmented RNA. Different species in different areas	broad range including macrophages, endothelium, hepatocytes and adrenal cortical cells	direct viral CPE (esp. liver & adrenal cortex), apoptosis (lymphocyte & splenic), DIC, minimal inflammatory	hypothermia	RBV has no-vitro or in-vivo effect. Small-interesting RNA under investigation
			FLAVIVIRIDAE		
Yellow fever	positive-sense, single-stranded, non-segmented RNA	Kupffer cells, hepatocytes, renal tubu-lar epithelium	biphasic illness. 1st phase = transient viraemia. 2nd phase = immune mediated. T-cell mediated hepatocyte apoptosis phase leads to coagulopathy, proinflammatory cytokines		no specific anti-viral/ immunomodulatory therapy
Dengue	positive-sense, single-stranded, non-segmented RNA (4 viruses, genetically & antigenically distinct)	circulating & tissue-resident mononuclear phagocytes (macrophages, Kupfer cells etc)	non-neutralising antibodies increases infection of macrophages leading to excessive pro-inflammatory immune response, vascular fragility & platelet dysfunction. Hepatitis mediated by CPE.	severe retroorbital headache, characteristic rash, generalised lymphadnopathy	no specific anti-viral/ immunodulatory therapy
Omsk	positive-sense, single stranded, non-segmented RNA	vascular & haematopeotic tissue	unclear, in animal models is related to viral repication and virus-induced hepatocyte and endothelial cell-damage		in-vitro evidence for RBV, IFN-a & interferon inducers
Kyasanur	positive-sense, single-stranded, non-segmented RNA	not clear	lymphocyte apoptosis, impaired myocardial contracility, splenic erythrophagocytosis	relative bradycardia, conjunctival injection, aseptic meningitis	not clear

Virus	Genome	Cell tropism	Pathogenesis	Clinical features	Treatment
Alkhumra	positive-sense, single-stranded, non-segmented RNA	not clear	not clear	aseptic meningitis	not clear
ARENAVIRIDAE					
Junin (*similar for other SAmerican HFs)	ambisense, single-stranded, bisegmented RNA	broad range including macrophages, endothelium, hepatocytes, astrolia and renal epithelium	Fatal disease due to persistent viraemia, but little CPE or inflammatory infiltrates. Likely due to disruption of intracellular function esp. in endothelium, hepatocytes & adrenal cortex. May induce high levels of IFNa, leading to platelet dysfunction.	effusions (pleural, pericardial, ascites)	immune plasma (proven efficacy, Junin only), RBV may be beneficial
Lassa	ambisense, single-stranded, bisegmented RNA	wide range: macrophages, endothelium, hepatocytes, renal epithelial cells & placental tissue		pharyngitis	clear evidence supporting RBV, esp. if given early
BUNYAVIRIDAE					
CCHF	negative sense, single-stranded, trisegmented RNA	macrophages, endothelium & hepatocytes	direct viral CPE (esp. hepatocytes), lymphocyte apoptosis, immune mediated damage (esp. endothelial damage & haemophagocytosis)	hepatomegaly	RBV has in-vitro effect, no clinical trials, but is generally given
Rift Valley	negative sense, single-stranded, trisegmented RNA	hepatocytes, myocytes, neurones	direct vial CPE (esp. hepatocytes, endothelium & neurones). Immune mediated post-infectious retinitis	encepjalities, retinal vasculitis (post-fever)	RBV, immunoglobulin & IFNa beneficial in animal studies
HFRS	negative sense, single-stranded, trisegmented RNA	vascular endothelium	direct viral CPE (esp. endothelium, renal, cardiac & anterior pituitary) and pronounced vascular permeability	back pain	RBV may be beneficial (1 trial), as immune-mediated antibody-blocking agents may be beneficial
SFTS	negative sense, single-stranded, trisegmented RNA	splenic macrophages & platelets	virus binds to platelets, engulfed by splenic macrophages & viral replication maintained spleen. Poor outcome associated with sustained viraemia & pro-inflammatory immune response.	GI upset and lymphadenopathy (esp. unilateral subinguinal lymphadenopathy)	RBV may be beneficial

> **✔ Evidence base**   Lassa epidemiology
>
> A key study in Sierra Leone by McCormick et al. [2] vividly demonstrates both how common Lassa is in endemic areas and how the majority of cases are either asymptomatic or mild.
>
> **Methods**
>
> - Combined cross-sectional seroprevalence and prospective cohort study in eastern Sierra Leone.
> - For cross-sectional study: anti-Lassa IgG measured in households, selected at random, from multiple villages.
> - For prospective cohort study: households selected at random received weekly visits, over a 15-month period, from surveillance officers. Episodes of fever recorded and anti-Lassa antibodies measured 2–3 weeks following febrile illness. Also, all individuals presenting to local health centre with fever were tested for Lassa.
> - Anti-Lassa antibodies detected using indirect immunofluorescence. Past infection = titre ≥1:16, recent infection = four-fold increase in titre [2].
>
> **Results**
>
> - Seroprevalence varied significantly between different locations (8–52%).
> - Mean seroprevalence across multiple sites was 22%.
> - Seroprevalence increased with increasing age.
> - Annual seroconversion rates varied geographically between 4 and 22 per 100 susceptible individuals.
> - Only 6–26% of people who seroconverted reported, or had a documented, febrile illness.
> - 5–15% of febrile patients seen at the local health centre seroconverted for Lassa. Only three individuals required hospitalization.
> - The rates of human infection closely mirrored rates of infection in local *Mastomys* rodent populations [2].

On admission the patient was mildly thrombocytopenic, lymphopenic, had an elevated creatinine and a mild transaminitis (Table 14.3). Cultures of blood and urine and investigations for malaria, HIV, syphilis, dengue virus, and hepatitis viruses A, B, and C were negative. Radiological imaging revealed small, bilateral pleural effusions. Typhoid and rickettsial infection were considered to be the two most likely diagnoses and the patient was commenced on intravenous ceftriaxone and oral doxycycline. The patient was nursed on an open ward without barrier nursing.

Table 14.3   **Blood results during admission**

Test	Local hospital		High-security ID unit	
	Day 1	Day 8	Day 15	Day 20
Haemoglobin (g/dL)	14.1	13.2	12.7	11.9
WCC (× 10^9/L)	1.6	6.5	7.2	6.7
Neutrophils (× 10^9/L)	1.1	4.3	4.4	3.9
Lymphocytes (× 10^9/L)	0.4	1.2	1.9	1.5
Platelets (× 10^9/L)	76	177	127	145
INR	1.2	0.8	1.3	1.1
APTT (s)	34	44	28	32
Urea (mmol/L)	18	5.5	4.2	2.3
Creatinine (µmol/L)	153	100	83	85
ALT (iu/L)	64	74	68	80
ALP (iu/L)	37	45	61	53
Bilirubin (µmol/L)	15	11	6	18
Albumin (g/L)	38	35	21	20
AST (iu/L)	75	98	186	155
GGT (U/L)	45	62	56	60
CRP (mg/L)	36	141	79	55

❝ Expert comment   General laboratory features in VHF

Akin to clinical presentation, general laboratory findings cannot be used to refute or confirm the diagnosis of Lassa infection or other VHFs; normal haematological and biochemical parameters do not preclude the diagnosis. Findings that support the diagnosis of VHF infection include thrombocytopenia, lymphopenia, and a transaminitis. However, these are common findings in viral infections of any type and also in the other differential diagnoses. Markers of haemoconcentration suggest increased vascular permeability and are a marker of severe disease.

> ✪ **Learning point** Haemorrhage in Lassa virus infection is rare
>
> Although the VHFs are grouped together by virtue of their capacity to cause fever and haemorrhage, the frequency and mechanisms by which they cause haemorrhage differ considerably [3]. Causes of haemorrhage include increased vascular permeability, due to viral infection of endothelial cells, an exuberant pro-inflammatory immune response, impaired production of clotting factors due to hepatocyte infection, and consumption of clotting factors and platelets in the setting of disseminated intravascular coagulation (DIC). Readers desiring a detailed description of VHF pathophysiology are directed to a review by Paessler and Walker [4]. Lassa is at one end of the spectrum, readily invading vascular endothelium but inducing neither cytopathic effect nor immune-mediated pathology. Impaired endothelial function following Lassa virus invasion can lead to increased vascular permeability, giving rise to refractory hypotension, but haemorrhage is rarely seen. Also, abnormal clotting is rare, DIC is almost never seen, and, as in this case, thrombocytopenia is mild, if present at all.

> ✚ **Clinical tip** Differential diagnosis
>
> One of the major challenges in managing febrile returned travellers is that the symptoms reported by the patient and signs elicited by the clinician are usually non-specific and do not permit an accurate diagnosis on clinical grounds alone. The VHFs fall into the category of 'undifferentiated fever', along with other important imported conditions such as malaria, rickettsial infection, typhoid, hepatitis, and leptospirosis. The protean manifestations of the VHFs and frequent absence of haemorrhage as a presenting feature mean that VHFs must be included in the list of differential diagnoses for all febrile returned travellers until either a risk assessment, based on a detailed travel history, and review of current epidemiology rules it out, or a negative VHF test result is obtained.

Despite receiving broad-spectrum antibiotics the patient remained intermittently febrile and became increasingly confused and disorientated, although biochemical and haematological parameters remained largely unchanged. Mantoux testing was negative, and echocardiography was normal. A contrast-enhanced CT scan of the patient's brain revealed small vessel disease, but no focal abnormalities and no meningeal enhancement. However, CSF examination revealed a normal opening pressure, elevated leukocyte count (31 cells/mm^3), erythrocyte count (119 cells/mm^3), protein (2.8 g/dL), and low glucose level (CSF 2.4 mmol/L, plasma 9.7 mmol/L). Gram and India ink stains were negative. Intravenous aciclovir and treatment for tuberculous meningitis (TBM) were commenced. No bacteria were grown from the CSF after 48 hours of incubation; PCR for HSV, VZV, enterovirus, and adenovirus was negative, and mycobacterial culture continued.

The patient was transferred to a different ward. After reviewing the case, the consultant now in charge of the patient's care undertook a viral haemorrhagic fever (VHF) risk assessment and, because this suggested a 'high possibility' of VHF, arranged for samples to be dispatched for urgent VHF testing (Figures 14.1 and 14.2). While awaiting the VHF result the patient was moved to a side room, barrier nursing was initiated, and local laboratories and the consultant in communicable disease control (CCDC) were notified (see Box 14.1). PCR testing for a panel of VHF pathogens revealed the presence of Lassa virus. Following this result the patient was transferred to the regional high-security infectious diseases unit (HSIDU) and both the CCDC and duty doctor on-call at the HPA were notified. An outbreak meeting was convened and all healthcare workers, laboratory staff, family, and friends who reported close contact with the patient or their clinical samples were placed under active surveillance.

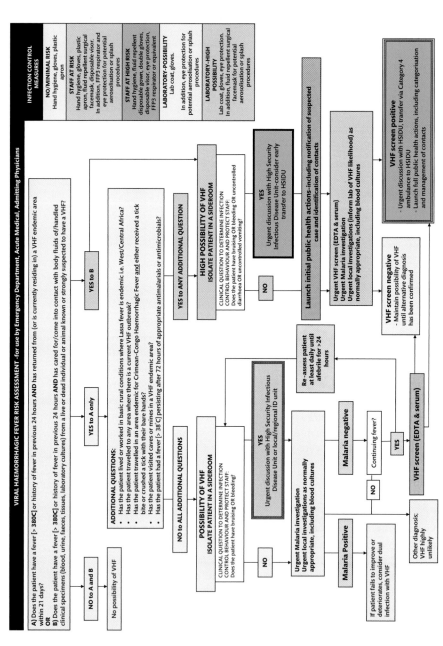

Figure 14.1 Risk assessment algorithm for viral haemohagic fevers in the UK.

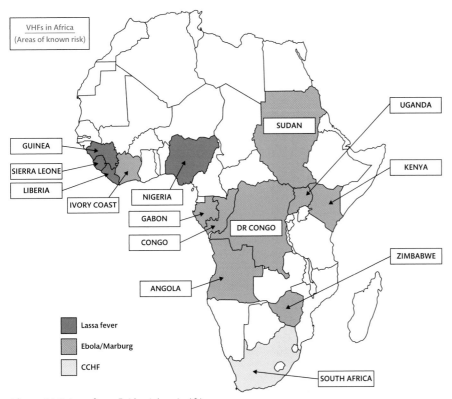

Figure 14.2 Lassa fever: Epidemiology in Africa.
Dark blue: The most severely affected countries are in the region known as the Manu River Union (Liberia, Sierra Leone, Guinea, and Nigeria). Light blue: There is evidence of Lassa virus infection in other African countries demonstrated either by sporadic human cases, or by rodent or human sero-prevalence studies.
Reproduced with permission from Health Protection Agency, *Maps of VHF regions*, © Crown copyright. Reproduced with permission of Public Health England, available from, available from http://www.hpa.org.uk/Topics/InfectiousDiseases/InfectionsAZ/ViralHaemorrhagicFever/VHFMaps/.

Box 14.1 Infection control

The potential for person-to-person transmission, the general lack of effective PEP, and the high mortality of some of the VHFs mean that initiating appropriate infection control measures is an essential part of managing every patient for whom, on the basis of an accurate risk assessment, VHF infection is considered a possibility. What precautions are required, for example with respect to patient accommodation, personal protective equipment (PPE), and how patient samples should be handled, varies depending on whether the potential for a VHF is 'possible', 'highly possible', or 'proven' and whether there is overt bleeding. Detailed guidance has been prepared by the Advisory Committee on Dangerous Pathogens (ACDP) [5].

Patient accommodation

All patients in whom VHF is suspected should be managed in a side room with its own toilet or commode and the number of staff tending the patient should be restricted. Patients with proven VHFs should ideally be transferred to a high-security ID unit (HSIDU). If transfer is not feasible, due to patient instability, a negative pressure side room should be used. In the UK, two centres have special isolators for managing patients with potential contagious VHFs: the Freeman Hospital in Newcastle, and the Royal Free Hospital in London. Transporting a patient with a VHF is logistically challenging. For example, only London and Newcastle ambulance crews, and the military, have the expertise required to safely transport patients with VHFs.

(continued)

Personal protective equipment

Standard 'droplet precautions' should be used for patients in whom VHF is a possibility, but who do not have overt signs of bleeding, i.e. gloves, plastic apron, and a fluid-repellent surgical facemask. Personnel undertaking aerosol or splash-inducing procedures, such as intubation, bronchoscopy, nebulizer use, and central line insertion should wear a disposable visor and FFP3 respirator. Enhanced droplet precaution should be used for patients with proven VHF, or those with possible VHF in whom there is overt bleeding, i.e. double gloves, fluid-repellent surgical gown, face visor, and FFP3 mask. Meticulous hand hygiene should be observed for all patients, irrespective of their VHF risk.

Testing of patient samples

It is imperative that samples from patients with possible or proven VHFs are tested locally while minimizing the risk to laboratory staff. Specimens from patients with a 'possibility of VHF' should be *handled as normal*; no special precautions are required.

Specimens from patients with a 'high possibility of VHF' or with proven VHF require extra care. For samples from patients that fall into these two categories, laboratories should be warned about incoming samples, samples should be transported by hand (not via 'air tubes') in appropriate packaging. Laboratory staff should wear appropriate PPE including face and eye protection during any sample-handling steps that are likely to create splashes or aerosols. Current guidance recommends that samples should be inactivated prior to analysis, but only if this does not interfere with the accuracy or interpretation of the assay. In practice, no suitable method for inactivating samples that allows routine analysis in clinical haematology and clinical chemistry laboratories has been identified. If inactivation is not possible, disinfection and decontamination procedures, which have been validated as effective against VHFs, should be used. Most automated analysers used in today's haematology and biochemistry laboratories fall into this category, being closed systems with waste directed into sealed containers and with cleaning cycles designed to inactivate VHFs. An alternative strategy is to use a dedicated blood gas analyser, either in the laboratory or at the patient's bedside. Extra care is required when manually handling samples, for example, during some coagulation and microbiological assays. Following testing, waste can be rendered safe by autoclaving on-site, using a 'destruct cycle'.

⊕ Expert comment VHF risk assessment

Imported viral haemorrhagic fevers are rare, but it is important to actively assess the risk of a patient having contracted one if they have visited an endemic country. The patient's travel destination, contacts, and activities all affect the likely risk of exposure. Key pieces of information required to make an accurate risk assessment include: nature of locations visited (town, shanty town, rural area), type of accommodation, close contact with any animals, ticks, or sick individuals, and any visits to caves or mines [5]. In this case, a VHF risk assessment should have been undertaken in the emergency department once it was established that he had a fever (>38°) and he had returned from Nigeria within the last 21 days. Performing a VHF risk assessment does not mean that other differential diagnoses should be ignored; malaria, typhus, enteric fever, etc. are common and, if they seem possible, must be tested for and treated while waiting for the results of additional tests. Use common sense in making a risk assessment and consider whether there is a credible route of infection. If a country has had 15 cases of VHF in a population of 10 million, and the patient has not been in the same region or has not been near a sick person, they are NOT likely to be a prime candidate for VHF. On the other hand, a history of caving in a VHF-endemic area and getting covered in bat guano is much more worrying!

✪ Learning point VHF epidemiology

A key component of the VHF risk assessment is determining whether the patient has travelled to an VHF-endemic area. VHFs vary in their distribution, from highly focal pockets of endemicity, such as Kyasanur Forest disease (limited to a small area in southwestern India), to Lassa, dengue, and yellow fever that have a wide geographic range. Up-to-date maps detailing the distribution of VHFs should be consulted as part of the risk assessment, and are feely available from a number of sources including the PHE (formerly the HPA) website (search 'VHF maps'). Lassa is endemic in West Africa, affecting Nigeria,

(continued)

Mali, Sierra Leone, Liberia, and Guinea. It is estimated that there are 300,000 cases and 5,000 deaths worldwide each year. In areas of endemicity, Lassa virus infection is considered alongside malaria and typhoid in the diagnostic workup of febrile patients. The patient described in the case study had travelled to Taraba state, an area of Nigeria in which Lassa is common. The varied epidemiology of the VHFs is determined by differences in their life cycles and mechanisms of transmission. The reservoir for Lassa is the *Mastomys* rodent species. Consequently Lassa is only found in areas inhabited by this rodent, with infection probably acquired by inhalation of fomites contaminated with rodent urine and faeces. This contrasts sharply with dengue virus. With humans as its reservoir, its geographic distribution is only limited by environmental conditions required to sustain its hardy mosquito vector, hence it causes infection in all continents except Antarctica.

⭐ **Learning point** Person-to-person transmission

Person-to-person transmission of VHFs requires inoculation of mucous membranes or broken skin with either infected blood and bodily fluids or with fomites contaminated by infected droplets. Needlestick injuries involving sharps used on viraemic patients are particularly associated with transmission. Aerosol transmission of VHFs does not occur. VHFs vary in their propensity to spread from person to person. This reflects differences in the degree and duration of viraemia and the frequency and mechanism(s) of haemorrhage. For example, person-to-person transmission does not occur with Hanta or dengue virus because haemorrhagic complications of these infections are immune-mediated and occur when blood and bodily fluids are devoid of viable virus. At the other extreme, Marburg, Ebola, and Crimean-Congo haemorrhagic fever (CCHF) viruses pose a real risk of transmission as haemorrhage is more common and is associated with high circulating VLs. In most cases of Lassa, viraemia is short-lived and low level; however, a significant number of healthcare professionals have died from nosocomial Lassa transmission, often from needlestick injuries. Following recovery from Lassa, viable virus may be shed in urine, breast milk, and genital secretions. Rare cases of sexual transmission have been reported. As a result, toilet bowls should be disinfected with bleach after use, breastfeeding should be temporarily avoided (unless there is no other way to support the baby), and condoms should be worn for 2–3 months after infection (or for 6 months if ribavirin (RBV) is given).

Combining the published reports describing surveillance efforts following Lassa cases from the UK [6], USA [7], and Germany [8], over 650 contacts have been investigated. No symptomatic secondary cases have been described and only one case of asymptomatic seroconversion was observed, in a doctor who examined and cannulated a patient without using PPE.

⊕ **Clinical tip** Laboratory features and diagnosis

Rapid diagnosis of VHF enables timely administration of both supportive and antiviral therapy, which improves survival *and* allows early initiation of effective infection control procedures, reducing the potential number of secondary cases. In acutely ill cases of VHF the PCR test is the most useful to detect the causative agent. In the UK an urgent testing service for all classes of VHF is available, 24 hours a day, for cases risk-assessed as 'high possibility' of VHF. The service is provided by the Rare and Imported Pathogens Laboratory (RIPL), HPA (PHE), Porton Down, and can be accessed by calling the Imported Fever Service (24-hour phone number 0844 77 88 990). With respect to Lassa virus, viraemia occurs throughout the febrile period. Reverse transcription-polymerase chain reaction (RT-PCR) is considered to be the most sensitive and specific assay, and is used in the UK.

⊕ **Clinical tip** Contact surveillance and PEP

Depending on the nature and duration of contact with the VHF patient, contacts are differentiated into 'high-risk' and 'low-risk'. High-risk contacts include those who have sustained direct exposure to blood or bodily fluids or had prolonged exposure while not wearing PPE. 'Low-risk' contacts are those who have had the same exposure but while wearing PPE, or those with lesser degrees of exposure. High-risk

(continued)

contacts undergo active surveillance; they are instructed to record their temperature daily and to call a nominated case manager before midday each day. Low-risk contacts undergo passive surveillance; they are instructed to measure their temperature each day and to contact their nominated case manager in the event of a temperature rise or development of any symptoms suggestive of infection. No restrictions with respect to travel, employment, and so on are imposed on contacts [6,9].

PEP using ribavirin (RBV) is advocated for many VHFs, but has been studied in few. With respect to Lassa, RBV should theoretically prevent infection. However, due to its side-effect profile, the low transmissibility of Lassa virus and lack of proven efficacy as PEP, a risk assessment is required prior to its use, balancing the risk of developing Lassa virus infection against the risk of ribavirin-associated toxicity. Generally prophylaxis is reserved for those individuals with proven high-risk exposures [10]. Prophylaxis should not be seen as a substitute for meticulous contact follow-up.

On arrival at the HSIDU the patient was commenced on intravenous ribavirin (Figure 14.3). Aciclovir, antibiotics, and anti-tuberculous therapy were stopped. The patient remained febrile and confused although haemodynamically and metabolically stable. Repeat blood tests confirmed a sustained viraemia despite intravenous ribavirin. Due to his relative immobility, prophylactic low-molecular-weight heparin was commenced. No further investigations into the cause of his neurological upset were performed because, following the ACDP guidelines, transferring the patient out of the isolation unit for repeat cerebral imaging and repeat LP was deemed to pose too high a risk to healthcare staff. The likely diagnosis was felt to be Lassa encephalitis. Unfortunately after 7 days in the isolation unit, and 25 days after arrival back in the UK, the patient suffered a cardiorespiratory arrest from which he could not be resuscitated. A post-mortem was not performed, but the cause of death was considered to be either a cardiac arrhythmia or pulmonary embolism as opposed to Lassa virus infection.

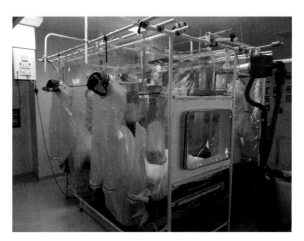

Figure 14.3 Inside a HSIDU.
Image courtesy of Ian Cropley.

✓ Evidence base Ribavirin in Lassa

Supportive therapy, including adequate fluid resuscitation and provision of blood products, is the mainstay of treatment for all patients with VHF infection and significantly reduces mortality. The efficacy of antivirals and immuno-modulatory therapy varies depending on the causative pathogen. Lassa is unusual among the VHFs in that antiviral therapy with ribavirin (RBV, a nucleoside analogue) has been clearly shown to be beneficial, with the first trial in humans conducted by McCormick et al. in 1986 [2].

Method

- Two hospitals in rural Sierra Leone
- 1st phase: observational cohort study of 441 patients with laboratory-confirmed Lassa virus infection
- 2nd phase: patients newly diagnosed with Lassa virus infection, complicated by AST level ≥150 iu/L randomized to receive either intravenous RBV and/or Lassa-convalescent serum (4 mL/kg, serum recovered from patients who had recovered from Lassa)
- Lassa diagnosed by viral culture and/or seroconversion
- Outcomes of patients in Phase 1 and Phase 2 compared
- Primary outcome: 30-day mortality
- Secondary outcomes: duration of viraemia [2]

Results

- Overall case fatality 16%
- Higher mortality associated with higher AST on admission (55% vs. 12% if AST >150 IU/mL vs. <150 IU/mL) and higher Lassa VL on admission (76% mortality if >5000 $TCID_{50}$/mL)
- RBV significantly reduced mortality irrespective of VL (from 76% to 32% and from 28% to 9% in patients with high and low Lassa VLs, respectively) and in patients with elevated AST (55% to 20%)
- No therapeutic benefit from Lassa-convalescent serum
- Starting RBV after day 6 of illness was associated with decreased survival benefit
- The most common and significant side effect of RBV therapy was anaemia, with as much as a 20% drop in haematocrit noted in some patients [2]

❝ Expert comment Patient management

The key features in managing the patient are to control blood sugar levels (hypoglycaemia is common), fluid balance (avoiding overhydration, which can be worse than hypoperfusion), acid–base balance, oxygenation, and clotting. Intravenous dextrose, fresh frozen plasma, and platelet infusions combined with controlled ventilation and inotropic drugs when required are the mainstay of supportive care. Ribavirin (RBV) therapy significantly reduces mortality from Lassa virus infection, although it remains an unlicensed indication. It has greatest activity against viral RNA polymerase but also impairs host DNA replication and commonly causes anaemia. RBV is also teratogenic and is present in semen, mandating the use of barrier contraception for 6 months after treatment. RBV has no proven value in other VHFs, even in those in which *in vitro* activity has been demonstrated, perhaps because small therapeutic effects are masked by the adverse reactions in the patient. An alternative explanation is that in sick people the drug PK are very different, and the dosage regimen may be subtherapeutic. In the future, it may be possible to tailor the dose of antimicrobials to a patient's condition by real-time monitoring of drug levels and adjusting the individual's regimen accordingly.

➕ Clinical tip Predictors of severe disease

In this case two poor prognostic factors were the sustained viraemia, despite administration of ribavirin, and the patient's older age. Other clinical and laboratory features predictive of fatal infection include elevated creatinine and AST, bleeding, and hypothermia [1]. Eradication of Lassa requires a cell-mediated immune response. In keeping with this, conditions associated with impaired cell-mediated immunity including advanced age, malnutrition, HIV infection, and pregnancy are associated with increased disease severity and mortality. Lassa infection in pregnancy is of particular

(continued)

concern as the virus readily infects the placenta, a site rendered 'invisible' to T cells in a bid to prevent immune activation against fetally expressed paternal antigens. Control of viral replication and maternal survival usually requires abortion of the fetus. The humoral immune response does not appear to be important. Antibodies generally appear late, if at all, and do not confer protection against re-infection.

> **⚖ Expert comment** Neurological consequences of Lassa infection
>
> Lassa, in contrast to the other Arenaviruses, is not overtly neurotropic. When CNS symptoms occur during Lassa, it is usually in the setting of shock, with associated cerebral hypoperfusion. However, the persistent encephalopathy exhibited by the patient in this case did not appear to be due to an obvious metabolic cause or haemodynamic compromise. It may have been due to CNS Lassa infection and bears a striking similarity to a case reported in Germany [11]. Repeated neuroimaging and CSF sampling might have helped confirm or exclude other causes of encephalopathy, but were not performed as the ACDP guidelines recommend that only bedside radiological investigations be performed in patients with proven VHF. One important, common complication of Lassa infection is sensorineural deafness. This occurs in 20% of cases, may be unilateral or bilateral, is permanent in two-thirds of cases, and its incidence does not correlate with the severity of the acute febrile illness or the level of viraemia; it is thought to be immune mediated.

Discussion

This case is characteristic of fatal Lassa infection and highlights some common misconceptions about viral haemorrhagic fevers (VHF) such as that haemorrhage is a common feature of all VHFs, death due to VHFs is usually rapid, and all VHFs are highly contagious and pose a serious risk to healthcare workers. In Lassa-endemic areas, with limited access to blood products, clotting factors and ribavirin, approximately 15% of patients hospitalized with Lassa infection die. Of the 13 cases imported to the UK since 1971, four have died (case fatality 31%), despite ready access to antivirals and supportive care. The higher case fatality in the UK may be because VHF testing is only performed in the most severe cases and suggests that a number of less severe cases go undiagnosed. The higher case fatality also raises two important questions with respect to this case: would an earlier diagnosis of Lassa infection and less stringent infection control measures following the diagnosis have been associated with a better outcome?

With respect to diagnostic delay, there is clear clinical evidence that ribavirin is effective against Lassa and that delayed initiation of RBV is associated with a worse outcome, likely because of prolonged viraemia and the consequences of disseminated infection and organ dysfunction. Rapid diagnosis requires early clinical suspicion and easily accessible diagnostic tests with a rapid turnaround time. In this case, the diagnosis of VHF was only suspected 10 days into the patient's admission. It is likely that the non-specific nature of the patient's presentation and the absence of heamorrhage or markedly deranged blood tests will have contributed to this delay. However, this presentation of an 'undifferentiated fever' is typical of Lassa and most of the other VHFs, and highlights the issue that VHFs cannot be diagnosed, or excluded, on the basis of clinical presentation and basic investigations. One could argue therefore that all febrile travellers should be managed as if they had a VHF pending a negative screen. This approach is inappropriate as it ignores the absolute requirement of a plausible route of acquisition. The ACDP risk assessment algorithm was designed to identify those patients with an appropriate epidemiological link to a VHF, either through travel in an endemic area or close contact with a possible case, and to assist clinicians in identifying those patients for whom VHF is of sufficiently high probability to justify VHF testing and initiation of infection control precautions. In this case, had a risk assessment been undertaken on arrival in the emergency department or on admission to the ward, the patient would have been classed as 'possibility of VHF', on the basis of fever and return from a VHF-endemic region. Once the first malaria film had been returned negative, VHF testing should have been performed. If Lassa had been diagnosed, and ribavirin commenced at this stage, it is possible that the patient's death might have been averted. Combining the ACDP algorithm with up-to-date epidemiological information, available from a variety of sources including PHE (previously the HPA) (https://www.gov.uk/government/organisations/public-health-england) and the National Travel Health Network and Centre (http://www.nathnac.org) should allow an accurate risk assessment to be completed in a matter of minutes. A VHF risk assessment should therefore be invoked for *all* febrile returned travellers. The second requirement for rapid diagnosis is ready access to laboratory services. Two laboratories in the UK have the capacity to test for VHFs, both run through the PHE; the RIPL, Porton Down and the Viral Zoonosis Unit in Colindale. Both laboratories can be contacted any time of day or night, ideally via the Imported Fever Service. Part of the drive to develop the Imported Fever Service was to act as a single point of contact to coordinate urgent on-call diagnostic services for molecular testing for viral haemorrhagic fevers and to provide round-the-clock telephone access to expert clinical and microbiological advice to support patient management, infection control, and public health interventions. It is important to remember that a risk assessment that suggests a patient has a 'possibility' or 'high possibility' of a VHF does not preclude the investigation of alternative diagnoses or the measurement of biochemical and haematological parameters.

   With respect to infection control in cases of VHF, there is a difficult balance between protecting healthcare workers and optimal management of the patient. If a VHF infection is suspected or diagnosed, regular haematology, biochemistry, microbiological, and radiological investigations are essential for directing supportive care, such as administration of blood products and clotting factors, and for ruling out alternative or coexistent diagnoses. For example, delaying a malaria film or processing a blood culture sample until a negative VHF screen has been returned is unnecessarily cautious and is likely to cause harm to the patient. Even in cases of proven VHF, blood films for malaria testing can be prepared. The samples should be handled in a safety cabinet, films should be disposed of by autoclaving as soon as they have been read, and work surfaces treated with 10,000 ppm chlorine. In this case, once the diagnosis of Lassa had been made, continued testing of hematology and biochemical parameters was possible because the patient was transferred quickly to a HSIDU. Both HSIDUs in the UK have a dedicated laboratory within the isolation unit. However, repeat LP and neuroimaging to investigate possible causes of the patient's ongoing encephalopathy were not performed. Given the duration of the patient's illness by the time they were transferred to their local HSIDU, it is unlikely that these further investigations would have altered the disease trajectory. However, it demonstrates the constraints within which clinicians care for patients with VHFs. It should be emphasized that not all VHFs have the capacity for person-to-person transmission and that those pathogens that can spread, vary significantly with respect to the rates, risks, and mechanisms of transmission and the efficiency of PEP. In some cases, the stringent infection control procedures advocated may ultimately be detrimental to the patient with VHF infection. With this in mind, the ACDP guidelines should be interpreted on a case-by-case or pathogen-by-pathogen basis (Table 14.2) and the stringency of infection control practices used should be commensurate with the risks and consequences of transmission. Advice from specialists in the clinical and infection control management of VHFs should be sought at the earliest opportunity.

A final word from the expert

Viral haemorrhagic fever is a descriptive term embracing over a dozen different diseases, with varying pathologies and risks of transmission to other persons and healthcare workers. The most dangerous fevers from a healthcare perspective are the Arenaviruses (principally Lassa fever), Ebola, Marburg, and CCHF.

The risk of VHF in a traveller must be seen in proportion, and other much more common diseases should be considered, sought for, and treated if necessary. Obtaining confirmation or exclusion of a VHF can take some time (depending on location, up to 16 hours with transport included) and withholding any investigation or treatment while waiting for a result may condemn a salvable patient to death. Always screen for malaria, and treat it if found. Consider the risk of enteric fevers, typhus, and leptospirosis, take blood cultures, and start empiric treatment with antimalarials, doxycycline, and ceftriaxone depending on your assessment. Isolate the patient and restrict staff access while you wait for the VHF results. Seek help early if you are concerned about a patient or their possible exposure.

If you have a confirmed case of VHF, you will need to liaise with your local public health officials for contact tracing and follow-up. You will also be bombarded by healthcare staff who are worried about implications for their own health. Reassure those who have no contact with the patient or his body fluids, inform those who have patient contact without body fluid contact that their risk is very low, and actively follow twice daily those with high-risk exposures such as eye splashes of blood or needlestick injuries. Seek expert advice on prophylaxis.

Acknowledgements

This case history combines details of several cases of Lassa infection imported into the UK in recent years. The authors would like to thank Dr Meera Chand and Dr Ian Cropley for reviewing previous drafts of this manuscript.

References

1 Asogun DA, Adomeh DI, Ehimuan J et al. Molecular diagnostics for Lassa fever at Irrua specialist teaching hospital, Nigeria: lessons learnt from two years of laboratory operation. *PLoS Negl Trop Dis* 2012; 6: e1839.

2 McCormick JB, King IJ, Webb PA et al. Lassa fever: Effective therapy with ribavirin. *N Engl J Med* 1986; 314: 20–26.

3 Peters CJ, Zaki SR. Role of the endothelium in viral hemorrhagic fevers. *Crit Care Med* 2002; 30: S268–73.

4 Paessler S, Walker DH. Pathogenesis of the viral hemorrhagic fevers. *Annu Rev Pathol* 2013; 8: 411–440.

5 Advisory Committee on Dangerous pathogens. Management of Hazard Group 4 viral haemorrhagic fevers and similar human infectious diseases of high consequence. London: Department of Health, 2012.

6 Kitching A, Addiman S, Cathcart S et al. A fatal case of Lassa fever in London, January 2009. *Euro Surveill* 2009; 14: 19117.

7 Holmes GP, McCormick JB, Trock SC et al. Lassa fever in the United States. Investigation of a case and new guidelines for management. *N Engl J Med* 1990; 323: 1120–1123.

8 Haas WH, Breuer T, Pfaff G, et al. Imported Lassa fever in Germany: surveillance and management of contact persons. *Clin Infect Dis* 2003; 36: 1254–1258.

9 Atkin S, Anaraki S, Gothard P et al. The first case of Lassa fever imported from Mali to the United Kingdom, February 2009. *Euro Surveill* 2009; 14: 19145.

10 Bausch DG, Hadi CM, Khan SH, Lertora JJ. Review of the literature and proposed guidelines for the use of oral ribavirin as postexposure prophylaxis for Lassa fever. *Clin Infect Dis* 2010; 51: 1435–1441.

11 Gunther S, Weisner B, Roth A et al. Lassa fever encephalopathy: Lassa virus in cerebrospinal fluid but not in serum. *J Infect Dis* 2001; 184:345–349.

15 Tropical liver abscess: diagnosis and management

Marcus Eder and Amber Arnold

🕮 Expert commentary Elinor Moore

Case history

A 52-year-old retired engineer attended the emergency department with a profound hypoglycaemic episode. A few days earlier, the patient had had several episodes of hypoglycaemia. His general practitioner had reduced the patient's insulin dosage. He had a past medical history of type 2 diabetes, hypertension, and hypercholesterolaemia for which he was taking insulin, metformin, and antihypertensives.

The patient reported a 2-month history of feeling generally unwell, which had started gradually at the end of a 4-month visit to India. He complained of lethargy, anorexia with a 10 kg loss of weight, and occasional shivering with sweats at night. Initially he felt well while in India, but had suffered from intermittent episodes of non-bloody diarrhoea.

> **✪ Learning point** Important causes of fever in the returning traveller; clinical features and key investigations [1]
>
> See Tables 15.1, 15.2, and 15.3.
>
> **Table 15.1 Important causes of fever according to timing**
>
> | Incubation period | Bacterial | Fungal | Protozoa and helminths | Viruses |
> |---|---|---|---|---|
> | **Short (<10 days)** | Respiratory tract infections, acute gastroenteritis, meningitis/sepsis, rickettsial infection, relapsing fever, melioidosis | Histoplasmosis | | Respiratory tract infections, acute gastroenteritis, West Nile virus, dengue, Chikungunya, Japanese encephalitis, viral haemorrhagic fevers |
> | **Medium (10–21 days)** | Enteric fever, brucellosis, Q-fever, leptospirosis, melioidosis | Coccidioidomycosis, histoplasmosis, paracocci-dioidomycosis | Malaria, trypanosomiasis, Chagas disease | Viral haemorrhagic fevers, CMV, EBV, HIV |
> | **Long (>21 days)** | Brucellosis, TB | | Malaria, amoebic liver abscess (ALA), acute schistosomiasis, African trypanosomiasis, visceral leishmaniasis | HIV, hepatitis A–E |
>
>
> (continued)

Table 15.2 Important causes of fever according to geographic area

Geographical area	Bacterial	Fungal	Protozoa and helminths	Viruses
Sub-Saharan Africa	Enteric fever, rickettsial infection, brucellosis, meningo-coccaemia, leptospirosis	Histoplasmosis, blastomycosis	Malaria, ALA, acute schistosomiasis, African trypanosomiasis, visceral leishmaniasis	Chikungunya, yellow fever, viral haemorrhagic fever (e.g. Lassa, Ebola, Marburg), HIV
North Africa, Middle East, & Mediterranean	Brucellosis, Q fever, rickettsial infection		Visceral leishmaniasis, (malaria)	Tuscan sandfly fever, Rift-Valley fever
Eastern Europe and Scandinavia	Lyme disease, tularaemia, brucellosis, Q fever			Hantavirus, TBE
South and Central Asia	Enteric fever, rickettsial infection, leptospirosis, brucellosis, Q fever		Malaria, ALA, opisthorchis	Dengue, Chikungunya, Japanese encephalitis Nipah, Crimean-Congo VHF
South East Asia	Enteric fever, leptospirosis, melioidosis, scrub typhus	Penicillinosis	Malaria, ALA, paragonomiasis, opisthorchis	Dengue, Chikungunya, Japanese encephalitis, Hantavirus
North Australia	Q fever, melioidosis, rickettsial infection			Dengue, Murray Valley, Ross River fever
South America and Carribean	Enteric fever, brucellosis, Q fever, leptospirosis	Coccidioidomycosis, histoplasmosis, paracocci-dioidomycosis	Malaria, ALA, Chagas disease	Dengue, Hantavirus, yellow fever
North America	Rocky Mountain spotted fever, Lyme disease, ehrlichiosis	Coccidioidomycosis, histoplasmosis	Babesiosis	West Nile virus, Hantavirus

Source: Data from *Journal of Infection*, Volume 59, Issue 1, Johnston V et al, Fever in returned travellers presenting in the United Kingdom: recommendations for investigation and initial management, pp. 1–18, Copyright © 2009 The British Infection Society. Published by Elsevier Ltd. All rights reserved.

(continued)

Table 15.3 Important causes of fever according focal symptoms

Focal symptoms	Bacterial	Fungal	Protozoa and helminths	Viruses
Undifferentiated fever	Enteric fever, sepsis, brucellosis, Q-fever, TB, leptospirosis, rickettsial infection		Malaria, ALA, acute schistosomiasis (= Katayama fever)	Dengue, Chikungunya, HIV, hepatitis B/C, viral haemorrhagic fever
& respiratory symptoms	Pneumonia, Legionella infection, melioidosis, TB	Coccidioidomycosis, paracocci-dioidomycosis, histoplasmosis	Paragonimus, Katayama fever, malaria	Influenza, tonsillitis, pharyngitis, sinusitis
& GI symptoms	Acute gastroenteritis/ traveller's diarrhoea, severe septicaemia, TB		Malaria, amoebic colitis/ALA	Acute gastroenteritis, viral haemorrhagic fever

Source: Data from *Journal of Infection*, Volume 59, Issue 1, Johnston V et al, Fever in returned travellers presenting in the United Kingdom: recommendations for investigation and initial management, pp. 1–18, Copyright © 2009 The British Infection Society. Published by Elsevier Ltd. All rights reserved.

The patient had stayed with relatives in urban northern India, none of whom were unwell. Except for a few mosquito bites, he denied any exposure to other insects or animals. He drank filtered water and most of his food was prepared at his relatives' house, with only occasional food from local restaurants. For many years, he had consumed significant amounts of alcohol (8 units daily).

On initial examination the patient appeared unwell with pallor and cool peripheries. His basic observations were as follows: temperature 39°C, pulse 100 bpm, blood pressure 110/50 mmHg, respiratory rate 32 breaths per minute, oxygen saturation 91% on air, capillary blood glucose 5.5 mmol/L (after intravenous glucose infusion), and Glasgow Coma Score (GCS) 15/15. Respiratory examination revealed stony dullness to percussion and reduced breath sounds throughout his right hemithorax. Abdominal examination revealed a distended abdomen with tenderness over his right upper quadrant but no signs of jaundice, peritonism, nor abnormal bowel sounds. The remainder of the examination was normal.

Malaria thick and thin films were negative. Basic blood tests revealed a moderate neutrophilia and thrombocytosis, a raised CRP and ALP, and a low albumin (Table 15.4). A chest radiograph showed air space opacification of the whole right lung, suggestive of pleural effusion, but normal findings on the left hemithorax (Figure 15.1). Urinalysis was normal.

❝ Expert comment Travel history

The most important part of diagnosing a tropical infection is to take a thorough travel history. This feature of the history might easily have been missed had the clinician only focused on the unstable diabetes, particularly as the travel is several months prior to presentation. The travel history should follow the time/person/place rule, i.e. a detailed description of when the person was overseas (time), what activities the patient undertook while abroad and what risks for disease the patient has (person), and exactly where the patient has been to (place).

❝ Expert comment Global ID update

For the latest information about ID outbreaks in different areas of the world the following web pages are suggested: PHE (formerly the HPA, http://www.hpa.org.uk), Promed (http://www.promedmail.org), NaTHNaC (http://www.nathnac.org), CDC (http://www.cdc.gov), or WHO outbreak data (http://www.who.int/csr/don/en). Also contact the HPA National Imported Fever Service for advice if needed, 0844 778 8990 (after discussion with local microbiology, virology or ID consultant).

> **✚ Clinical tip** Think malaria!
>
> Malaria is always the first infection to consider in any febrile patient with a history of travel to the tropics within the last few years. A negative malaria film does not exclude malaria, especially when performed in laboratories unfamiliar with looking at malaria blood films. It is therefore suggested that three malaria films are taken on successive days to rule out malaria. The newer rapid diagnostic tests (RDTs) should not replace blood films but they have a high sensitivity for FM, almost comparable to expert malaria microscopy, so if this test is also negative at admission to hospital, an alternative diagnosis needs to be considered immediately. The high platelet count and neutrophilia also would go against malaria in this case.

Table 15.4 **Admission and follow-up blood test results**

Parameter (units)	Admission	Day 8 (deterioration)	Week 6 (outpatient follow-up)
WBC (/mm^3)	14.7	24.2	7.8
Neutrophils (/mm^3)	12.3	23.5	4.5
Lymphocytes (/mm^3)	1.6	0.3	2.5
Eosinophils (/mm^3)	0.01	0.00	0.09
Hb (g/dL)	9.5	10.2	11.4
Platelets (/mm^3)	599	447	371
CRP (mg/L)	147	131	16
Creatinine (µmol/L)	63	153	67
Albumin (g/L)	17	12	22
Aspartate transaminase (iu/L)	6	20	11
Bilirubin (µmol/L)	8	15	5
ALP (iu/L)	520	644	287
Blood cultures	Negative		
Malaria thin & thick film and RDT	No parasites seen; negative		

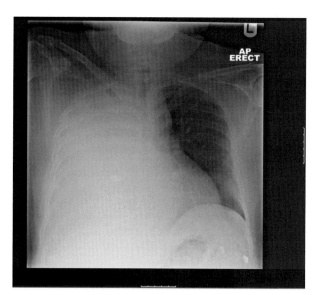

Figure 15.1 Chest radiograph showing air space opacification of the whole right lung, suggestive of pleural effusion, but normal findings on the left hemithorax.

The initial management included fluid resuscitation, tight blood glucose control, and empirical antibacterial treatment with intravenous co-amoxiclav for presumed respiratory tract infection. A Seldinger chest drain was inserted into the right pleural space, which drained 2 litres of straw-coloured fluid. This was a lymphocytic transudate (Table 15.5).

On day 2 of his admission, a contrast CT scan of thorax, abdomen and pelvis showed a 10 × 9 cm homogeneous fluid collection in segments 5 and 6 of the liver, and residual pleural effusion with lower lobe consolidation in the right hemithorax (Figure 15.2).

An 8F pigtail drain was inserted into the liver abscess under ultrasound guidance, revealing anchovy-coloured fluid (Table 15.6). A blood-borne viruses screen (including HIV and hepatitis B/C) was negative.

High-dose metronidazole (800 mg three times a day) was added to the co-amoxiclav to cover for both possibilities of pyogenic and ALAs (Table 15.8). The following day, the amoebic serology results suggested active amoebic infection while admission urine, faeces, and blood cultures were negative. The antibiotic regimen was rationalized to metronidazole alone.

Table 15.5 Pleural fluid results

Test (units, where relevant)	
Glucose (mmol/L)	4.7
Protein (g/L)	30
Microbiology	Macroscopic appearance: yellow-coloured fluid
	Microscopy result: few lymphocytes seen
	Culture: no growth on routine culture
	Microscopy for AFB and TB culture: negative (3 samples)
Cytology	No malignant cells on cytology

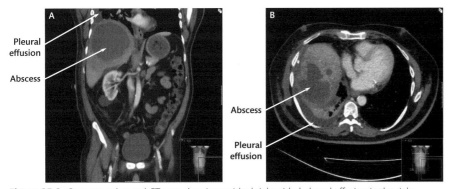

Figure 15.2 Contrast-enhanced CT scan showing residual right-sided pleural effusion in the right lower lobe and a 10 × 9 cm lobulated, mostly homogeneous fluid collection in segments 5 and 6 of the liver, with subtle rim enhancement and reduced attenuation involving approximately a 2 cm rim of surrounding liver.

Table 15.6 Liver abscess investigations

Test	Result
Liver abscess fluid microbiology (day 1 + day 8)	Macroscopic appearance: thick, brown-coloured Microscopic appearance: debris Culture: no growth on routine culture Microscopy for AFB and TB culture: negative
Liver abscess fluid cytology	No malignant cells seen
Amoebic serology: CAP test and IFAT*	Both positive
Faeces routine culture and microscopy	No pathogens isolated; ova, cysts, parasites not seen

* Cellulose acetate precipitation (CAP) test and immunofluorescent antibody test (IFAT).

⭐ **Clinical tip** Examples of microorganisms known to cause liver abscesses

See Table 15.7.

Table 15.7 Pathogens associated with liver abscesses

Group of pathogens		Examples
Protozoa, helminths		*Entamoeba histolytica, Echinococcus* spp
Bacteria	Gram-negative	*Klebsiella* spp, *Escherichia coli, Pseudomonas* spp, *Salmonella* spp, *Proteus* spp, *Citrobacter* spp, *Serratia* spp; *Burkholderia pseudomallei* (melioidosis); *Fusobacterium, Bacteroides* spp (anaerobes)
	Gram-positive	*Enterococcus, Streptococcus, Staphylococcus; Actinomyces* spp, *Nocardia* spp, *Clostridium* spp
	Mycobacteria	*Mtb*, atypical mycobacteria
Fungi (rare)		e.g. *Candida* spp (in immunosuppressed patients)

Adapted from Johannsen et al, Infections of the liver and biliary system, pp. 951–9, in Mandell GL, Bennett JE, and Dolin R (eds), *Principles and Practice of Infectious Diseases*, 6th edition, Elsevier Health Sciences Division, Copyright © 2004, with permission from Elsevier.

⭐ **Learning point** Amoebic serology (IFAT and CAP test)

There are multiple different serological tests [2] for ALA and in general most perform similarly. They all may produce false-negative results in early disease and can remain positive for many years, making positive results in patients from endemic countries harder to interpret. A minimum of 0.5 mL of serum is required for testing at the reference laboratory. An indirect fluorescent antibody test (IFAT) is used as a screening assay for suspected ALA. It measures amoebic antibodies bound to fluorescent goat anti-human antibodies, detectable on fluorescent microscopy. The test is positive at high titres between 1/160 and 1/320, which occurs in over 95% of cases of ALA by the end of the first 14 days (and in 75% of cases of colitis, at a low titre). A positive IFAT is confirmed with a cellulose acetate precipitation (CAP) test, which uses soluble amoebic antigen showing precipitation with the patient's serum in the presence of amoebic infection. Compared to the IFAT, the CAP test is less sensitive but more specific, since it does not have the drawback of false-positives in non-amoebic liver disease. It becomes negative after infection (may take up to a year), which can help in differentiating between past and current infection [3].

➕ **Clinical tip** Microscopy analysis issues

Faecal microscopy for amoebic cysts has a low sensitivity in ALA (8–44% of cases), even in diarrhoeal disease [4]. Furthermore, stool microscopy has a high false-positive rate because *E. histolytica* is microscopically indistinguishable from non-pathogenic *E. dispar* or *E. moshkovskii* [4,5,6,7]. In endemic

(continued)

countries, *E. dispar* was found to be up to 10 times more common than *E. histolytica* [5]. Enzyme-linked immunosorbent assay (ELISA) methods are available to differentiate between *E. histolytica* and *E. dispar* in stool specimens. New PCR techniques provide higher diagnostic sensitivity and specificity in stool samples, and also in tissue and liver abscess aspirate samples [6] (see Table 15.8).

Table 15.8 Sensitivity of tests

Test	Colitis	Liver abscess
Microscopy of stool	25–60%	10–40%
of abscess fluid	NA	<20%
Antigen detection stool	90%	~40%
serum	65% (early)	~100% (before treatment)
abscess fluid	NA	~40%
Multiplex PCR on stool	>94%	NA
on abscess fluid	NA	87%

Source: Data from Anjana Singh et al, Rapid diagnosis of intestinal parasitic protozoa, with a focus on *Entamoeba histolytica, Interdisciplinary Perspectives on Infectious Diseases*, Volume 2009, Article ID 547090, Copyright © 2009 Anjana Singh et al; and Rashidul Haque et al, Amebiasis, *New England Journal of Medicine*, Volume 348, Issue 16, pp. 1565–73, Copyright © 2003 Massachusetts Medical Society. All rights reserved.
NA = not applicable

During the first week the patient showed a satisfactory response to treatment. He started feeling better and his febrile episodes resolved. His vital signs normalized and the serum inflammatory markers improved. By day 8 of his admission, only a small amount of fluid (200 mL) had drained from the liver abscess, therefore both chest and liver abscess drains were removed. Two hours after drain removal the patient developed an acute deterioration with a high temperature (39.2°C), sinus tachycardia (120 bpm), hypotension (80/50 mmHg), tachypnoea (38 breaths per minute), and hypoxia (oxygen saturation of 90% on air). Venous blood gas analysis showed a metabolic acidosis (base deficit of –5.8 mmol/L, lactate of 3.6 mmol/L). Urgent blood tests showed significantly raised inflammatory response (Table 15.4). An urgent CT scan of chest and abdomen ruled out a pulmonary embolism or rupture of the ALA into the pericardium, pleural space, or peritoneal cavity as a cause for the rapid deterioration. The size of the abscess appeared unchanged. The cause of the acute deterioration was thought to be bacterial superinfection of the ALA, exacerbated by removal of the pigtail drain, resulting in acute septicaemia although no organisms were isolated in the blood cultures.

✪ Learning point Epidemiology

Invasive amoebiasis (IA) occurs due to intestinal or extra-intestinal infection with the protozoan organism *Entamoeba histolytica*. IA occurs throughout the world but is most common in developing countries, because of poor hygiene and sanitation. It is associated with a high morbidity and mortality, causing an estimated 70,000 deaths per year worldwide [5]. In industrialized countries, IA is most commonly found in migrant populations, returning travellers, in sexually active MSM, and institutionalized individuals [4]. Whereas the reported incidence of IA is equal in men and women, the incidence of ALA is found to be around ten times higher in men than in women [7,8]. Environmental factors (such as differences in alcohol consumption) and genetic factors have been postulated for this sex bias [8], and an association between susceptibility for ALA and HLA-DR3 has been observed [7].

❝ Expert comment
Treatment

Treatment for ALA comprises either oral metronidazole 800 mg three times per day for 10 days, or alternatively, oral tinidazole 2 g od for 5 days. Cysts remain in the intestinal lumen in 40–60% of patients receiving metronidazole or tinidizole treatment, and so the initial treatment must be followed by a course of oral diloxanide furoate, 500 mg, three times per day for 10 days, or paromomycin, to eradicate cysts [5].

✛ Clinical tip
Infection control and public health [10]

Cyst excretion in asymptomatic carriers and patients treated without cyst active agents represents an infective risk to others. Household contacts of patients with amoebic dysentery should be screened and treated with cyst active agents. It is good practice to screen and treat household contacts of those with liver abscess as well.

❝ Expert comment
Complications

It is important to rule out rupture of the ALA, as this is the most important cause of rapid clinical deterioration during treatment. However, bacterial superinfection of the ALA is common, especially after instrumentation. Efforts should be made to obtain cultures of blood, urine, and abscess fluid, but if they are negative, this should not put you off this diagnosis [9].

The patient was managed in the HDU with inotropic support, and broad-spectrum antibacterial cover restarted. A further drain was inserted into the liver abscess under ultrasound guidance and 750 mL of fluid was drained from the liver abscess. He stabilized over subsequent days and completed 10 days of metronidazole followed by a course of diloxanide furoate. He was discharged after 24 days in hospital and the family were screened for cysts in the stool by the GP.

Discussion

This case illustrates the presentation of a patient with ALA complicated by a reactive pleural effusion and subsequent bacterial superinfection secondary to instrumentation.

The parasite, *Entamoeba histolytica*, is typically acquired through ingestion of food or water contaminated by faeces from amoebic cyst-carrying humans (see Figure 15.3).

The cyst travels to the large bowel where excystation occurs, converting into eight trophozoites. Most of the trophozoites settle in the mucin layer of the bowel and form new cysts by binary fission leading to asymptomatic carriage (80% of infections) or diarrhoeal disease. New cysts may pass through the bowel and out in faeces to infect others [4,5,7]. Asymptomatically infected individuals can go on to develop invasive disease, with one study showing 4% of children with asymptomatic infection later developing diarrhoea or dysentery [11]. Less commonly the trophozoites invade the colonic epithelium via attachment to a specific lectin, leading to epithelial cell death (causing dysentery) or absorption into the portal venous system and subsequently settling in the liver. Direct extension of a liver abscess can occur into the abdomen, pleural space, and pericardium or very rarely haematogenous spread to the brain. Rupture of ALA or any other foci can cause severe or life-threatening disease as the amoebic pus is highly immunogenic and can lead to shock and collapse. Extra-intestinal disease is thought to occur in less than 1% of infections [5,7,8].

There are no animal reservoirs so human excretions represent the only source of ongoing transmission of infection. Cysts can live in the environment for months and are relatively stable in chlorine at the levels that are used in drinking water. Cysts can be destroyed by hyperchlorination, iodine, and boiling, and filtered out by certain filtration methods. Outbreaks in drinking water have been reported. One example of a large outbreak was in Tblisi, Republic of Georgia, in 1998, where interruptions of the drinking water supply and changes to water pressure were thought to be the cause. A total of 177 cases of suspected amoebiasis were identified, of which 52 were diagnosed with liver abscess (predominantly men) and 53 with intestinal infection. ELISA seropositivity was 71% in those diagnosed with ALA, 21% in those diagnosed with GI infection, and 9–13% in controls, suggesting that there was a high rate of asymptomatic infection [12].

Typically, ALA presents a few weeks to months after exposure [8] with a short history (2–4 weeks) of fever and right upper quadrant pain [4,7,8]. The pain may be referred into the chest or shoulder [5,7]. Concurrent GI symptoms with ALA are unusual (only occurring in 10–35% of patients) [4,7,8]. Abdominal ultrasound will detect most cases of ALA. Usually ALA presents as a solitary hypoechoic area contiguous to the liver, most commonly in the right lobe (80% of cases) [5,7,8,9]. Pus from aspiration of an ALA is classically described as an odourless, non-purulent, sterile fluid of a pink-brown colour ('anchovy sauce' coloured). It contains cellular debris

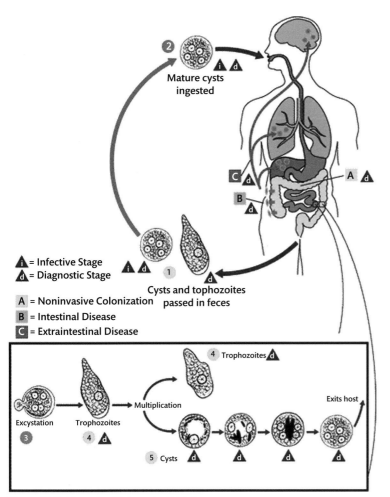

Figure 15.3 Life cycle of *Entamoeba histolytica*.

Cysts and trophozoites are passed in feces (1). Cysts are typically found in formed stool, whereas trophozoites are typically found in diarrhoeal stool. Infection by *Entamoeba histolytica* occurs by ingestion of mature cysts (2) from faecally contaminated food, water, or hands. Excystation (3) occurs in the small intestine and trophozoites (4) are released, which migrate to the large intestine. The trophozoites multiply by binary fission and produce cysts (5), and both stages are passed in the faeces (1). Because of the protection conferred by their walls, the cysts can survive days to weeks in the external environment and are responsible for transmission. Trophozoites passed in the stool are rapidly destroyed once outside the body, and if ingested would not survive exposure to the gastric environment. In many cases, the trophozoites remain confined to the intestinal lumen (A: noninvasive infection) of individuals who are asymptomatic carriers, passing cysts in their stool. In some patients the trophozoites invade the intestinal mucosa (B: intestinal disease), or, through the bloodstream, extraintestinal sites such as the liver, brain, and lungs (C: extraintestinal disease), with resultant pathologic manifestations.

Reproduced from DPDx, CDC Division of Parasitic Diseases and Malaria (DPDM), Parasites and Health, Amebiasis; Life Cycle, 2009, available from http://www.cdc.gov/dpdx/amebiasis/

with very few white cells and only rarely evidence of amoeba [4,5,9]. *Entamoeba histolytica* PCR has been shown to be a useful test when used on pus but is not currently available [3,4,6]. Pyogenic liver abscess (PLA) often presents in a patient who is very unwell with swinging fevers and sepsis [4,8]. Lesions are often multiple and are usually associated with hepatobiliary or GI pathology and/or trauma, instrumentation, and diabetes [8]. This patient's history with the finding of a single lesion and pleural effusion suggested ALA over PLA. Serology can take a few days for results to become available but a diagnostic aspirate can be performed to rule out a pyogenic abscess. The diagnostic yield is higher if antibiotics are withheld until the aspirate is performed, but this may not be possible if the patient is critically unwell. However, standard blood cultures should always be undertaken before starting the antibiotics.

⚙ **Learning point** Epidemiology and clinical presentation of ALA vs. PLAs

See Table 15.9.

Table 15.9 Comparison of epidemiological and clinical aspects of amoebic vs. PLAs

	ALA caused by *E. histolytica*	PLA
Epidemiology	Worldwide; endemic in developing countries (poor hygiene/sanitation) Men > women; adults > children Risk factors: immunosuppression (including steroid use), malnutrition, alcohol Migrant, returning traveller Sexually transmitted (rectal, genital); institutionalized (faecal-oral spread)	Worldwide occurrence Often underlying hepatobiliary or GI pathology Increased risk at older age, diabetes or any other forms of immunosuppression
Clinical presentation	Symptoms develop a long time after exposure (weeks to months) Fever (tends to be more constant than in PLA), RUQ pain, malaise, sweats, anorexia, weight loss, cough, tender hepatomegaly, reactive right-sided pleural effusion. Diarrhoea uncommon Odourless anchovy-coloured pus with very few white cells and no organisms Usually right side of the liver (80% cases) + single abscess Ultrasound: no hyperechoic rim	Shorter latency period Classically swinging high pyrexia. Other symptoms may include right upper abdominal pain. Patient typically systemically unwell or critically ill more frequently than in ALA Green/yellow pus, often with an offensive smell, with many white cells and organism usually identifiable on standard cultures Any location in liver, frequently multiple Ultrasound: usually hyperechoic rim
Complications	ALA rupture through diaphragm (reported in 15% of ALA cases) may lead to formation of hepato-bronchial fistula (expectoration of brown sputum = ALA fluid) or pericardial involvement (1%), presenting as pericarditis/tamponade Rupture into peritoneum → peritonitis Very rare: Involvement of CNS (↑mortality risk), genitourinary tract (rectovaginal fistulae), perianal or cutaneous tissues Bacterial superinfection of the abscess; ALA mortality 0.2–2% (adults)	Locally expanding PLA, involving other organs or leading to peritonitis Bacteraemia with haematogenic spread into other organs or sites High mortality risk from severe septicaemia

Source: Data from Johannsen et al, Infections of the liver and Biliary System, pp. 951–9, in Mandell GL, Bennett JE, and Dolin R (eds), *Principles and Practice of Infectious Diseases*, Sixth edition, Elsevier Health Sciences Division, Copyright © 2004; Petri WA Jr., et al, Enteric Amebiasis, pp. 967–8, in Guerrant RL, Walker DH, and Weller PF (eds), *Tropical Infectious Diseases: Principles, Pathogens and Practice*, Second Edition, Elsevier Health Sciences, Copyright © 2011 and Farthing MJ, and Cevallos, Ana-Maria, Intestinal Protozoa, pp. 1375–406, in Cook GC, and Zumla A (eds), *Manson's Tropical Diseases*, Twenty Second Edition, Saunders, Elsevier, Copyright © 2008.

✔ Evidence base Amoebic serology comparison [2]

A serodiagnosis study in the Netherlands [2] assessed the performance of in-house ELISA and dipstick assays and a commercial latex agglutination test.

Each test showed a high overall sensitivity (93.3% for each test) when evaluated with serum from radiologically proven/CAP test positive cases of ALA (n = 27), amoebic colitis patients (n = 7) or cases with *Entamoeba histolytica* passage (n = 11). ELISA and dipstick showed 100% diagnostic sensitivity for ALA.

Specificity of the tests was evaluated on a range of samples (n = 238) from patients with other infectious and non-infectious conditions, and showed 97.1%, 98.1%, and 99.5%, for ELISA, dipstick, and LAT, respectively. Of great importance, the ELISA showed 96.7% specificity and the dipstick and LAT each 98.4% specificity when tested on sera of patients with PCR-confirmed *Entamoeba dispar* infection.

The importance of this study lies in demonstrating the high diagnostic quality of the ELISA test, which is one of the most frequently used tests in European laboratories, as well as for the easy-to-use dipstick test and the commercially available latex test. In particular these tests correctly differentiated carriers of *Entamoeba histolytica* from those of the non-pathogenic *Entamoeba dispar*.

Complications have been reported in a varying number of patients undergoing needle aspiration or percutaneous drain insertion of ALA, including pain, bleeding into the catheter, subcapsular haematoma, and rupture of abscess [9,13]. Episodes of shaking and chills after drain insertion are described [9]. It was postulated that our patient deteriorated because of super-added infection in the abscess as his condition worsened when the drain was removed. Alternatively it may have been that drug therapy alone had not been effective and further drainage was required. Most patients with ALA recover without aspiration or drainage on metronidazole alone [4,5,7,8]. A recent Cochrane review compared image-guided percutaneous needle aspiration (PNA) plus metronidazole versus metronidazole alone for uncomplicated ALA. There was inadequate evidence for a firm conclusion but in seven poor-quality trials there was no additional benefit of aspiration in terms of clinical recovery or radiological resolution [14].

However, one trial in larger liver abscesses more than 10 cm in diameter of either amoebic or pyogenic origin suggests that there is a benefit to more extensive drainage compared to just aspiration [9]. It has been suggested that poor response to antimicrobial therapy (after 5 days), diagnostic uncertainty, large lesions at risk of rupture, or left-sided lesions are all indications for percutaneous aspiration [5,7,8]. Lesions on the left lobe of the liver are more dangerous because they can rupture into the pericardium [8]. Open surgical rather than radiologically guided drainage is indicated in cases of ruptured abscess or unsuccessful percutaneous procedure [5].

✔ Evidence base Randomized, prospective study of catheter drainage compared to needle aspiration in the management of large liver abscesses [13]

Study design: Patients presenting with a large liver abscess to a surgical centre in India over a period of 3 years were randomly allocated to either percutaneous catheter drainage (PCD) or needle aspiration (PNA) of the abscess, after initiation of empiric intravenous antibiotics. Treatment progress was monitored with regular ultrasound scans up to 6-month follow-up.

Both groups (36 patients each) were reported as having similar baseline characteristics, although there was a lower proportion of amoebic abscesses in the PNA group, compared to PCD (61.1% vs. 78.9%, respectively). Outcomes included the number of days to clinical recovery based on relief of pain and fever, duration of antibiotic use (days), the number of days in hospital, the occurrence of complications, failure of the intervention, and death.

(continued)

Results: Successful treatment' was reported for 97% of patients receiving PCD, compared to 86% receiving PNA (a non-significant difference). Five patients with unsuccessful PNA required surgical procedures, one of whom died from a ruptured abscess. There was a faster clinical relief (p = 0.04) and shorter duration of antibiotics (p = 0.02) with the PCD group compared to the PNA group. There was no difference for length of stay between the two groups. Complete abscess cavity resolution on ultrasound was observed in a higher proportion of PCD cases, compared to PNA.

Conclusion: The authors concluded that PCD and PNA were equally effective when managing large liver abscesses, with slightly better performance of PCD. However, PCD was more likely to be acceptable for patients with large abscesses, or multiple abscesses, who would then not require repeat PNA interventions [13].

A final word from the expert

This case highlights the importance of taking a full travel history when patients present unwell to the acute medical services. Many general physicians are unsure about the diagnostic possibilities when considering infections acquired in the tropics. Physicians must focus on the timing (i.e. the possible incubation period of the disease), the person (i.e. risk factors for acquiring disease), and the place (i.e. exact geography of travel) to make a realistic differential diagnosis. The first tropical infection to consider is malaria, as it is common and early diagnosis and treatment saves lives. There are now many resources (some listed here) for obtaining the latest epidemiological information on disease outbreaks overseas. In this case, ALA is not an unusual diagnosis to make in a diabetic man who drinks excessive alcohol and has been for a lengthy trip to India, staying with relatives. The clinical features of ALA can be very non-specific, however, and it can be difficult to distinguish it from a PLA. There may be clues from the imaging or from the nature of the pus to distinguish the two, but clinical presentation and basic blood parameters may be very similar. The stool microscopy is often unhelpful, and therefore the crux of the diagnosis relies on interpretation of the amoebic serology. The amoebae are exquisitely sensitive to metronidazole or tinidizole, requiring relatively short courses of treatment, with little need for drainage of the pus compared to PLAs. Mortality rates in patients with PLA are high in some of the older literature, mostly from late diagnosis and then subsequent rupture of the abscess into the pericardium, pleural cavity or abdominal cavity. This is a very rare phenomenon these days in developed countries, with the availability of imaging and a recognition of the need for intervention in some cases to avoid rupture. Complications from instrumentation, in particular, super-added BI, is a more common occurrence these days.

References

1 Johnston V, Stockley JM, Dockrell D et al. Fever in returned travellers presenting in the United Kingdom: recommendations for investigation and initial management. *J Infect* 2009; 59: 1–18.
2 Van Doorn HR, Hofwegen H, Koelewijn R et al. Use of rapid dipstick and latex agglutination tests and enzyme-linked immunosorbent assay for serodiagnosis of amebic liver abscess, amebic colitis, and *Entamoeba histolytica* cyst passage. *J Clin Microbiol* 2005; 43: 4801–4806.
3 Health Protection Agency. *User Manual*; HPA Parasitology Reference Laboratory, 2011.
4 Petri WA Jr., et al. Enteric Amebiasis. In: Guerrant RL, Walker DH, Weller PF (eds.), *Tropical Infectious Diseases: Principles, Pathogens and Practice*, 2nd edition. Elsevier Health Sciences, 2011; pp. 967–983.

5 Farthing MJ, Cevallos, A-M. Intestinal protozoa. In: Cook GC, Zumla A (eds.), *Manson's Tropical Diseases*, 22nd edition. Saunders, 2008; pp. 1375–1406.

6 Singh A, Houpt E, Petri WA. Rapid diagnosis of intestinal parasitic protozoa, with a focus on *Entamoeba histolytica*. *Interdiscip Perspect Infect Dis* 2009; 2009.

7 Haque R, Huston CD, Hughes M, Houpt E, Petri Jr WA. Amebiasis. *N Engl J Med* 2003; 348: 1565–1573.

8 Johannsen EC, Madoff, Lawrence C. Infections of the liver and biliary system. In: Mandell GL, Bennett JE, Dolin R (eds.), *Principles and Practice of Infectious Diseases*, 6th edition. Elsevier Science Health Science Division, 2004; pp. 951–959.

9 van Sonnenberg E, Mueller PR, Schiffman HR et al. Intrahepatic amebic abscesses: indications for and results of percutaneous catheter drainage. *Radiology* 1985; 156: 631–635.

10 PHLS Advisory Committee on Gastrointestinal Infections. Preventing person-to-person spread following gastrointestinal infections: guidelines for public health physicians and environmental health officers. *Commun Dis Public Health* 2004; 7: 362–384.

11 Haque R, Mondal D, Kirkpatrick BD et al. Epidemiologic and clinical characteristics of acute diarrhea with emphasis on *Entamoeba histolytica* infections in preschool children in an urban slum of Dhaka, Bangladesh. *Am J Trop Med Hyg* 2003; 69: 398–405.

12 Barwick RS, Uzicanin A, Lareau S et al. Outbreak of amebiasis in Tbilisi, Republic of Georgia, 1998. *Am J Trop Med Hyg* 2002; 67: 623–631.

13 Singh O, Gupta S, Moses S, Jain DK. Comparative study of catheter drainage and needle aspiration in management of large liver abscesses. *Ind J Gastroenterol* 2009; 28: 88–92.

14 Chavez-Tapia NC, Hernandez-Calleros J, Tellez-Avila FI, Torre A, Uribe M. Image-guided percutaneous procedure plus metronidazole versus metronidazole alone for uncomplicated amoebic liver abscess. *Cochrane Database Syst Rev* 2009; 1.

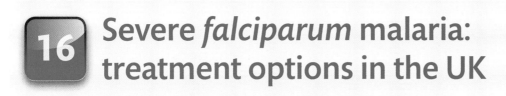

Severe *falciparum* malaria: treatment options in the UK

Marcus Eder and Amber Arnold

Expert commentary Elinor Moore

A 44-year-old male construction worker collapsed at home 2 weeks after returning from a 3-month stay in Nigeria. He had felt generally unwell with profound sweating, abdominal pain, headaches, and intermittent diarrhoea for one week. There was no significant past medical history of note or regular medication use. The patient did not drink alcohol to excess or smoke. He was born in Nigeria but had been resident in the United Kingdom for 20 years. He worked in construction and every few years would spend several months in Nigeria working with a mining company. During the latest trip to Nigeria he had worked in rural areas, living with other mining workers in simple container accommodation. The patient had not taken precautions against malaria as he felt that he would be 'immune' to malaria, given that he had grown up in Nigeria.

> ⭐ **Learning point** Immunity to malaria [1]
>
> **Acquired immunity**
>
> Individuals resident in countries with endemic FM develop immunity to disease after repeated childhood infections. The immunity that develops is not sterilizing, and infection still occurs without the symptoms and consequences of severe disease. Individuals with acquired immunity may present with few symptoms despite heavy parasite infections. Parasites can also be found incidentally when patients are well. In both situations the patient should be treated for malaria and, even if the patient is well, many suggest that they should be admitted to hospital for treatment [2].
>
> Adult immunity is dependent on continued exposure to malaria and is usually lost within a year or two of living outside an endemic country. Therefore, expatriates living in countries that are not endemic with malaria should be advised to take malaria prophylaxis and undertake bite preventative measures (for example, sleeping under impregnated bed nets and using insect repellent) on return to a malaria-endemic area. The need for continued exposure in maintaining immunity also explains why those living in areas where malaria is only transmitted seasonally do not develop a high level of immunity and are at risk of severe disease into adulthood.
>
> **Genetic factors**
>
> Individuals heterozygous for various haemoglobinopathies are less susceptible to FM infection. This is most evident in heterozygous sickle cell disease. Once the sickled red blood cells are infected with the malaria parasite there is enhanced clearage of the damaged cells in the reticulo-endothelial system. This advantage is not seen in homozygous sickle cell disease. The resistance to malaria parasites is present but less evident in glucose-6-phosphate dehydrogenase (G6PD) deficiency and thalassaemia trait. A large number of genetic polymorphisms exist that confer susceptibility or resistance to severe FM [3].

One month into his stay in Nigeria, the patient spent 3 days at a local hospital receiving treatment for malaria. He reported getting some mosquito bites but no other significant exposure to insects or animals. He drank bottled water only and ate in local restaurants. He denied any high-risk sexual activity.

> **🄰 Expert comment**
>
> Reports of malaria episodes in the tropics may represent true infection, but equally may be illness secondary to an alternative pathogen, as malaria is often overdiagnosed in many tropical healthcare institutions. The report of receiving mosquito bites while in the tropics, or lack of them, is generally unhelpful. Some patients may have very little skin reaction to mosquito bites and therefore may not recall bites. Malaria still needs to be considered in those taking malaria prophylaxis, as this will not be fully protective in all cases. Questioning about sexual contacts is important to consider concurrent STIs, in particular, HIV.

On initial examination the patient appeared unwell and was confused (GCS 14/15). He was pyrexial at 38.4°C, tachycardic with a pulse rate of 120 bpm but not hypotensive (BP 126/87 mmHg). He had mild respiratory distress with a raised respiratory rate of 24 breaths per minute and oxygen saturation of 96% on air. The blood glucose (6.9 mmol/L) was in normal range.

He had a non-blanching, petechial rash over his shins but no clinical evidence of jaundice, lymphadenopathy, or peripheral oedema. Cardiovascular and respiratory examinations were normal. There was a palpable spleen at 4 cm on abdominal examination. There was no evidence of meningism or focal neurological changes.

Arterial blood gas analysis showed a compensated metabolic acidosis with a base deficit of –5.7 mmol/L and a lactate of 2.9 mmol/L. Urinalysis was negative for nitrates, blood, and leucocytes. Initial management in the emergency department included supplemental oxygen, intravenous fluids, and an intravenous dose of 2 g of ceftriaxone, to cover meningococcal infection in view of the rash.

A blood film showed parasites of *Plasmodium falciparum* with an estimated 3.6% of the red blood cells infected. A rapid diagnostic antigen test was also positive for *Plasmodium falciparum* and negative for other *Plasmodium* species.

> **⊕ Clinical tip** Malaria laboratory diagnosis [3,4]
>
> The malaria blood film (or 'smear') remains the gold standard in diagnosing malaria, providing information on:
>
> 1. identification of infecting malaria species (*Plasmodium falciparum* versus non-falciparum *Plasmodium* species);
> 2. parasite count (i.e. density of infection, 'parasitaemia': % of total red blood cells infected);
> 3. stage of infection (i.e. the presence of schizonts, a marker for poor prognosis).
>
> The blood films are only as good as the microscopist reviewing the films. For this reason it is recommended to perform three blood films 12–24 hours apart to safely rule out malaria. Blood samples can be tested at any time in relation to the fever periods.
>
> RDTs are increasingly used in laboratory practice. They use qualitative immunochromatographic methods detecting malaria-specific antigens (e.g. histidine-rich protein 2, HRP2) and species-specific lactate dehydrogenase. They are easy to use, resembling a pregnancy testing kit. For those unfamiliar with looking at blood films, they show increased sensitivity and specificity compared to a blood smear. False-positive results can occur with recently treated malaria, or in the presence of heterophile antibodies or rheumatoid factor. False-negative results can occur with insufficient antigen, in the presence of *P. falciparum* with HRP2 variants, or with a damaged test kit.

✪ Learning point Imported malaria: UK epidemiology

Malaria remains the most common potentially life-threatening imported tropical disease in Western travellers. In the UK between 1,500 and 2,000 cases of FM are reported annually with on average 5–10 deaths [2].

In a survey of 20,488 cases of imported malaria to the UK (from a total of 39,300) between 1987 and 2006, 64% of cases were travellers visiting friends and family (VFR) in Africa and Asia from which they or a family member had migrated, 19% of cases were holidaymakers, 16% were foreign visitors to the UK, 13% new immigrants to the UK, and 10% people undertaking business abroad. Only 7% of those visiting family undertook recommended prophylaxis [5].

Over the same 20-year period, 25,054 cases of FM were reported, 96% of which were in individuals who had travelled to Africa, with Ghana and Nigeria accounting for just over half; 65% of cases were seen in London; and rates were higher in September and January, the months during which most travel occurs.

In the same 20-year period there were 183 deaths from FM in the UK with a mortality rate of 7.4 (95% CI 6.3–8.5) per 1000 cases [5].

❝ Expert comment

In experienced hands, the malaria blood film is a sensitive method for malaria diagnosis. The RDTs are extremely useful, however, for those not familiar with looking at blood films for malaria parasites. For this reason, if the initial blood film and RDT is negative at presentation, an alternative diagnosis should immediately be considered. In cases of diagnostic uncertainty, however, it is safest to treat as FM until an expert has reviewed the blood film. The specialized parasitology laboratory at the Hospital for Tropical Diseases in London can review blood films in difficult cases. A reliable estimation of the parasite count and malaria stage can also be difficult in inexperienced hands; therefore decisions about the type and route of administration of treatment should be based on clinical assessment as well as laboratory information.

✚ Clinical tip Symptoms and presentation in FM [1,3]

The shortest time between mosquito bite and symptoms is 7 days and this is increased in those with malaria immunity or taking malaria prophylaxis. Of non-immune travellers 95% will present within a month of return, but reports of onset up to one year after last possible exposure to malaria do occur.

Non-specific symptoms are common and may include headaches, body aches, 'flu-like' symptoms, malaise, and abdominal pain with nausea, vomiting, and diarrhoea. The fever pattern can be unremmitting or with acute attacks (paroxysms) of fever and shivers. Anaemia, jaundice, postural hypotension, and hepatosplenomegaly may be identified on examination.

Clinical features of severe disease include prostration, circulatory collapse, respiratory distress, altered consciousness, multiple convulsions, pulmonary oedema, abnormal bleeding, haemoglobinuria, and jaundice.

Many patients can present with confusion and reduced GCS. However, fever, hypoglycaemia, and seizures can cause many of these features rather than cerebral malaria. Cerebral malaria is defined as occurring in a patient who is deeply unrousable or with GCS ≤8 once other causes have been ruled out [1].

Chronic malaria, common in immune individuals, may present with very non-specific symptoms, such as breathlessness and generalized weakness due to anaemia (often found in pregnant women).

> **⊘ Evidence base** Risk factors for death in the UK [6]
>
> **Study design:** A retrospective study by Checkley et al. looked at 25,054 cases of FM (including 483 cases of mixed infection) with known outcome reported to the UK reference laboratory between 1987 and 2006.
>
> **Results:** A total of 184 FM-associated deaths (case fatality of 0.05%) were identified; 18% of fatalities occurred at home, 3.4% in an ambulance, and 75% in hospital. Most of the deaths were early with the median time to death being 2 days. Mortality was found to increase steadily with age (case fatality of 4.6% in those aged >65 years) and patients aged >65 years had a 10.68 times greater likelihood of death from FM compared to 18–35-year-old patients (95% CI 6.4; 17.8, p <0.001). Low mortality was observed in young patients 5–18 years (fatality 0.33%), and no deaths were seen in children ≤5 years. The odds of death associated with tourism were higher than the odds of death associated with VFR (OR 8.2, 95%CI 5.1–13.3, p <0.001); fatality was lower in patients born in an African endemic country compared to those born outside such countries (0.4% vs. 2.4%; p <0.001). There was an inverse relationship between the number of cases seen in each region of the UK and the death rates [6].

A CXR showed interstitial shadowing in the left midzone and in the bases consistent with pulmonary oedema. Blood results showed a raised serum creatinine of 579 µmol/L, thrombocytopenia with a platelet count of 34×10^9/L, and a normocytic anaemia with a haemoglobin of 10.4 g/dL (Table 16.1). An unenhanced CT of the head showed no intracranial abnormalities.

Table 16.1 Blood results from admission and day 2

Parameter	On admission	On day 2 (after 2 platelet transfusions)
Parasitaemia (%)	3.6	10.7
Neutrophils (× 10⁹/L)	4.6	3.5
Lymphocytes (× 10⁹/L)	1.7	1.2
Eosinophils (× 10⁹/L)	0.02	0.09
Hb (g/dL)	10.4	10.0
Platelets (× 10⁹/L)	34	45
CRP (mg/L)	380	260
Urea (mmol/L)	34.5	38.6
Creatinine (µmol/L)	579	607
ALT (iu/L)	24	71
Albumin (g/L)	23	22
Bilirubin (µmol/l)	22	31
ALP (iu/L)	35	44
Random glucose (g/dL)	6.7	5.5
Prothrombin time (sec)	14	13

> **❝ Expert comment** Interpretation of blood results
>
> The malaria blood film parasite count frequently rises on days 2 and 3 after commencing appropriate treatment. This particularly occurs if schizonts are seen on the original blood film, as this represents red blood cells full of many matured parasites, ready to burst and infect many new red blood cells (see Figure 16.1). For this reason it is useful to follow daily blood film parasite counts until the film is negative. The haemoglobin level is usually only slightly reduced, but if less than 8 g/dL may require blood transfusion, particularly in pregnant women and in those with immunity and a more chronic presentation. The platelet count is universally low, and not a marker of severity. The bilirubin level is usually mildly raised, but if very high can indicate severe haemolysis. The CRP can be very high in some cases. If it continues to be high despite appropriate treatment and improvement in parasite count, a concurrent BI may be present.

The diagnosis at this stage was severe FM as well as a possible coexisting bacterial sepsis.

> **❝ Expert comment**
>
> The use of empirical broad-spectrum antibacterials in all severe FM patients is debatable. In adult patients with malaria there seems to be a propensity for Gram-negative bacteraemias, possibly due to a defective gut wall from parasite damage to the gut capillary. In children there may be concurrent pneumococcal infection. In patients seen in the UK with severe malaria, blood culture evidence of concurrent bacteraemia at the time of malaria diagnosis is very rare. However, those who undergo prolonged hospitalization with intensive care may succumb to hospital-acquired infections later in their course of illness. The UK malaria treatment guidelines suggest use of concurrent antibiotics if there is evidence of shock [2]. The WHO guidelines suggest the need for a low threshold to start broad-spectrum antibiotics [7]

> **✚ Clinical tip** Severe malaria
>
> FM can be classified as uncomplicated or severe, based on clinical and laboratory findings. Patients classified with severe malaria are at higher risk of death, as are those with a parasitaemia >2%, pregnant women, and children. These groups plus those unable to swallow should receive parenteral antimalarials. Table 16.2 summarizes the main features of severe malaria that should be looked for according to the UK's British Infection Society guidelines [2]. The WHO definition includes further clinical features of prostration, respiratory distress due to acidosis, and jaundice [1]. In a UK retrospective study of 75 patients classified as suffering from severe malaria, 6 (8%) died, 6 (8%) had cerebral malaria, 31 (41%) had impaired consciousness level, 8 (11%) had renal failure with creatinine level over 265 µmol/L, 7 (9%) developed ARDS of whom 4 died, 1 had DIC, and 1 (1%) had blackwater fever [8]. A number of clinical and laboratory features (≥1) may be observed in severe FM. See Table 16.2.

Table 16.2 Presence of at least one of the following clinical and laboratory abnormalities indicates severe FM

Clinical manifestations	Comment
Circulatory collapse (shock: BP <90/60 mmHg)	'Algid' malaria; consider coexisting bacterial sepsis
Impaired consciousness or seizures	Reduced consciousness may be caused by hypoglycaemia or seizures as well as cerebral FM
Acute respiratory distress (ARDS), pulmonary oedema	↑capillary permeability due to FM or consider iatrogenic fluid overload
Abnormal/spontaneous bleeding	May be result of DIC or severe thrombocytopenia
Haemoglobinuria (blackwater fever)	Must be in the absence of G6PD deficiency. Haemolysis caused by FM or drugs

Laboratory tests	Comment
Severe anaemia (haemoglobin ≤8 g/dL)	
Hypoglycaemia (blood glucose <2.2 mmol/L)	May be a complication from severe FM or from treatment with quinine
Renal impairment (oliguria <0.4 mL/kg BW/ hr, Creat >265 µmol/L)	Pre-renal/renal causes are most common
Acidosis (pH <7.3); hyperlactataemia	

⊛ Learning point Life cycle and pathophysiology of severe malaria

See Figure 16.1.

All the symptoms of malaria are due to the asexual erythrocytic stage of infection. Rupture of blood schizonts induces host leucocyte and cytokine responses leading to the fever and non-specific features of infection. Infected and uninfected erythrocytes become less deformable, inducing haemolysis and splenic clearance, contributing to anaemia. The severe features are due to a complex interaction of the immune factors, metabolic changes (including glucose consumption by the parasites), and abnormal microcirculation due to blood schizonts which become 'sticky' and adhere to capillaries in peripheral organs. The exact mechanism that explains how the coma in severe malaria is so reversible with normally no residual effects is not fully understood [1].

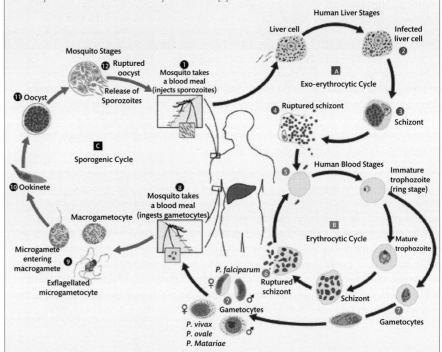

Figure 16.1 Schizonts are rarely seen in peripheral blood of *Plasmodium falciparum* infections, except in severe cases. When seen, schizonts contain anywhere from 8 to 24 merozoites. Image shows schizonts of *P. falciparum* in a thin blood smear.

The malaria parasite life cycle involves two hosts. During a blood meal, a malaria-infected female *Anopheles* mosquito inoculates sporozoites into the human host (1). Sporozoites infect liver cells (2) and either mature into schizonts (3a), which rupture and release merozoites (4), or enter a dormant hypnozoite state (3b). After this initial replication in the liver (exo-erythrocytic schizogony; A), the parasites undergo asexual multiplication in the erythrocytes (erythrocytic schizogony; B). Merozoites infect red blood cells (5). The ring stage trophozoites mature into schizonts, which rupture releasing merozoites (6). Some parasites differentiate into sexual erythrocytic stages (gametocytes) (7). Blood stage parasites are responsible for the clinical manifestations of the disease.

The gametocytes, male (microgametocytes) and female (macrogametocytes), are ingested by an *Anopheles* mosquito during a blood meal (8). The parasites' multiplication in the mosquito is known as the sporogonic cycle (C). While in the mosquito's stomach, the microgametes penetrate the macrogametes, generating zygotes (9). The zygotes in turn become motile and elongated (ookinetes) (10) which invade the midgut wall of the mosquito where they develop into oocysts (11). The oocysts grow, rupture, and release sporozoites (12), which make their way to the mosquito's salivary glands. Inoculation of the sporozoites (1) into a new human host perpetuates the malaria life cycle.

Reproduced from DPDx, CDC Division of Parasitic Diseases and Malaria (DPDM), Parasite Image Library: Malaria, 2009, available from http://www.dpd.cdc.gov/dpdx/HTML/ImageLibrary/Malaria_il.htm

Initial management at the local hospital included oral Malarone (atovaquone/proguanil, 4 tablets) and close monitoring of vital signs and blood glucose. After discussion with the local ID unit, the patient was given intravenous quinine (loading dose 20 mg/kg and subsequent doses 8-hourly at 10 mg/kg).

The patient was transferred to the ID centre and admitted to the intensive care unit. He was immediately given intravenous artesunate and, in view of the worsening acidosis, preventative haemofiltration was started via a central venous catheter line inserted after platelet transfusion.

> **✪ Learning point** Renal impairment and FM [9]
>
> Acute renal impairment is common in severe FM in adults and adolescents (though not in children), with rates of 10–50% reported in different series of patients with severe FM. There tend to be two groups of patients that develop renal impairment. The first group develop renal impairment as part of multi-organ failure and tend to have a high mortality, often within 24 hours of presentation. The second group are patients in whom the FM has been treated successfully but still go on to suffer renal impairment. The second group have a good prognosis if dialysis is available and the majority recover with a renal function back to baseline [1]. The histological picture is a mixture of acute tubular necrosis (ATN), interstitial nephritis, and glomerulonephritis. Clinically oliguria is common and in 60% of patients there is an associated proteinuria (<1 g/24 h normally) which recovers with renal function. Of the patients with renal impairment, 50–80% require dialysis. Peritoneal dialysis is less effective but has been shown to save lives in areas where haemofiltration is not available.

> **❝ Expert comment**
>
> In many hospitals there may be difficulties getting the antimalarial treatment to the patient in time. It is therefore worth checking with the pharmacist what medication is available so that, once prescribed, there is minimal delay for the patient to receive the drug. Any antimalarial is better than no antimalarial (i.e. by preference, IV quinine or IV artesunate if intravenous treatment is indicated; otherwise adequate oral regimen).

Within the first 3 days after admission, the patient remained haemodynamically stable, with his initial confusion fully resolving and urine output slowly improving. He had continuous veno-venous haemofiltration (CVVH), and was managed with administration of 40% oxygen via a face mask, and administration of two units of red blood cell concentrates. A chest radiograph on day 2 suggested upper lobe diversion but no frank pulmonary oedema. An HIV test was negative. Full additional laboratory results are listed in Table 16.1.

> **❝ Expert comment** Management of severe FM
>
> A common misperception is that the renal impairment seen in patients with FM is secondary to dehydration, and that excessive intravenous fluid replacement is required. In fact it is important to keep patients euvolaemic, as the malaria parasite damage to the pulmonary capillaries means that patients are at high risk of developing pulmonary oedema/ARDS. If patients are able to maintain their own fluid intake orally, then they should be left to do so. Blood transfusions for anaemia are appropriate, if the haemoglobin is low, but exchange transfusions are little used these days. This is in part due to the rapid efficacy of intravenous artesunate. The patient should be monitored for ARDS and renal impairment despite adequate parasite clearance from the blood.

On day 4 of his stay, the patient continued to improve and haemofiltration was discontinued. His malaria film was negative and treatment with IV artesunate was changed to oral agents. In view of the resolving acute kidney injury, in order to avoid accumulation of proguanil from Malarone administration (atovaquone/proguanil), doxycyline 100 mg BD (7-day course) was given instead. The patient continued to improve during the second week of his stay, with satisfactory improvement of renal function.

➕ **Clinical tip** Treatment of severe malaria

Intravenous artesunate and quinine are both effective in the treatment of severe FM. Drug regimens are outlined in Table 16.3.

Table 16.3 Treatment regimens of intravenous artesunate and quinine, both effective in the treatment of severe FM

Drug	Dosage	Duration	Followed by (oral)
Quinine dihydrochloride	Intravenous: quinine dihydrochloride Loading dose: 20 mg/kg in 5% dextrose or dextrose saline over 4 h Followed by: 10 mg/kg every 8 h for first 48 h, reduce to 12-hourly if intravenous therapy continues >48 h Oral: quinine sulphate (switch when patient can swallow): 600 mg oral 3 times a day	5–7 days	Doxycycline 200 mg od for 7 days Or Clindamycin 450 mg 3 times a day for 7 days (pregnancy)
Artesunate	Intravenous: 2.4 mg/kg given as an intravenous injection at 0, 12, and 24 h then daily thereafter Switch to oral quinine as above or other oral agent, see below	5–7 days	

Both intravenous options can be followed by oral Malarone (atovaquone/proguanil) 4 tablets for 3 days; the follow-on course of doxycycline/clindamycin is not required

Source: Data from *Journal of Infection*, Volume 54, Issue 2, David G. Lalloo et al, UK malaria treatment guidelines, pp. 111–121, Copyright © 2006 The British Infection Society. Published by Elsevier Ltd. All rights reserved.

Discussion

The challenges faced in the management of FM in the UK compared to malaria-endemic countries are often very different. The most common stumblingblock in the UK is not considering the diagnosis for areas where little malaria is seen. In this case the patient was slow to present but on admission the diagnosis was made very quickly. The original team looking after the patient started antimalarial treatment quickly but did not consult guidelines or specialist advice initially, and so started oral rather than parenteral treatment. Any treatment is better than no treatment, but the severity of this case required intravenous therapy and the patient to be transferred to a local ID unit. Here, the patient switched from intravenous quinine treatment to intravenous artesunate in the belief that parasite clearance from the blood may be quicker with artesunate. However, many hospitals do not have access to artesunate but they do have intensive care facilities. It is vital to undertake careful fluid balance, regular blood glucose monitoring, and appropriate management for ARDS/pulmonary oedema and renal impairment. This patient had a good outcome but it is not clear whether this was because of artesunate use.

For many years, intravenous quinine has been the standard treatment for severe FM, despite its narrow therapeutic index and its potential to induce cardiac arrhythmias, hypoglycaemia, and cinchonism (tinnitus and deafness). Unfortunately quinine is only active against the early trophozoites stage of infection, not the schizont stage, which explains why the parasite count may rise on days 2 and 3 of treatment. The primary regime is then followed by a secondary regime, such as doxycycline or clindamycin. A loading dose for intravenous quinine is recommended in most current national and international guidelines. Use of a loading dose has demonstrated faster action, but no mortality benefit or difference in other outcome measures when compared to quinine used without a loading dose, according to a Cochrane literature review. Higher rates of hearing loss are seen with the use of a loading dose [10].

Over recent years, the alternative antimalarial drug, artesunate, an artemisinin derivative, has been evaluated as an alternative treatment. Artemisinin derivatives have been shown *in vitro* to work on all the erythrocytic forms and also are considered the most potent and fast-acting of the antimalarial compounds [11]. Artesunate is administered at a dose of 2.4 mg/kg body weight 12-hourly for 2 doses, then 24-hourly until an oral switch can be initiated. The side effects of artesunate include cardiotoxicity, a transient rise in the transaminases, reticulocytopenia, headaches, and dizziness. However, it is generally better tolerated than quinine.

Artesunate treatment for severe FM has been evaluated in two large RCTs on adults and children in Asia and Africa, respectively [12,13]. In both studies shorter parasite clearance time, fewer side effects, and lower mortality were observed in cases treated with artesunate compared to those treated with quinine (see Evidence base: The SEAQUAMAT trial). Similar conclusions were reached in a meta-analysis looking at treatment for severe FM [14]. The analysis covered eight trials including 1,664 adults and 5,765 children, all conducted in endemic regions of Africa and Asia. Findings concluded that artesunate treatment reduced the risk of death by 39% in adults (95% CI 25–50%) and by 24% in children (95% CI 10–35%). It also reduced episodes of hypoglycaemia during treatment by 45% (95% CI 26–59%).

✅ Evidence base The SEAQUAMAT trial [12]

The aim of this landmark trial was to assess whether artesunate therapy could reduce mortality from severe malaria in resource-poor settings.

Study design: The trial is an open-labelled RCT conducted in five centres in Bangladesh, India, Indonesia, and Myanmar and compared intravenous artesunate to quinine therapy for FM. A total of 730 patients in the artesunate group (70% severe) received 2.4 mg/kg bolus at admission, and at 12 hours and 24 hours, followed by every 24 hours after that. When they were ready they were switched to an oral version of artesunate to complete a 7-day course. A total of 731 patients in the quinine group (74% severe) received 20 mg/kg loading dose followed by 10 mg/kg 3 times a day. They were switched to oral quinine when recovered sufficiently to complete a 7-day course.

Results: Mortality in the artesunate group was 15% (107 of 730) compared with 22% (164 of 731) in the quinine group (intention-to-treat analysis). This corresponded to an absolute reduction of 34.7% (95% CI 18.5–476%; p = 0.0002). It was noted that the mortality benefit was significantly improved with artesunate for deaths 48 hours after arrival rather than death in the first 48 hours. The benefit of artesunate was also significantly more important in hyperparasitaemic patients than non-hyperparasitaemic (parasites over 10%) (OR 0.34, CI 0.17–0.69, p = 0.001). However, no significant difference was seen in time to discharge from hospital, neurological sequelae, or a number of other clinical parameters.

Concerns: There is concern that the difference between the two groups has been overestimated in this study. Only 3% of patients in the quinine arm were classified as being hypoglycaemic, which some authorities feel is very low compared to other studies. It is postulated that hypoglycaemia was not detected and therefore not treated, contributing to the higher mortality in the quinine-treated group [15].

In light of the evidence stated above, current WHO guidelines recommend artesunate as first-line treatment in severe FM [16]. However, in the UK guidelines, quinine remains the drug of choice and artesunate is listed as an alternative. The UK preference for quinine is largely because artesunate remains an unlicensed drug, with its formulation not having met good manufacturing practice (GMP) requirements. Another reason is that limited data are available from centres in developed countries regarding safety and efficacy of artesunate in severe imported malaria. One retrospective case series of 24 patients at a London treatment centre found that artesunate was effective and safe in all but one patient. This patient developed transient late-onset haemolysis, which is a potential side effect of artesunate [17].

In the UK retrospective analysis, a shorter median length of stay was found in patients treated with artesunate (3.5 vs. 5 days, $p = 0.017$) compared to 167 historic controls treated with quinine. Also, although not statistically significant, no fatalities or hypoglycaemic events were seen in the artesunate group (vs. five of each in the quinine group); in addition, fewer ICU admissions and faster parasite/fever clearance were observed in patients treated with artesunate compared to quinine. Despite the limitations of this small retrospective study, it supported the use of artesunate as an effective and safe alternative to quinine in the UK [17].

One of the reasons that the data in SEQUAMAT from the low-income countries may not be transferable to all patients in high-income countries is that much of the increased mortality in the quinine group could have been due to its significant side effects, especially hypoglycaemia, that can be easily monitored and treated with resources. Another reason is that when causes of death are looked at in the UK, a large proportion of excess deaths are not due to inadequate (quinine) treatment but rather due to no treatment at all, with delayed presentation and delayed diagnoses contributing significantly [6]. Also the Checkley et al. study showed that deaths occur early with a median of 2 days [6] whereas artesunate was shown to be more effective at preventing later deaths [12] (often these are due to hypoglycaemia in resource-poor settings). For these reasons artesunate and quinine are both good treatments for severe malaria in the UK.

A final word from the expert

Malaria is the first consideration in any unwell patient who has been in a malaria-endemic area within the last year. In the UK, poor outcomes come from a delay in the diagnosis, therefore the most important step in improving outcomes is to remember this common tropical disease. Although malaria blood films are the gold standard in diagnosis and give additional information beyond just the diagnosis, RDTs are extremely useful, particularly in laboratories unfamiliar with looking at a malaria film. It is important to make an assessment of the severity of infection. Although for many the treatment course is uneventful, with excellent outcomes, a small proportion will have severe and life-threatening disease and it is vital to identify this group. There has been some discussion here about the choice of antimalarial agent, but equally important is good supportive care, in particular strict fluid balance, managing ARDS/pulmonary oedema and renal impairment, and being vigilant for hypoglycaemia. For this reason it is often appropriate for severe cases to be managed in a high-dependency setting. It is useful to seek early advice from the local ID unit as the UK malaria mortality data does suggest worse outcomes in centres unfamiliar with managing this condition. They may also be able to assist with the choices of antimalarial therapy. Although evidence is mounting for the use of artesunate for severe disease, the availability is patchy and quinine has a long track record as an effective treatment. What is key is that malaria treatment is not delayed, and any antimalarial agent is better than none. There are areas in the world, in particular certain areas in South East Asia, where FM is resistant to a range of antimalarial agents. If resistance is suspected, then discussion with experts from the Hospital for Tropical Diseases in London is required. However, the majority of FM patients seen in the UK will have acquired it in Africa, which has little evidence of resistance to either quinine or artesunate.

References

1 World Health Organization (WHO). Severe falciparum malaria. *Trans Roy Soc Trop Med Hyg 2000*; 94 Suppl 1: S1–90.

2 Lalloo DG, Shingadia D, Pasvol G et al. UK Malaria treatment guidelines. *J Infect* 2007; 54: 111–121.

3 Day N. Malaria. In: Andrew Brent, Robert Davidson, and Anna Seale (eds.), *Oxford Handbook of Tropical Medicine*, 4th edition, Oxford University Press; 2014; pp. 33–68.

4 Cheeseborough M. Parasitological tests. In: *District Laboratory Practice*, 2nd edition. Cambridge University Press, 2005; pp. 239–258.

5 Smith AD, Bradley DJ, Smith V et al. Imported malaria and high risk groups: observational study using UK surveillance data 1987–2006. *BMJ* 2008; 337: a120.

6 Checkley AM, Smith A, Smith V et al. Risk factors for mortality from imported falciparum malaria in the United Kingdom over 20 years: an observational study. *BMJ* 2012; 344 doi: 10.1136/bmj.e2116.

7 World Health Organization. *Guidelines for the Treatment of Malaria*, 2nd edition, 2010. Accessed online 20/09/2012, at http://whqlibdoc.who.int/publications/2010/9789241547925_eng.pdf

8 Phillips A, Bassett P, Zeki S, Newman S, Pasvol G. Risk factors for severe disease in adults with falciparum malaria. *Clin Infect Dis* 2009; 48: 871–878.

9 Barsoum, RS. Malarial acute renal failure. *J Am Soc Nephrol* 2000; 11: 2147–2154.

10 Lesi AFE, Meremikwu MM. High first dose quinine regimen for treating severe malaria. *Cochrane Database Syst Rev* 2004. Issue 3.

11 Rosenthal PJ. Artesunate for the treatment of severe falciparum malaria. *N Engl J Med* 2008; 358: 1829–1836.

12 Dondorp A, Nosten F, Stepniewska K et al. South East Asian Quinine Artesunate Malaria Trial (SEAQUAMAT) group. Artesunate versus quinine for treatment of severe falciparum malaria: a randomised trial. *Lancet* 2005; 366: 717–725.

13 Dondorp AM, Fanello CI, Hendriksen ICE et al., for the AQUAMAT group. Artesunate versus quinine in the treatment of severe falciparum malaria in African children (AQUAMAT): an open-label, randomised trial. *Lancet* 2010; 376: 1647–1657.

14 Sinclair D, Donegan S, Lalloo DG. Artesunate versus quinine for treating severe malaria. *Cochrane Database Syst Rev* 2011, Issue 3.

15 Woodrow CJ, Planche T, Krishna S. Artesunate versus quinine for severe falciparum malaria. *Lancet* 2006; 367: 110–111.

16 World Health Organization. *Guidelines for the Treatment of Malaria*, 2nd edition – Rev. 1, 2011. Accessed online 20/09/2012, at http://www.who.int/malaria/publications/atoz/mal_treatchild_revised.pdf

17 Eder M, Farne H, Cargill T, Abbara A, Davidson RN. Intravenous artesunate vs. intravenous quinine in the treatment of severe falciparum malaria: a retrospective evaluation from a UK centre. *Pathog Glob Health* 2012; 106: 181–187.

17 Imported *Plasmodium vivax*

Emily Wise

Expert commentary Tom Doherty

Case history

A 26-year-old man, originally from Pakistan, presented to his local emergency department in London with a 4-day history of irregular paroxysms of high fever, accompanied by myalgia, arthralgia, and a dry cough. This episode was preceded by prodromal symptoms of mild malaise, headache, and anorexia, lasting approximately 48 hours.

He had moved to the United Kingdom 4 months earlier. In Pakistan he mainly ate food prepared at home, kept halal, and drank tap water. He was unsure of his immunization history. He denied any significant medical history but had experienced one episode similar to his current illness while still in Pakistan. At that time, his local hospital had diagnosed malaria and typhoid and had given him a 3-day course of antimalarials and a 7-day course of antibiotics.

> **✚ Clinical tip** Regard diagnoses from other hospitals and laboratories with scepticism when quality control cannot be assured
>
> When assessing a returned traveller or recent immigrant who has already presented to an alternate healthcare provider, do not assume given diagnoses to be definitive, particularly where you cannot be sure of the diagnostic tools used or vouch for quality control of their laboratories. In resource-poor settings, patients may be empirically treated for malaria in the absence of blood film confirmation, as a default diagnosis for a febrile illness. Many laboratories worldwide still employ the Widal test as a presumptive test for enteric fever. This serological test needs to be interpreted with caution as it is neither sensitive nor specific and previous infection with typhoid or administration of the typhoid vaccination may produce a positive result in the absence of disease. Definitive diagnosis of enteric fever requires isolation of *Salmonella* Typhi or *S.* Paratyphi from blood, stool, or bone marrow culture.

The patient had been afebrile and looked clinically well on initial assessment at triage and so had been placed in a cubicle in the minors department. When the emergency department doctor reviewed the patient 2 hours later, she found him on the trolley looking pale and unwell, vigorously shivering with his teeth chattering, and reluctant for the three blankets covering him to be removed. Observations at this point were a temperature of 39°C, a respiratory rate of 26 breaths per minute, and the patient had a sinus tachycardia at 115 beats per minute (bpm). However, his blood pressure and oxygen saturation were in the normal range. The patient was fully alert and orientated and had no rash, lymphadenopathy, nor meningism. He had palmar and conjunctival pallor and HSV vesicles on his right upper lip. His chest was clear and his heart sounds normal on auscultation. His abdomen was soft and non-tender and his spleen was just palpable. At the end of the history and examination, the patient threw off the blankets and experienced a drenching sweat before falling asleep. Initial blood tests revealed he was anaemic (haemoglobin 9 g/dL) and mildly thrombocytopenic (platelet count 109×10^9/L) but had a normal white cell differential.

➕ Clinical tip Thrombocytopenia and anaemia is highly suggestive of malaria but there is a broad differential diagnosis

A low platelet count is almost universally present in patients with *Plasmodium* infections, particularly if they are non-immune (for example, a person non-resident in a malaria-endemic area experiencing their first episode of malaria). A full blood count result is often more quickly available to clinicians than the result of a malaria blood film, and the platelet count may help direct the clinician as to what the diagnosis will be. However, the demonstration of thrombocytopenia is not sufficient grounds to commence empirical treatment for malaria, and thick and thin blood film confirmation should be awaited.

Differential diagnosis of returning traveller with fever and thrombocytopenia

- **Viral:** dengue, HIV (seroconversion), CMV, EBV, viral haemorrhagic fever viruses (Lassa, Ebola, etc.)
- **Parasitic:** malaria (*Plasmodium*), visceral leishmaniasis (*Leishmania*), human African trypanosomiasis (*Trypanosoma brucei*)
- **Rickettsial:** scrub typhus (*Orientia tsutsugamushi*), epidemic typhus (*Rickettsia prowazekii*), other rickettsial infections
- **Spirochaetes:** leptospirosis (*Leptospira*)
- **Other bacterial:** haemolytic uraemic syndrome (HUS) secondary to *Escherichia coli* 0157:H7, DIC secondary to bacterial sepsis

> **🎙 Expert comment**
>
> Each paroxysm of fever characteristically takes 48 hours for *P. falciparum*, *P. ovale*, and *P. vivax* (hence the classic name for *P. vivax*: 'benign tertian malaria') and 72 hours for *P. malariae*. In practice, this 'classical' pattern of fever is seldom seen.

> **🎙 Expert comment**
>
> In addition to thrombocytopenia, most patients with imported malaria have a slightly elevated bilirubin as a result of haemolysis, although clinical jaundice is unusual.

The patient's CRP was elevated at 43 mg/L, his creatinine was raised considering he had a slight build, at 140 μmol/L; however, liver function and blood glucose were both normal. A chest radiograph was normal. A blood gas analysis was performed and his lactate was in the normal range. An HIV test was not offered to the patient. A thick and thin blood film for malaria was requested.

➕ Clinical tip Opportunistic HIV testing

The current (2008) British HIV Association (BHIVA) testing guidelines include advising to offer an HIV test to:

- Any general medical admission from a local population with an estimated HIV prevalence of above 2 in 1000;
- All patients where HIV enters the differential diagnosis;
- All persons from a country where the HIV prevalence is above 1%;
- All persons who report sexual contact abroad with individuals from countries where the HIV prevalence is above 1% [1].

Travellers returning from the tropics or sub-tropics presenting to healthcare providers should be opportunistically offered screening for HIV as:

- They may have had unprotected sexual intercourse or participated in other high-risk behaviours in countries with high HIV rates;
- They may be otherwise normally fit and well and therefore be unlikely to have contact with a healthcare provider again in the near future;
- An early diagnosis of HIV and the commencement of antiretroviral therapies is associated with a better prognosis than if HIV is not diagnosed until it has become symptomatic.

Do not allow your embarrassment about making an enquiry into an individual's sexual behaviour prevent you from offering them HIV testing. Although consent for HIV testing should always be sought, it is not necessary to involve a specialist counsellor or to explore all risk factors. An HIV test can be introduced to a patient as a 'routine test done for all patients with a febrile illness that can be sent with the blood samples already being sent'.

After a delay of 2 hours the blood film had not been reported. The patient continued to be tachycardic and experienced another rigor despite antipyretics. The clinician made enquiries and was told by the duty haematology technician that he did not feel he had the expertise to read a blood film for malaria and that it would be performed by the lead technician the following day, but an immunochromatographic (ICT) antigen test for *Plasmodium falciparum* had been performed and was negative. Following considerable pressure from the clinician a blood film was read and reported as positive for *P. falciparum* with a parasitaemia of 1%. The patient was admitted and oral quinine was commenced.

⊗ **Learning point** Correct and timely diagnosis of malaria by microscopy is of critical importance

P. falciparum infection may rapidly become life-threatening and a patient who reports a fever and a history of travel in a malaria-endemic country within the last year, whether or not they have undertaken prophylaxis, should have a blood film performed and reported (by telephone if positive) ideally within 4 hours of being requested, and certainly on the same day as the test is performed [2]. Microscopy of Giemsa-stained, thick and thin films of peripheral blood is specific, enables identification of the *Plasmodium* species, allows quantification, and is also relatively cheap and easy to perform. Blood film examination is operator dependent but can be an extremely sensitive diagnostic tool; an experienced laboratory technician may be able to detect a parasitaemia as low as 0.0001%. Malaria cannot be excluded until thick and thin films, prepared from three separate blood specimens, have been examined by an experienced microscopist, the repeat films being performed at 24-hour intervals after the initial negative test. Empirical treatment for malaria should not be commenced until diagnostic confirmation of infection, and supportive treatment should be provided to patients in the meanwhile. If the patient has recently taken antimalarial drugs, the parasites may be too few in number to be detected in a peripheral film. If malaria is still suspected the patient should stop antimalarials and repeat blood films should be performed.

Immunochromatographic RDTs are dipstick, cassette or card-based malaria-antigen detection assays designed for use 'in the field' in endemic areas. In such settings, where good-quality microscopy may not be accessible, RDTs may help reduce the over-use of antimalarial drugs. Positivity indicates an active infection.

RDTs utilize bound antibodies to one or more parasite-derived specific antigens, such as HRP2 (present only in *P. falciparum*), species-specific *Plasmodium* lactate dehydrogenase (pLDH) or aldolase (found in *P. falciparum*, *P. vivax*, *P. malariae*, and *P. ovale*). In 2011 the World Health Organization (WHO) reported that there were over 200 different commercially available RDTs for malaria and published its third round evaluation of RDTs, including 35 designed to detect *P. vivax*. The study found that the majority of RDTs designed to detect *P. vivax* had a high sensitivity (≥95%) at higher parasite concentrations (2,000 or 5,000 parasites/μL). However, at low parasite density (200 parasites/μL), sensitivity for *P. vivax* detection varied widely between products and only 20% had panel detection scores ≥90%. Overall false-positive rates were low, although six tests had rates >10% on clean-negative samples. Higher false-positive rates were seen with some RDTs testing parasites-free samples containing human antibodies such as rheumatoid factor [3]. In resource-rich settings, RDTs may be used in addition to, but not as a substitute for, microscopy, which remains the gold standard technique for malaria diagnosis.

If, as in the case described, there is uncertainty as to which is the infecting species of *Plasmodium*, it is safest to treat for *P.* FM in the acute setting, while awaiting confirmation. In all cases where malaria parasites are identified, an aliquot of blood should be sent to the UK Malaria Reference Laboratory (MRL) for surveillance and identification confirmation (this is a free service).

The following day the patient was much improved. His creatinine normalized and he was no longer suffering with rigors. The medical team was contacted by the laboratory and informed that the patient's films had been reviewed by the MRL and had been reported as positive for *P. vivax* and negative for *P. falciparum* parasites.

✪ **Learning point** Epidemiology of *P. vivax*

P. vivax occurs throughout both most of the world's temperate zones and in large areas of the tropics and is estimated to cause 80–300 million of the 250–500 million cases of clinical malaria a year. *P. vivax* is the dominant species of malaria outside the African continent, accounting for more than 50% of cases in the Middle East, Asia, Western Pacific, and Central and South America. *P. vivax* occurs much less frequently than *P. falciparum* in eastern and southern Africa (where *P. vivax* represents around 10% of malaria cases) and *P. vivax* occurs very rarely in West Africa (where it is the cause of less than 1% of recorded malaria cases) [4].

P. vivax occurs only infrequently in West Africa due to the lack of the red blood cell surface Duffy antigen among West Africans. The merozoite stage of *P. vivax* uses the Duffy molecule on the surface of the erythrocyte to attach to and enter the cell (whereas *P. falciparum* uses multiple mechanisms to achieve red cell entry). Most people of West African origin lack Duffy blood group antigen alleles Fy^a and Fy^b required for erythrocyte invasion, thus making them resistant to *P. vivax* infection. It remains controversial whether Duffy antigen negativity became established in West Africa due to its aiding survival (the relatively benign nature of *P. vivax* infections may be a quite recent phenomenon) or whether it was already established in those populations and selected against the parasite invading those areas.

❝ **Expert comment**

Malaria acquired in South Asia is very unlikely to be *P. falciparum*, while *P. ovale* can only be contracted in West Africa.

✓ **Evidence base** Imported malaria and high-risk groups: observational study using UK surveillance data 1987–2006, [5]

A retrospective observational study using the UK National MRL surveillance data:

- 39,300 cases of malaria reported to MRL as imported to UK during 1987–2006.
- Median age of cases was 31 years, 38% female.
- *P. falciparum* accounted for 24,859 (63%) cases, *P. vivax* 10,904 (28%), *P. ovale* 6%, *P. malariae* 1.5%, and one case of *P. knowlesi*.

With regard to *P. vivax*:

- Reports of *P. vivax* declined from 3,954 (years 1987–1991) to 1,244 (years 2002–2006).
- The proportion of patients with malaria being infected with *P. vivax* also declined over these time periods: ratio of *P. falciparum* to *P. vivax* infections 1.3 to 1 in years 1987–1991, ratio of *P. falciparum* to *P. vivax* infections 5.4 to 1 in years 2002–2006.
- 80% of *P. vivax* malaria came from South Asia. Imported cases from South Asia declined significantly for all species of malaria despite a sustained increase in volume of travel.

Of all malaria reported, most cases (13,215 out of 20,488 cases, 64.5%) were acquired by travellers VFR, usually in a country in Africa or Asia from which members of their family had migrated. People travelling for this reason were at 7.9 times higher risk of acquiring malaria than other travellers.

Cases of malaria in the UK were concentrated in areas where African and South Asian migrants had settled.

The patient was given a 600 mg dose of chloroquine and discharged with three further 300 mg doses to be taken 6, 24, and 48 hours after the initial dose.

✪ **Learning point** Chloroquine therapy

Chloroquine is the drug of choice for the erythrocytic stage of drug-sensitive *P. vivax*. Chloroquine is active against the *Plasmodium* food vacuoles, interfering with the parasite's mechanism for detoxifying the byproducts of the digestion of haemoglobin, leading to the accumulation of toxins.

Chloroquine is generally well tolerated. Side effects include GI disturbances, headache, and hypotension, and ECG abnormalities may occur after parenteral administration. West African people may experience

(continued)

pruritus. Rare, more serious effects include bone marrow suppression and hypersensitivity reactions. Chloroquine is safe in pregnancy but should be avoided in patients with a history of psoriasis or epilepsy as it may exacerbate these conditions.

While there is now extensive worldwide resistance to chloroquine in *P. falciparum*, much of the world currently remains free from chloroquine-resistant *P. vivax* strains. Chloroquine resistance was first identified in *P. vivax* in 1989 in Papua New Guinea (30 years after it was first described in *P. falciparum*), and the majority of individuals with *P. vivax* infection from the island now fail chloroquine therapy. Chloroquine resistance has been reported in isolated and sporadic cases including in Indonesia, Myanmar, South Korea, Thailand, India, Turkey, Ethiopia, Madagascar, Brazil, Peru, and Colombia. Monitoring is hampered by the inability to culture *P. vivax* and a lack of genetic markers for resistance [6]. The Advisory Committee on Malaria Prevention in UK Travellers (part of PHE) still currently advocates using chloroquine as first-line treatment for *P. vivax* infections, regardless of geographical origin. In the event of chloroquine failure in *P. vivax*, the acute infection may be treated with quinine, atovaquone–proguanil (Malarone) or artemisinin combination therapies (ACTs) [2].

The patient's serum G6PD level was tested and he was given a prescription for primaquine (required to eradicate the dormant hypnozoite stage responsible for *P. vivax* relapses), but was asked to wait to hear from the medical team before commencing this treatment. Two days after the patient was discharged his G6PD level was reported as within the normal range. A member of the team attempted to ring him to tell him that it was safe to take the course of primaquine but was unable to reach him and this was not followed up further.

Nine months later the patient re-presented to his general practitioner complaining of a recurrence of his symptoms and fevers over the preceding 10 days. He had not left the UK since his first admission. He was re-referred to his local hospital and a recrudescence of the *P. vivax* malaria was confirmed on a blood film. He was re-treated with a course of chloroquine and further relapse was prevented with a course of 30 mg primaquine for 14 days. The patient made a full recovery.

> ✪ **Learning point** Relapses
>
> The *P. vivax* life cycle includes a dormant stage. In *P. vivax* and *P. ovale* infections, a small fraction of the sporozoites entering the pre-erythocytic liver stage will deviate from the primary path of schizont development and will differentiate into dormant forms in the hepatocytes, referred to as hypnozoites, after the Greek god of sleep, *Hypnos*. The dormant stages give rise to the 'relapses' as occurred in the case.
>
> The stimuli that activate latent hypnozoites to provoke relapse currently remain unknown, but may include other febrile illnesses. The time interval between the primary attack and relapses (and also for initial incubation period) predominantly depends on the infecting strain of *P. vivax*, and number of sporozoites injected by the infecting mosquito. Geographical variation in climate and vector availability is thought to have exerted evolutionary pressure on *P. vivax* strains. *P. vivax* acquired in tropical areas, where the vectors may be omnipresent and year-long transmission is feasible, have a short incubation period (e.g. 10–17 days) and short relapse periods (e.g. every 3 weeks). In contrast, strains from more temperate regions (for example, the Russian strain of *P. vivax hibernans*) may have long incubation and relapse periods of 8 months or more to coincide with the summer availability of the vector. Systemic illness as well as other unknown factors are likely to play a large role in the relapse of *P. vivax* infection [7].
>
> In patients with *P. vivax* infections in whom the hypnozoite stage is not treated, more than 25% will relapse with the disease. Primaquine is currently the only effective drug available to eradicate the hypnozoite stages. After acute *P. vivax* has been treated with chloroquine, relapse should be prevented with the administration of 30 mg primaquine as a daily single dose for 14 days. This is double the dose used in *P. ovale* (15 mg/day), as certain strains of *P. vivax* have been demonstrated to possess innate
>
> (continued)

resistance to primaquine. The mechanism of action of primaquine is thought to be on the parasite mitochondria by deregulating electron transport.

Primaquine is generally well tolerated. However, in people with inherited G6PD deficiency (the most common inherited enzyme deficiency), primaquine ingestion may precipitate acute intravascular haemolysis and methaemoglobinaemia. Primaquine should therefore only be prescribed once the patient's G6PD status is known. Primaquine is contraindicated in pregnancy because of the risk of neonatal haemolysis. Any woman who has contracted *P. vivax* (or *P. ovale*) while pregnant should first be treated with chloroquine and then receive weekly chloroquine prophylaxis until after delivery, when hypnozoite eradication may be offered.

If relapse occurs, re-treatment with chloroquine followed by primaquine is indicated. Relapse in patients who are diagnosed with presumed mono-infection with *P. falciparum* has been observed which is due to undiagnosed co-infection with *P. vivax* at the time of the *P. falciparum* diagnosis [2].

ⓘ Expert comment

In patients who are deficient in G6PD, several strategies can be used. One is to do nothing, as not every patient with benign relapsing malaria will have hypnozoites. In patients with mild G6PD deficiency, a lower dose of primaquine may be administered, but for longer, for example 45–60 mg primaquine as a single weekly dose for 8 weeks. In patients with more pronounced G6PD deficiency, the haemolysis may be progressive and fatal, and hypnozoite eradication with primaquine should not be attempted. Instead the patient may be offered chloroquine prophylaxis for a period of several months, which may be enough to suppress any blood-stage infection emerging from the hypnozoites, or relapses should be awaited and promptly treated with chloroquine.

Discussion

The main challenge in this case was diagnosis. Difficulty in obtaining diagnostics out-of-hours is not unusual in hospitals where malaria is not commonly seen, taking into consideration the time pressures on laboratory staff and the relative inexperience of some laboratories in making this diagnosis. Discrepancies between the blood film and RDTs, as in the case described, may arise in inexperienced hands. The key lessons are to wait for laboratory confirmation of presence of malaria before commencing treatment, and to treat for *P.* FM in the acute setting if there is any uncertainty regarding which species of *Plasmodium* is present or if dual infection is suspected (currently recommended treatments for *P. falciparum* also adequately cover acute *P. vivax* (but not for the hypnozoite stage).

Another interesting feature in the case was that the patient appeared to be relatively unwell on initial presentation, despite being infected with *P. vivax* rather than *P. falciparum* (the species more commonly associated with end-organ complications). Indeed, patients with *P. vivax* often may appear to be disproportionately unwell for their actual clinical state, as a result of fevers and rigors induced by the high levels of inflammatory cytokines released in *P. vivax* infections, in particular, tumour necrosis factor-alpha TNF-α.

Furthermore, it is always worth bearing in mind that a patient with *P. vivax* may still develop severe disease. *P. vivax* was traditionally referred to as 'benign tertian malaria' as it was felt not to be associated with life-threatening complications (as well as being a reference to the fever pattern seen in *P. vivax*) and, from an evolutionary standpoint, it is suspected that *P. vivax* has caused human infections for a longer period than *P. falciparum* and therefore may have evolved ways to replicate without being fatal to the host [8]. However, the patient described did have a dry cough and a slightly raised creatinine and these may have been early markers of progression to more severe disease. In the majority of cases of *P. vivax*, the infection is indeed benign, but patients may develop severe disease due to undetected dual infection with *P. vivax* and *P. falciparum,* or may be developing the less common, but increasingly recognized, complicated *P. vivax*. Indeed, many of the recognized complications of severe *P. falciparum* infection have also been observed, albeit much less frequently, in *P. vivax* infection. Severe anaemia, non-cardiac pulmonary oedema, and in severe cases acute respiratory distress syndrome (ARDS), renal impairment, and cerebral malaria have all been associated with infection with *P. vivax*. It is possible that in some such cases diagnostic facilities may not be available to reliably rule out co-infection with *P. falciparum*. However, in some cases in which severe *P. vivax* disease has been reported, PCR molecular testing was utilized to rule out co-infection [9].

Multiple reasons have been proposed for the typically less severe clinical course in *P. vivax* compared with *P. falciparum*. First, the parasitaemia in *P. vivax* is typically lower than in *P. falciparum,* rarely reaching more than 2% of infected red blood cells. Reasons for the lower parasitaemia include the preference of *P. vivax* to invade reticulocytes (immature red blood cells), and the slower replication rate of *P. vivax* relative to *P. falciparum*. Second, red blood cells infected with *P. vivax* are thought to lack the ability to cyto-adhere and sequestrate and do not display the same reduction in deformability, mechanisms considered essential in the pathogenesis of severe *P. falciparum* infection [10].

> **⊘ Evidence base** Is benign tertian malaria actually benign? [11]
>
> This paper is a retrospective review of case records of all confirmed malaria cases in a single hospital in India in one year to determine incidence of complications of *P. vivax*.
>
> - 121 cases of *P. vivax* and two cases of *P. falciparum-P. vivax* co-infection identified
> - Thrombocytopenia was seen in 113 patients but there were no major bleeding complications
> - Renal dysfunction was seen in 21 patients
> - 3 deaths were attributed to acute respiratory distress syndrome (ARDS) [11]

A final word from the expert

The case described highlights many of the challenges that may occur in the management of a case of imported *P. vivax* malaria. First, difficulty may be experienced by the clinician in trying to obtain a malaria blood film in a timely manner in a district general hospital, and a RDT is not an adequate substitute in such circumstances. A further issue explored in the case and following discussion is how to manage the possibility of severe *P. vivax*, which is increasingly being recognized. The main learning points here are that suspected malaria should not be empirically treated without confirmatory diagnostics and severe malaria should be treated as infection with *P. falciparum* in the first instance.

References

1 British HIV Association, British Association of Sexual Health and HIV and British Infection Society. *UK National Guidelines for HIV Testing,* 2008.

2 Lalloo DG, Shingadia D, Pasvol G et al. UK malaria treatment guidelines. *J Infect* 2007; 54: 111–121.

3 Malaria Rapid Diagnostic Test Performance. *Results of WHO product testing of malarias RDTs: Round 3* (2010–2011).

4 Mendis K, Sina BJ, Marchesini P, Carter R. The neglected burden of *Plasmodium vivax* malaria. *Am J Trop Med Hyg* 2001; 64: 97–106.

5 Smith AD, Bradley DJ, Smith V et al. Imported malaria and high-risk groups: observational study using UK surveillance data 1987–2006. *BMJ* 2008; 337: a120.

6 Price RN, Douglas NM, Anstey NM et al. New developments in *Plasmodium vivax* malaria: severe disease and the rise of chloroquine resistance. *Curr Opin Infect Dis* 2009; 22: 430–435.

7 White NJ. Determinants of relapse periodicity in *Plasmodium vivax* malaria. *Malaria Journal* 2011; 10: 297.

8 Anstey NM, Russell B, Yeo TW, Price RN. The pathophysiology of vivax malaria. *Trends Parasitol* 2009; 25: 220–227.

9 Tan LKK, Yacoub S, Scott S et al. Acute lung injury and other serious complications of *Plasmodium vivax* malaria. *Lancet Infect Dis* 2008; 8: 449–454.

10 Warrell D, Gilles H. *Essential Malariology*, 4th edition. London: Arnold, 2002.

11 Gogia A, Kakar A, Byotra SP et al. Is benign tertian malaria actually benign? *Tropical Doctor* 2012; 42: 92–93.

18 Typhoid fever: antibiotic treatment choices

Nicholas Feasey

Expert commentary Chris Parry

Case history

A 24-year-old woman was referred to hospital by her general practitioner complaining of a 7-day history of worsening fevers, headache, and mild, generalized abdominal pain. She felt nauseous, but had not vomited and had no change in bowel habit. She had previously been fit and well and had no recent history of travel. She was in full-time education and was living with her parents. Although born and raised in the United Kingdom, her parents originally came from Bangladesh. When she first presented 3 days previously she was treated symptomatically, with a presumptive diagnosis of influenza. Following persistent high fevers, she was referred to hospital for further investigation.

> **Learning point** Clinical features of typhoid fever
>
> Incubation period varies from 1 to 2 weeks, although may be up to 2 months, while in paratyphoid fever it ranges from 1 to 10 days. The duration of uncomplicated, untreated illness is approximately 4 weeks. Initially, patients complain of headache, malaise, and fever. Abdominal discomfort, constipation, and a mild non-productive cough are common. As the infection progresses, the fever becomes sustained. By the second week there may be abdominal distention and splenomegaly. Rose spots, crops of 2–4 mm-diameter pink papules which fade on pressure are a hallmark of typhoid; however, they have been found to be uncommon in some series and are difficult to detect in dark-skinned individuals. They are caused by bacterial embolization and may be culture positive, although culture is rarely performed. If the disease is allowed to progress, abdominal distension becomes pronounced and diarrhoea may occur; a delirious confusional state may ensue followed by coma, shock, and respiratory distress—crackles may develop over the lung bases. Death may occur from overwhelming toxaemia, myocarditis, intestinal haemorrhage, or perforation. Convalescence is often lengthy.
>
> If untreated, mortality is approximately 10–20%, but with the use of antibiotics should be <1%. Variation in the clinical picture is common, and mild and unapparent infections are frequent. Diarrhoea may occur even during the first week and young children may present with a high fever and febrile convulsions.
>
> There are numerous intestinal and extra-intestinal complications of typhoid, but prompt diagnosis and treatment should help to prevent them. The two most serious complications of enteric fever are intestinal haemorrhage and perforation. Clinical signs of haemorrhage include circulatory collapse and lower GI bleed. Recognition of perforation may be difficult as it often occurs on a background of a tender or already-distended abdomen with scanty bowel sounds. Clinical features include worsening of pain, change in findings on abdominal examination, and air under the diaphragm on an erect CXR. Either should prompt urgent fluid resuscitation, CT scan of the abdomen, and surgical referral. In the case of perforation, antimicrobial cover should be broadened to cover GI flora including anaerobes.
>
> (continued)

> **Clinical tip**
> Differential diagnosis
>
> The differential diagnosis of typhoid is wide and dependent on the travel history. It includes non-focal causes of fever (i.e. malaria, dengue, influenza, HIV seroconversion, leptospirosis, rickettsial disease, trypanosomiasis, brucella, and tularaemia). In some cases the signs are more focal and pneumonia, TB, meningitis, encephalitis, viral hepatitis or liver abscess should be considered. Rarely the disease can be confused with connective tissue disease or lymphoproliferative conditions.

Other extra-intestinal manifestations include the following:

- Hepatobiliary: jaundice, cholangitis, and cholecystitis. Biochemical changes indicative of a mild hepatitis are a common feature of the acute stage. Pancreatitis has also been reported.
- Neurological: a toxic confusional state is common in late-stage typhoid. Bacterial meningitis is rare. Encephalomyelitis may develop.
- Cardiac: toxic myocarditis and endocarditis occur in 1–5% of cases, often in association with toxic confusion, and represent a significant cause of death in endemic countries.
- Respiratory: rarely, lobar consolidation may develop.
- Renal: subclinical DIC occurs commonly in typhoid fever; this rarely manifests as HUS.
- Other: abscess formation in bones, joints, spleen, and ovaries has been reported.

The patient was alert but looked unwell; her temperature was 39.5°C, heart rate was 95 bpm, and blood pressure was 100/60 mmHg. Her heart sounds were normal and her chest was clear. Abdominal examination revealed 1 cm hepatomegaly, with general abdominal tenderness, but no guarding. There was no meningism or rash. The admitting team performed routine biochemical and haematological investigations (Table 18.1), blood and urine culture, and requested a CXR and abdominal ultrasound scan. She was empirically commenced on intravenous co-amoxiclav as per the hospital guidelines for non-focal sepsis.

Table 18.1 Baseline blood tests

IFull blood count		ILiver function tests	
Haemoglobin	9.7 g/dL	Bilirubin	16 µmol/L
MCV	80.2 fL	Alk Phos	140 iu/L
WCC	6.4 × 10⁹/L	ALT	100 iu/L
Neutrophils	3.1 × 10⁹/L	Albumin	30 g/L
Lymphocytes	2.7 × 10⁹/L		
Platelets	167 × 10⁹/L	CRP	157 g/dL

Over the following 2 days, a high swinging fever was documented and the patient remained unwell. The CRP had started to fall, but the ALT climbed to 150 iu/L. Her CXR was normal and ultrasound confirmed mild hepatomegaly. At this time the admitting team received a call from the microbiologist saying her blood culture was positive with Gram-negative rods visible on microscopy. In view of the persistent pyrexia, intravenous gentamicin was added to broaden the Gram-negative cover.

On day 3 the team was informed that *Salmonella* Typhi had been identified, indicating a diagnosis of typhoid fever. The isolate was reported to be susceptible to all first-line antibiotics by disc testing, including ampicillin, trimethoprim, cefotaxime, and gentamicin, and a ciprofloxacin MIC would follow. As typhoid had not been suspected, the isolate had not been tested for nalidixic acid (Na) resistance, a laboratory marker of decreased ciprofloxacin susceptibility (DCS). The patient was switched to intravenous cefotaxime 2 g three times a day and was isolated in a side room with full enteric precautions. The local health protection unit was informed of the diagnosis, triggering contact tracing and an investigation into the possible source.

The nomenclature of the genus Salmonella is complex. The genus consists of two species, *Salmonella bongori* and *Salmonella enterica*. *Salmonella enterica* is further divided into six subspecies. Most clinically important *Salmonella* isolates are from a single subspecies: *Salmonella enterica* subspecies *enterica*. Salmonellae are further typed according to somatic O (lipopolysaccharide) and flagellar H antigens which gives rise to over 2,500 serotypes or 'serovars' (Kaufmann–White scheme). Typhoid (or enteric) fever is caused either by *Salmonella enterica* subsp *enterica* serovar Typhi, abbreviated to *S*. Typhi and distinguished by the presence of the Vi capsular antigen, or by *S*. Paratyphi A which has no Vi antigen.

Salmonella serovars are often grouped together on the basis of their clinical behaviour as being either invasive/typhoidal (*S*. Typhi and *S*. Paratyphi A) or as non-typhoidal salmonellae (NTS). Typhoid fever classically presents as non-focal sepsis, as was the case in our patient [1]. NTS infections, in contrast, are typically associated with self-limiting enterocolitis. NTS serovars associated with human disease, such as *S*. Typhimurium and *S*. Enteritidis, tend to be zoonotic in their transmission and are found in a range of hosts such as poultry, cattle, pigs, and reptiles. This simplistic distinction breaks down in immunocompromised individuals, including the very young and very old, among whom NTS may cause severe invasive disease. Bloodstream infection with NTS is particularly common in sub-Saharan Africa where immune compromise secondary to malaria, malnutrition, and the HIV pandemic is common. The clinical presentation is similar to that of typhoid fever in many respects, including frequent absence of prominent diarrhoeal illness, and indeed constipation is often a clinical feature [2].

✪ **Learning point** Laboratory diagnosis

Although a mild leucocytosis may develop initially, as the disease progresses, a normal WCC or leucopenia and neutropenia can be seen. Even in uncomplicated cases, low-grade normocytic anaemia, mild thrombocytopenia, modestly elevated serum transaminases, and mild proteinuria are common. A patient with a persistent high fever, a normal WCC, mildly abnormal liver transaminases, and a relevant travel history is suggestive of typhoid.

Isolation of the organism by culture of blood or bone marrow remains the best way of diagnosing typhoid. While *S*. Typhi may also be cultured from stool or (less commonly) urine, this may reflect carriage. In the absence of prior antimicrobial therapy, the sensitivity of blood culture is 60–80% [1]. The median number of bacteria in the blood of patients with typhoid is 1 CFU/mL and so a good volume of blood for culture (5–10 mL) is needed. The viable blood counts are higher in children than in adults so that the lower volume of blood taken in children can still be sufficient. The bacterial load is approximately tenfold higher in bone marrow, hence the higher sensitivity of culture at 80–90%. Furthermore marrow often remains culture positive despite antibiotic therapy. Nucleic acid amplification tests (NAATs) are under development to detect *S*. Typhi DNA, but they do not yet outperform blood culture, probably because of the low number of organisms.

Serology has historically been performed using the Widal test, but this test has many limitations and cannot be recommended. Raised antibodies may result from previous typhoid immunization or earlier infection(s) with NTS which share common O antigens with *S*. Typhi or *S*. Paratyphi. In endemic countries, cross-reactivity with NTS and numerous other pathogens and/or past exposure to *S*. Typhi mean that the Widal test lacks specificity. Moreover, some patients show a poor or negligible antibody response to active infection. Newer tests that directly detect IgM or IgG antibodies to a wide range of *S*. Typhi antigens have been developed which compare favourably with the Widal test, but none of them performs well enough to be recommended for routine use.

✪ **Learning point** Epidemiology

Most developed countries continue to report a small numbers of typhoid fever cases each year. Many, but not all, are in travellers returning from countries where the disease remains endemic. Typhoid is an important cause of morbidity and mortality in areas of the developing world where clean water and adequate sanitation are lacking. The incidence is highest (>100/100,000 p.a.) in the Indian subcontinent, South-East and south-central Asia, and at medium incidence (10–100/100,000 p.a.) in the rest of Asia,

(continued)

Africa, and Central and South America. In 2011, 257 cases of *S*. Typhi and 215 cases of *S*. Paratyphi A were confirmed by the UK HPA, 82% of which were UK residents returning from travelling overseas. The majority of these cases were associated with travel to see friends and relatives in countries in the Indian subcontinent [4]. Another 5–10% of cases were imported by non-residents from these endemic countries. Of interest in relation to this case is that between 5% and 10% of UK cases had no history of overseas travel. Such cases are difficult to diagnose and have important implications for public health management by PHE (formerly the HPA) [5].

⭐ **Learning point** Pathophysiology

The infecting dose of *S*. Typhi needed to produce illness in healthy individuals is large, with a dose of 10^7 organisms required to cause a 50% attack rate. Gastric acidity is an important defence against enteric infections, and gastric hypoacidity from any cause (e.g. antacids, H_2 antagonists, and PPIs) will probably reduce the infective dose required for invasive disease. In order to cause systemic infection, typhoid invades small intestinal epithelial cells and Peyer's patches without eliciting an inflammatory immune response, and is then able to survive in an intracellular niche principally in macrophages. In this intracellular location the organism travels to mesenteric lymph nodes and then to the liver, spleen, and bone marrow. Here the organisms multiply for a period of usually 1–2 weeks, before re-entering the bloodstream, marking the onset of clinical illness. Dissemination in the bloodstream facilitates metastatic infection, and the involvement of the gallbladder and Peyer's patches is especially important. Biliary infection renders stool cultures positive and pre-existing gallbladder disease predisposes to chronic biliary infection and thus chronic faecal carriage. Infection and inflammation of Peyer's patches may lead to the formation of ulcers, usually in the terminal ileum but occasionally in the colon, which in turn may erode into a blood vessel causing severe haemorrhage or through the gut wall leading to intestinal perforation and peritonitis.

On day 4, the patient was still febrile at 39°C and unwell. The CRP had fallen to 124 g/dL but ALT and ALP continued to rise. The ciprofloxacin MIC was reported as 0.25 microgram/mL and the microbiologist suggested that ciprofloxacin was not an appropriate oral option for treatment. By day 5, the patient was starting to feel better, the fever settled, liver function test results had plateaued and the patient was switched to oral azithromycin 500 mg od. As the patient was keen to go home she was discharged to complete a 10-day course of antibiotic treatment.

Three days later the patient returned, complaining that her fever had returned (see Clinical tip: Recurrent fever in typhoid). On this occasion, her fever was 38.0°C, heart rate was 130 bpm, and blood pressure was 102/75. Blood was re-cultured and she was re-started on intravenous cefotaxime in addition to the oral azithromycin. The blood culture was negative on this occasion. The microbiologists checked the cefotaxime and azithromycin MIC of the original isolate and found it to be 0.1 microgram/mL and 8 microgram/mL, respectively. Her temperature settled again within 24 hours, but, in view of the recurrent fever she was continued on cefotaxime (2 g three times a day) and azithromycin (500 mg od) for 10 days. At clinic follow-up 6 weeks later she reported no further symptoms. Arrangements were made for three stool samples to be submitted and they were culture negative for *S*. Typhi.

⭐ **Learning point** Carriage

Challenge studies in normal human volunteers have demonstrated that the stool may become culture positive for a few days after initial infection, reflecting gut replication, but then becomes negative. GI shedding recommences following secondary bacteraemia and infection of the biliary tree and Peyer's patches. With successful antibiotic treatment shedding in the stool then declines and normally stops

(continued)

within 6 weeks of this peak. However 1–3% of individuals become chronic carriers, with long-term shedding in faeces (occasionally urine) which may be intermittent. Chronic carriers are defined as those who excrete the organism for more than one year although in practice if still positive at 3 months after acute infection they are likely to continue carriage. Workers from the food industry and healthcare or childcare workers should have three consecutive negative faecal cultures, prior to returning to work [5].

Antibiotic treatment of the initial illness does not always prevent chronic carriage, although fluoroquinolones are more effective than older agents in this regard if the initial infection is susceptible to fluoroquinolone. Should chronic carriage occur, antibiotic treatment should be guided by the susceptibility tests. Ciprofloxacin (750 mg twice daily for 4 weeks) has a reported cure rate of 83%. Pre-existing biliary disease favours chronic carriage and cholecystectomy may be necessary, but is not always successful, because of persisting hepatic infection. Chronic urinary carriers should be investigated for urinary tract abnormalities, including schistosomiasis.

⊕ **Clinical tip** Prevention of typhoid

Typhoid is an exclusively human disease with infection transmitted by ingestion of food or water contaminated with the faeces of a patient or carrier who is excreting the organism. It is common in overcrowded conditions, including informal settlements and refugee camps, and poor human sanitation plays a major role in disease transmission. Raw fruit and vegetables are important vehicles in some countries where human faeces are used as a fertilizer or where contaminated water is used to make fruit look attractive in the market. Contaminated water sources have been implicated in large outbreaks. Measures should be taken to protect travellers from infection and to prevent onward transmission from index cases in hospital, in the laboratory, and in the community.

- Typhoid vaccination (Typherix [VI antigen, oral Ty21a]) is recommended for travellers to highly endemic areas in Asia and Africa. However, the protection is partial and travellers should be made aware of this and encouraged to pay close attention to personal, food, and water hygiene.
- While in hospital, patients with typhoid should be isolated and managed with attention to adequate hand washing and safe disposal of faeces and urine.
- S. Typhi is a hazard group 3 pathogen, which has in the past caused infection and death of laboratory staff, and there are rules governing its safe handling within the laboratory.
- Cases of typhoid should be notified to PHE who have guidelines on when to take further action [5].

⊕ **Clinical tip** Recurrent fever in typhoid

The clinical response to appropriate antibiotic treatment in typhoid is slow and the patient may feel better before their temperature settles. In this case the patient was discharged on the first day that the temperature returned to normal. But the temperature may have continued to rise and fall for several more days with fever recurrence just representing a slow recovery. The other alternative is a relapse, but this typically occurs a week or more (up to 2 months) after full recovery and stopping therapy. Relapses are generally milder and shorter than the initial illness although can sometimes be more severe. Relapse after treatment with fluoroquinolones (1.5%) or broad-spectrum cephalosporins (5%) is less common than after treatment with chloramphenicol, trimethoprim-sulfamethoxazole, and ampicillin but is increased if the treatment duration is short [6]. Rarely, second or even third relapses may occur. In endemic areas, recurrent fever may also be due to re-infection with a different strain of *Salmonella* Typhi.

Discussion

This case illustrates a number of the challenges in managing a case of typhoid fever, including some uncommon features. A positive blood culture revealed the diagnosis, which would otherwise have been difficult in the absence of a history of foreign travel. Even when typhoid is suspected, confirming the diagnosis can be difficult. Choosing the optimum antibiotic for treatment can be challenging and reflects the lack of a good evidence base from RCTs.

S. Typhi and *S.* Paratyphi A, like other Gram-negative pathogens, have a propensity to evolve resistance to antibiotics. Chloramphenicol was first used to treat typhoid fever in 1948. It was effective in accelerating recovery to a week or less and reduced the incidence of complications and death. Relapse and chronic faecal carriage were a problem with chloramphenicol therapy, but less so if therapy was given for 2–3 weeks. The haematological side effects of chloramphenicol were a concern although they appeared to be uncommon in endemic areas. Chloramphenicol resistance appeared in the early 1970s but co-trimoxazole and amoxicillin were equally effective alternatives.

Plasmid-mediated resistance to chloramphenicol, ampicillin, and co-trimoxazole (referred to as multidrug resistant or MDR phenotype) emerged rapidly in the late 1980s in the Indian subcontinent and parts of South-East Asia, in some areas causing large outbreaks. Although the proportion of strains with the MDR phenotype has subsequently declined in many areas, in only very few have they disappeared. Extended-spectrum cephalosporins, fluoroquinolones, and azithromycin have been the main alternatives in the face of resistance to the older agents. Drugs such as the aminoglycoside gentamicin are active *in vitro* but not *in vivo* because they lack intracellular penetration.

Oral ciprofloxacin and ofloxacin were found to be very effective for treating typhoid with short recovery times (3–5 days) and low rates of relapse and post-treatment faecal carriage. Oral ciprofloxacin and ofloxacin at 10–20 mg/kg daily yield peak levels and an area under the plasma concentration curve (AUC) value considerably above the MIC of wild-type *S.* Typhi and *S.* Paratyphi A (≤0.03 microgram/mL). Furthermore, the antibiotics are bactericidal and concentrate intracellularly where the bacteria reside in the host. Even very short courses of therapy of 5 days or less at a dose of 10 mg/kg were found to be acceptably effective in non-severe disease and are potentially employable in outbreak situations.

Unfortunately, after 2–3 years of widespread use of ciprofloxacin and ofloxacin as empiric therapy for febrile illness, typhoid isolates with decreased susceptibility to ciprofloxacin and ofloxacin emerged, particularly in South and South East Asia. Isolates with decreased ciprofloxacin (and ofloxacin) susceptibility (DCS) have MICs ranging between 0.1 and 0.5 microgram/mL and are usually nalidixic acid resistant (NaR). These are usually spontaneous mutants that are naturally present within the wild-type population that have been selected by widespread antibiotic use. These strains have single point mutations at position 83 and 87 of the *gyrA* gene encoding amino acid changes that lead to impaired binding of ciprofloxacin or ofloxacin to DNA gyrase. Ciprofloxacin or ofloxacin treatment of infection with these strains is associated with prolonged fever clearance times, high clinical failure rates, and increased post-treatment faecal carriage when compared with the response to infections with wild-type strains [6,7]. These differences are particularly evident when lower doses and short durations of the antibiotics are used.

Expert comment
Older drugs

Chloramphenicol, amoxicillin, and cotrimoxazole have all had an important role in the management of typhoid fever, especially chloramphenicol—do they still have a role today? There are few head-to-head comparisons with the newer agents. However, the longer treatment courses required, the spread of resistance, and a less favourable side-effect profile mean that none of these drugs should now be regarded as first-line therapy for typhoid and paratyphoid fever.

Expert comment
Fluoroquinolones and children

Typhoid is common in children whereas fluoroquinolones have been considered to be contra-indicated in children because of concerns over damage to developing joints and tendons. The evidence for this is from the effects of fluoroquinolones on the growing joints of young beagle dogs. The compassionate use of fluoroquinolones in children with drug-resistant infections suggests that this is not a problem, particularly when used for the relatively short durations required to treat typhoid. However, some paediatricians still recommend avoiding this group of drugs if there is a suitable alternative.

The new generation fluoroquinolone, gatifloxacin, remains effective for infections with DCS strains [9]. In three RCTs conducted in areas where the proportion of DCS strains is over 80%, the cure rates have been >90% with fever clearance times of 3–4 days and very low relapse rates. The drug retains its activity because of binding with topoisomerase IV, usually not modified in DCS strains, as well as DNA gyrase. Gatifloxacin has been associated with dysglycaemia in the elderly and those being treated with corticosteroids and this has led to restrictions on its use in some countries. Although the population at risk of typhoid, children and young adults, is different from the group at risk of this side effect, glucose levels should be monitored if this drug is employed.

The parenteral extended-spectrum cephalosporins are the principal choice for patients sick enough to require hospital admission. Cefotaxime (1 g IV three times a day) and ceftriaxone (2 g IV od) retain useful activity against *S.* Typhi and other salmonellae. Reports of resistance to this group of drugs are currently rare in *S.* Typhi and *S.* Paratyphi A, although are emerging in NTS. Treatment with these antibiotics is associated with slow recovery times and relapse, and must be given for a sufficient duration which is probably at least 10 days. The oral third-generation cephalosporins, in particular cefixime, have been used in in typhoid with variable results and cannot be recommended as a first-line choice. Second-generation cephalosporins are also not effective either orally or intravenously.

Azithromycin, an azalide antibiotic, is an effective oral option in typhoid fever. It is concentrated within cells, making it ideal for the treatment of this intracellular infection. It has fever clearance times of less than a week and very low rates of relapse and re-infection. Resistance appears to be uncommon although there are anecdotal reports of increasing resistance in South Asia. As yet there are no clearly defined disc susceptibility breakpoints so the laboratory is unable to report antibiotic susceptibility to the clinician. BSAC and Eucast comment that wild-type isolates of S. Typhi should have an MIC ≤16 microgram/mL. In this case the MIC was 8 microgram/mL and should be associated with a satisfactory response. In the randomized clinical trials that have included azithromycin, the dose used has varied between 10 and 20 mg/kg and the duration of treatment varied between 5, 7, and 10 days. There is no clear evidence as to which is best although many recommend a dose of 20 mg/kg/day for 7 days.

There have been no comparative antibiotic trials for the management of severe and complicated typhoid fever. Third-generation cephalosporins are often started when patients present with severe sepsis and before a diagnosis is established. In a confirmed, fully susceptible infection, whether a fluoroquinolone would be better than an extended-spectrum cephalosporin is not known, and the role of combination therapy is also undefined. Azithromycin should be avoided as a single agent in severe disease. In patients with intestinal perforation, surgery is necessary with a widening of the antibiotic spectrum to cover the GI flora. In the subset of patients with an altered consciousness level (delerious, obtunded, stuporose, or comatose) or shock (defined as a systolic blood pressure of less than 90 mmHg in adults or less than 80 mmHg in children), with evidence of decreased skin, cerebral, or renal perfusion, where the mortality can be up to 50%, adjunctive therapy with high-dose dexamethasone (initially 3 mg/kg body weight, followed by eight doses of 1 mg/kg 6-hourly) significantly reduced mortality in a placebo-controlled randomized trial. Limitations of this study were that patients were treated with chloramphenicol rather than more modern agents and the number included was small.

Evidence base Quantitation of bacteria in blood of typhoid fever patients and relationship between counts and clinical features, transmissibility, and antibiotic resistance [10]

- 369 cases of S. Typhi in Vietnam
- The median S. Typhi count in blood was 1 CFU/mL, of which a mean of 63% were intracellular
  - Children had higher median blood bacterial counts than adults
  - Patients who excreted S. Typhi in faeces had higher bacteremias
- Blood bacterial counts were higher in infections caused by MDR S. Typhi, suggesting a relationship between resistance and virulence

---

Evidence base Quantitation of bacteria in bone marrow from patients with typhoid fever: relationship between counts and clinical features [11]

- 81 Vietnamese patients with confirmed S. Typhi, 93% MDR
- Median of 9 CFU/mL in bone marrow compared to 0.3 CFU/mL in simultaneously sampled blood

(continued)

- The number of bacteria in blood correlated inversely with the duration of preceding fever
- Effective antibiotic pretreatment had a significantly greater effect in reducing blood counts compared to bone marrow counts (p <0.001)
- The bacterial load in bone marrow may reflect the clinical course of the infection, and high levels may suppress neutrophil proliferation

Treatment

Evidence base Fluoroquinolones for treating typhoid and paratyphoid fever (enteric fever) [8]

The most recent Cochrane review serves to highlight the paucity clinical end-point data to inform treatment decisions in S. Typhi infection.

- 26 studies, involving 3033 patients included
- Fluoroquinolones performed well in treating typhoid, and may be superior to alternatives in some settings
  o Authors unable to draw firm general conclusions on comparative contemporary effectiveness, given changing resistance pattern and small study size
- Some evidence that gatifloxacin remains effective where resistance to older fluoroquinolones has developed; however, the different fluoroquinolones were not compared directly

Evidence base A multi-center RCT of gatifloxacin versus azithromycin for the treatment of uncomplicated typhoid fever in children and adults in Vietnam [9]

This is an example of one of several recent well-conducted RCTs in areas where MDR and DCS typhoid strains are common.

- Azithromycin (20 mg/kg/day (maximum 1 g) od for 7 days) vs. gatifloxacin (10 mg/kg/day orally od for 7 days) in an open randomized study in children and adults
- 358 patients enrolled; 287 had blood culture confirmed typhoid
- 96% of the *Salmonella enterica* serovar Typhi isolates were resistant to Na and 58% were MDR
- MIC range of azithromycin was 12 (1.5–16) microgram/mL
- MIC range of gatifloxacin was 0.19 (0.004–0.5) microgram/mL
- Median time to resolution of fever was 4.4 days in both treatment arms (95% CI 3.9–4.9 days for gatifloxacin vs. 3.7–4.7 days for azithromycin)
- No significant difference in the overall treatment failure in each arm: 13/145 (9.0%) patients in the gatifloxacin group and 13/140 (9.3%) patients in the azithromycin group

A final word from the expert

The extended-spectrum cephalosporins remain a suitable choice for the empiric therapy of typhoid when patients are sick enough to require admission to hospital. When the diagnosis is confirmed and the patient is beginning to improve, an oral stepdown to azithromycin or ciprofloxacin (if the isolate is susceptible) is a reasonable strategy. Oral azithromycin or ciprofloxacin (if the isolate is susceptible) can be used from the outset if the disease is non-severe and can be managed on an outpatient basis. Gatifloxacin is a further option in the presence of DCS strains although it is unclear if it will remain active against strains, increasingly reported from cities in the Indian subcontinent, with full ciprofloxacin resistance (MIC ≥1.0 microgram/mL).

Can ciprofloxacin or ofloxacin still be used in infections from isolates with DCS? The data to address this issue are incomplete. There is clear evidence that they should not be used at low doses or for short durations. There is some evidence that if they are used at a dose of 20 mg/kg for 7 days or longer, many patients with non-severe disease will recover, albeit slowly. Less clear is what proportion will not recover and whether the proportion of patients with post-treatment positive faecal carriage will still be high, thus encouraging further spread.

The value of the routine use of combinations of these drugs, and their role in the management of severe disease, is currently undefined and must await future prospective studies. Similarly, the role of high-dose steroids in combination with modern antibiotics is a topic that would benefit from further study.

References

1 Parry CM, Hien TT, Dougan G, White NJ, Farrar JJ. Typhoid fever. *N Engl J Med* 2002; 347: 1770–1782.

2 Feasey NA, Dougan G, Kingsley RA, Heyderman RS, Gordon MA. Invasive non-typhoidal salmonella disease: an emerging and neglected tropical disease in Africa. *Lancet* 2012; 379: 2489–2499.

3 Parry CM, Thuy CT, Dongol S et al. Suitable disk antimicrobial susceptibility breakpoints defining Salmonella enterica serovar Typhi isolates with reduced susceptibility to fluoroquinolones. *Antimicrob Agents Chemother* 2010; 54: 5201–5208.

4 Health Protection Agency. *Enteric fever (Salmonella typhi and paratyphi)—2011 update.* HPA, 2012.

5 Health Protection Agency. *Public Health Operational Guidelines for Typhoid and Paratyphoid (Enteric Fever).* HPA Typhoid and Paratyphoid Reference Group, 2012.

6 Parry CM, Vinh H, Chinh NT et al. The influence of reduced susceptibility to fluoroquinolones in *Salmonella enterica* serovar Typhi on the clinical response to ofloxacin in typhoid fever. *PloS Neglect Trop Dis* 2011; 5: e1163.

7 Crump JA, Kretsinger K, Gay K et al.; Emerging Infections Program FoodNet and NARMS Working Groups. Clinical response and outcome of infection with *Salmonella enterica* serotype Typhi with decreased susceptibility to fluoroquinolones: a United States foodnet multicenter retrospective cohort study. *Antimicrob Agents Chemother* 2008; 52: 1278–1284.

8 Effa EE, Lassi ZS, Critchley JA et al. Fluoroquinolones for treating typhoid and paratyphoid fever (enteric fever). *Cochrane Database Syst Rev* 2011; CD004530.

9 Dolecek C, Tran TP, Nguyen NR et al. A multi-center randomised controlled trial of gatifloxacin versus azithromycin for the treatment of uncomplicated typhoid fever in children and adults in Vietnam. *PLoS One* 2008; 3: e2188.

10 Wain J, Diep TS, Ho VA et al. Quantitation of bacteria in blood of typhoid fever patients and relationship between counts and clinical features, transmissibility, and antibiotic resistance. *J Clin Microbiol* 1998; 36: 1683–1687.

11 Wain J, Pham VB, Ha V et al. Quantitation of bacteria in bone marrow from patients with typhoid fever: relationship between counts and clinical features. *J Clin Microbiol* 2001; 39: 1571–1576.

19 Hospital-acquired *Legionella* pneumonia

Catherine Roberts

🕐 **Expert commentary** William Newsholme

Case history

A 59-year-old man with squamous cell carcinoma of the vocal cords was admitted to hospital with a progressive history of stridor. He was found to have supra-epiglottic fibrosis. He therefore underwent surgical epiglottectomy and had a routine 2-day stay on the intensive care unit before returning to the ward for further postoperative care.

One week postoperatively, he developed bilateral pneumonia with right upper zone and left middle zone changes visible on CXR (Figure 19.1). He developed diarrhoea and was moved to a side room. He was initially commenced on co-amoxiclav and gentamicin for hospital-acquired pneumonia according to the hospital protocol. Despite antibiotic therapy, 2 days later he developed marked hypoxia with deteriorating CXR changes (Figure 19.2) and was transferred to the intensive care unit for intubation and ventilation. As part of the investigation for late-onset hospital-acquired pneumonia, a urinary *Legionella* antigen test was performed and was positive. His antibiotic therapy was changed to intravenous clarithromycin and RIF. The local health protection unit was informed and an infection control meeting was called.

⊗ **Learning point** Diagnosis

Classically, respiratory samples were cultured on buffered charcoal yeast extract (BCYE) agar as the main method of diagnosis. Sensitivity is reported as ranging from 20% to 95% with more severe disease leading to higher sensitivity rates.

Specific diagnosis is usually made by urinary antigen testing. The rapid immunochromatographic enzyme assay has an approximate sensitivity of 80% and specificity of 95–100% for *L. pneumophila* serotype 1 which causes the majority of cases. False-negative results may occur in those with non-serotype 1 disease and in 20% of cases of serotype 1 disease.

Sensitivity and specificity have been shown to be dependent on the severity of the disease, with a sensitivity of 86% being reported in more severe disease and as low as 38% for mild disease [1]. Antigen testing remains positive for several days after antibiotic initiation.

For patients in whom diagnosis cannot be made by antigen testing, diagnosis can be made with either an increase in serum IFAT titres, or direct fluorescence (DFA) by mAbs from clinical samples. The latter tests are performed in the reference laboratory. PCR of clinical samples looking for *L. pneumophila* DNA can be used in the detection of outbreaks [1].

When investigating a case of *Legionella*, PHE (formerly the Health Protection Agency) uses the following definitions [2]:

(continued)

❝ Expert comment

Urinary antigen excretion occurs
as early as day 1 of infection, and is
detectable in about 80% of cases by
day 3. A small proportion of patients
take longer to develop antigenuria
and in some cases it has been
reported to persist up to a year.

Confirmed case

- Isolation (culture) of *Legionella* species from clinical specimens
- Seroconversion (a fourfold or greater increase in titre) determined using a validated indirect immunofluorescent antibody test (IFAT)
- The presence of *L. pneumophila* urinary antigen

Presumptive case

- A single high titre of 128 using IFAT as above (or a single titre of 64 in an outbreak)
- A positive DFA on a clinical specimen using validated mAbs

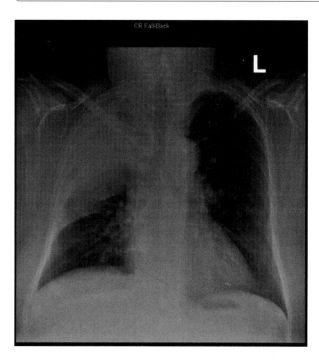

Figure 19.1 CXR showing right upper zone and early left lower zone consolidation.

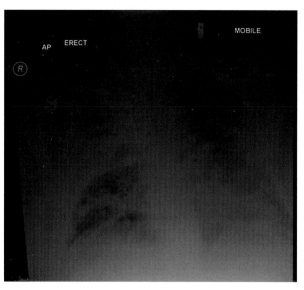

Figure 19.2 CXR showing diffuse consolidation and some early cavitation.

> **✪ Learning point** Case definition
>
> The incubation period for *Legionella* is between 2 and 16 days [3]. However, the incubation period in the majority of cases in most outbreaks is 1–10 days, on which the PHE bases its definitions, as follows [2]:
>
> 1. Definitely nosocomial
>   Patients who spent all of the 10 days in hospital before onset of symptoms
> 2. Probably nosocomial
>   a. Patients who spent between 1 and 9 of the 10 days in hospital prior to onset of symptoms and either became ill in a hospital associated with one or more cases of legionnaires' disease
>   OR
>   b. yielded an isolate that was indistinguishable by mAb subgrouping or by molecular typing methods from isolates obtained from the hospital water system at about the same time
> 3. Possibly nosocomial
>   Patients who spent between 1 and 9 of the 10 days in hospital prior to onset of symptoms, in a hospital not known to be associated with any other cases of legionnaires' disease and where no microbiological link has been established between the infection and the hospital

❝ Expert comment

Calling an MDT meeting as early as possible in the outbreak is crucial.

It is important to set a case definition early in the investigation process to allow rapid identification of the at-risk population, other possible cases, and environmental sources.

The patient's clinical condition deteriorated. He required maximal ventilation with 100% oxygen via an oscillator and continuous haemofiltration for renal failure. He subsequently developed bilateral pneumothoraces and worsening consolidation. At this point his therapy was changed to levofloxacin intravenously. The patient had a prolonged intensive care admission of over 2 months complicated by a bronchopleural fistula and recurrent pseudomonal ventilator-associated pneumonias. However, the patient slowly improved and was subsequently discharged home.

At the initial infection control meeting, it was established that the patient had developed pneumonia 9 days after admission and so could have acquired *Legionella* at home or following admission to hospital. The hospital Estates Department provided records of the hot and cold water maintenance and testing for the clinical areas attended by the patient. Routine *Legionella* testing was performed as per national guidelines, every 6 months, with the last check being 5 months previously. This assessment had shown low levels of *Legionella* colonization in the hospital area under investigation. As such, the system had been pasteurized and subsequent routine cleansing with chlorine dioxide was introduced.

A number of possible *Legionella* sources were identified. Diagrams of the ward water supply were assessed by the maintenance team and no 'dead legs' were identified. The showers, taps, a faulty hot drinks machine, the ice machine, and nebulizer/humidifier machines were considered as sources. The operating theatres were felt to be of low risk as the patient was intubated for most of his stay and the theatre used did not have a stand-alone air conditioning system. The patient had a 2-day postoperative stay on the intensive care unit; for most of this period he was ventilated and was given bed baths; no significant risks were identified on the ICU. Investigation at the patient's home revealed only a shower that had been used infrequently by the patient. Five other patients with hospital-acquired pneumonia were identified on the ENT ward and were tested for *Legionella*.

As a result of the above information, the following actions were taken. Sampling for all possible sources of *Legionella* was to be performed both at home and in the hospital. Filters were to be attached to all showers. Ice machines and hot drinks dispensers on the ward were taken out of service. A log of nebulizer use was created. The identified patients with a respiratory illness were to be tested for *Legionella* and all patients from the ICU and ENT wards who developed a subsequent respiratory illness were to be tested for *Legionella*. Of the five patients who had been identified as having a

❝ Expert comment

To provide appropriate infection control advice it is important to have some understanding of hospital water supply and maintenance systems and some understanding of the relevant Healthcare Technical Memoranda, e.g. *HTM 04-01* [4]. The day-to-day running of hospital water systems is undertaken by Estates personnel, but Infection Control personnel should have oversight of routine monitoring of microbiological standards.

respiratory illness, none tested positive for *Legionella*. Four further patients developed respiratory symptoms during the possible incubation period (10 days); again no cases of *Legionella* were identified. Testing of the home revealed no *Legionella*. Testing of the hospital water systems revealed two taps that the patient had used as having *Legionella* colony counts of greater than 10,000 CFU/L. When the engineers investigated, they found that a valve within a pipe had broken and created stagnant water behind it. There had been no reported problems related to this valve. The engineers replaced the valve and pasteurized the system. A second cycle of *Legionella* sampling was performed after pasteurization and no *Legionella* was detectable.

> ⊕ **Clinical tip** What to do when you, as microbiologist, receive *Legionella* sampling results
>
> *Legionella* sampling and management of detectable levels is routinely managed by Estates Departments. However, it is useful to understand bacterial load levels in case you are asked for interpretation within an outbreak setting. Within a cooling tower, levels of 100 CFU/L or less are considered satisfactory. With levels of 100–1,000 CFU/L, the count should be confirmed, a risk assessment made, and a review carried out of bacterial control measures. With levels of more than 1,000 CFU/L, the system should be immediately re-sampled and cleansed with a biocide. A risk assessment should then be performed to identify any system failures [5].

Discussion

This case demonstrates a number of important points in both patient management and infection control. Hospital acquisition is rare, but can occur even in the setting of exemplary estates maintenance practice. Therefore, a high index of clinical suspicion is needed to identify cases.

The first difficulty with management of this case was to identify *Legionella* as a cause of pneumonia. The ENT clinicians had understandably commenced treatment for nosocomial pneumonia. However, the dramatic clinical deterioration led the intensive care physicians to question the aetiology. The presence of non-respiratory symptoms, such as GI symptoms in this case, may raise the possibility of *Legionella* infection. Patients with underlying immunosuppression, in this case malignancy and smoking history, are at higher risk not only of acquisition, but also of more severe disease. In this case, there were no biochemical abnormalities to guide the diagnosis.

> ⊛ **Learning point** Epidemiology
>
> *Legionella* is a Gram-negative bacillus (GNB) that was first identified as a cause of pneumonia in 1976 following a hotel-associated outbreak in Philadelphia at an American Legion convention. It is now estimated to cause between 2% and 8% of community-acquired pneumonia cases in the United Kingdom and on average about 200 cases are reported to PHE each year. There has been a steady increase in the number of cases reported over the last 20 years, which is likely due to a number of features including increased testing. The majority of cases are community (49%) and travel associated (41%), with a much smaller proportion linked to nosocomial acquisition (7%) [3].
>
> *Legionella pneumophila* is responsible for 90% of human *Legionella* infections. There are several serogroups of *L. pneumophila* associated with human disease, with groups 1, 4, and 6 being the most common in causing disease. Where the agent has been isolated, 70–90% of UK cases are serogroup 1. There are, to date, 17 other *Legionella* species that have been associated with human disease. Some of these species have a distinct geographical distribution. In particular, *L. longbeachae* is the predominant *Legionella* organism in Australia and New Zealand.

➕ **Clinical tip**   Clinical features of *Legionella* and laboratory findings

Legionella has two clinical manifestations: Pontiac fever and legionnaires' disease. Pontiac fever is an acute self-limiting undifferentiated febrile illness usually occurring 36 hours after exposure. Legionnaires' disease has a broad range of presentations.

Although a respiratory component to the illness is usually present, non-respiratory symptoms, especially predominant GI symptoms, can be suggestive of *Legionella* disease [6,7], as follows:

- Fever >38.8°C (88–92%)
- Cough (40–90%)
- Chest pain (13–35%)
- Dyspnoea (25–60%)
- Myalgia/arthralgia (20–40%)
- Diarrhoea (20–50%)
- Nausea/vomiting (8–50%)
- Headache (40–48%)
- Neurologic abnormalities (4–53%)

Laboratory findings associated with *Legionella* are non-specific, but may include renal and hepatic dysfunction, thrombocytopenia, hyponatraemia, hypophosphataemia, high ferritin, haematuria, and proteinuria. These biochemical abnormalities are unusual in other forms of pneumonia.

➕ **Clinical tip**   Risk factors [6,7]

Host risk factors—factors that result in decreased local or systemic cellular immunity

- Chronic lung disease
- Smoking history (2×–7× increased risk)
- Male gender (2×)
- Age >40 years
- Glucocorticoid usage
- Cytotoxic chemotherapy
- SOT
- Treatment with TNFα

In HIV, cavitatory pneumonia, disease relapse, and prolonged bacteraemia have occurred.

Exposure [3]

- Air conditioning systems
- Hot and cold water systems
- Living near cooling towers
- Use of spa or whirlpools
- Humidifiers
- Air washers
- Emergency showers
- Indoor ornamental fountains

🔾 **Expert comment**

There are suggestions that *Legionella* may also be more common in long-distance drivers, exposed to windscreen washer water [8].

In our case, the urinary antigen test was positive. However, it is worth remembering that false-negative results may occur in 20% of serotype 1 disease and also in non-serotype 1 disease (10% of cases). Therefore, if the clinical picture is suggestive and the urinary antigen test is negative, it may be worth discussing the case with the reference laboratory. In our case, the diagnosis was rapidly confirmed by the reference laboratory using urinary immunochromatographic tests (ICT).

Treatment should be commenced in all presumed cases while the diagnosis is confirmed. In this case, *Legionella* was not considered likely and treatment was commenced a few hours later based on the results of the urinary antigen test. A number of antibiotics have been shown to be effective against *Legionella*; these include quinolones, macrolides, tetracyclines, tigecycline, trimethoprim-sulphamethoxazole, clindamycin, and imipenem. However, the most effective agents are macrolides and quinolones.

Two major studies have compared the efficacy of quinolones and macrolides, both in the setting of large community *Legionella* outbreaks in Spain. In the first study, the use of a macrolide (either clarithromycin or erythromycin) was compared with a fluoroquinolone (either ofloxacin or levofloxacin). The authors found that time to defervescence and duration of hospital stay were shorter when the patient was treated with a fluoroquinolone [9]. The second study was an observational study of patients being treated with a number of agents according to the physician's choice. The antibiotics used included azithromycin, clarithromycin, and levofloxacin. In the levofloxacin group, additional RIF and clarithromycin were used in some cases. The study found that when levofloxacin was compared with a macrolide, there was a lower duration of hospital stay and a lower risk of complications. This study also assessed the effects of additional RIF. There was no reduction in the time to defervescence. The duration of hospital stay and the number of complications seen was greater in the group treated with combination therapy. However, this finding probably reflects selection bias. There was also an increase in hepatotoxicity in those treated with a combination of levofloxacin and RIF [10].

✅ **Evidence base** Comparison of fluoroquinolones and macrolides [9,10]

There are no RCTs comparing quinolones to macrolides. However, there are uncontrolled observational studies, which show that fluoroquinolones are superior in terms of time to defervescence, length of hospital stay, and complications, but not mortality.

Fluoroquinolones vs. macrolides in the treatment of Legionnaires disease [9]

- Spanish multi-centre prospective observational study (including Murcia outbreak)
- *Legionella* Ag serogroup 1 positive (100%)
- 130 patients included
- 76 received macrolide (33 erythromycin/43 clarithromycin) vs. 54 received fluoroquinolone (4 ofloxacin/50 levofloxacin) for longer than 14/7
- Dosage: levofloxacin 500 mg twice daily IV until apyrexial when it was switched to od oral; clarythromycin 500 mg twice daily or erythromycin 500–1000 mg four times daily either IV or oral
- Equivalent severity of patients and background conditions
- Time to fever defervescence: 77 hours macrolides, 48 hours fluoroquinolones, p = 0.000
- Duration hospital stay: 9.9 days macrolides, 7.6 days fluoroquinolones, p = 0.09
- There was a non-significant trend (p = 0.4) towards more complications in those treated with a macrolide (23.6 %) compared to those treated with a fluorquinolone (16.65%). There was no difference in mortality or rates of ventilation.

Antimicrobial chemotherapy for Legionnaires disease: levofloxacin versus macrolides [10]

- 2001 Murcia outbreak: contaminated cooling tower, >800 suspected cases, 449 confirmed
- Observational, prospective, non-randomized
- 292 patients, of whom 69 outpatients, 38 patients excluded
- Pneumonia and culture/*Legionella* Ag positive/increase in serotitre
- Antibiotics according to admitting physician
- Azithromycin (n = 35), clarithromycin (n = 32), levofloxacin (dose not stated in paper) (n = 187, of whom additional RIF in 45, additional clarithromycin 2)
- Complications : n = 3 macrolide, n = 1 levofloxacin, p = 0.08
- Hospital stay: 7.2 days macrolides vs. 4.4 days levofloxacin, p = 0.03
- Duration of fever: macrolide 4.6 days vs. levofloxacin 4.4 days, p = 0.5: levofloxacin alone 4.3 days vs. levofloxacin plus RIF 5.7 days, p = 0.03
- Cure rate: macrolide 65 (100%) vs. levofloxacin 142 (99.3%) , p = 0.4: levofloxacin alone 44 (97.7%) vs. levofloxacin plus RIF 45 (100%), p = 0.3
- Hospital stay: macrolide 7.2 days vs. levofloxacin 4.4 days, p = 0.03: levofloxacin alone 5.4 days vs. levofloxacin plus RIF 8.9 days, p = 0.002 [10]

The patient was initially commenced on clarithromycin and RIF. However, following a detailed review of the evidence, the patient's immunosuppressed state and the clinical deterioration led the team to switch her therapy to intravenous levofloxacin.

Infection control

When faced with a case of *Legionella*, the possible source of infection should be identified and public health authorities notified (Box 19.1). In this case, as a result of the timing of infection, it was not clear whether the patient had acquired the infection in the community or in the hospital. It was therefore necessary to investigate both foci as a matter of urgency. Whether community or hospital acquired, investigation follows along similar lines. A detailed exposure history should be obtained, potential sources identified, maintenance records examined where appropriate, and environmental sampling performed. In our case, the infection control measures focused on five areas: identification of other potentially infected patients, widespread sampling of the water systems, making the ward safe, heightened awareness for other developing cases taking into account the incubation period, and information dissemination. We liaised with the HPA, the reference laboratory, and notification services, at an early stage. This gave us support in management of a potential outbreak and home testing. This case also illustrates that a good maintenance record does not rule out the potential for a new fault to occur and become a source of infection.

Box 19.1 Infection control

Legionella is a bacterium of aquatic environments living usually within free-living protozoa or in biofilms. Human infections are most commonly acquired following amplification of the bacteria in water systems containing stagnant pools, in the presence of scale or sediment, or in water kept at temperatures between 25°C and 42°C. Infection usually occurs following aerosolization. The Health and Safety Executive (HSE) therefore requires that all wet cooling systems and hot and cold water systems within institutions meet a number of standards [5]. These include: checking the performance of the system and its component parts, and inspecting the accessible parts of the system for damage and signs of contamination. Routine testing of the water quality and bacterial numbers should also be performed. The precise requirements vary according to water system and water chemistry. However, sampling is usually performed 6-monthly.

The bacterium can be eradicated by heat (above 60°C), biodispersants, oxidizing and non-oxidizing biocides, and UV radiation. The appropriate method to be applied varies according to the system [5].

Person-to-person spread has not been reported and so there is no need for source isolation of the patient while in hospital. Legionnaires' disease is notifiable under the Heath Protection Notification Regulations 2010.

HSE assessment of risk of *Legionella* contamination of water source [5]

- Water is stored or recirculated as part of your system.
- The water temperature in all or some parts of the system is between 20°C and 45°C.
- There are sources of nutrients such as rust, sludge, scale, and organic matter.
- The conditions are likely to encourage bacteria.
- It is possible for water droplets to be produced and, if so, whether they can be dispersed over a wide area, e.g. showers and aerosols from cooling towers.
- It is likely that any of your employees, residents, visitors, etc. are more susceptible to infection due to age, illness, a weakened immune system, etc. and whether they could be exposed to any contaminated water droplets.

A final word from the expert

Legionellosis provides a classic example of the need for an understanding of the ecology of an organism, as well as its clinical behaviour, in order to identify possible sources of infection. It is important to question the patient about less commonly thought-of exposures such as home spa baths, dental surgery water supplies, visits to garden and DIY stores/shows, car and pressure washers, as well as the more obvious exposures in public spaces to fountains, cooling towers, etc.

The case highlights the importance in a nosocomial setting of viewing the potential exposure sites to identify all water-using systems in the area. It also highlights the importance of a good working relationship between Infection Control and hospital Estates. Water system plans should be reviewed with Estates and all maintenance protocols and logbooks should be examined, as well as conducting staff interviews with those involved with system use and maintenance. Extensive water sampling may prove necessary, and must be conducted promptly to allow rapid instigation of emergency controls.

Remember to get the hospital communications team involved early in the investigation; the case is likely to trigger media interest.

Legionella should be considered in the differential diagnosis of any hospitalized patient with an enigmatic community- or hospital-acquired pneumonia, especially in those severe enough to require HDU/ITU input.

Despite the relative ease of diagnosis using urinary antigen detection, it remains important to obtain respiratory specimens, be they sputum, BAL, or biopsy, to allow for serotyping and molecular confirmation of associated cases in an outbreak setting.

While macrolides and fluoroquinolones are effective monotherapies for less severe *Legionella*, the role of adjunctive RIF, particularly in severe disease, remains less clear. Despite several studies, evidence remains conflicting due to the limitations of these studies; however, the addition of RIF to treatment regimes is recommended for severe disease and for patients with significant co-morbidities [11].

References

1 Blázquez RM, Espinosa FJ, Martínez-Toldos CM et al. Sensitivity of urinary antigen test in relation to clinical severity in a large outbreak of Legionella pneumonia in Spain. *Eur J Clin Microbiol Infect Dis* 2005; 24: 488.

2 http://www.hpa.org.uk/Topics/InfectiousDiseases/InfectionsAZ/LegionnairesDisease/CaseDefinitions/.

3 Lee JV, Joseph C; PHLS Atypical Pneumonia Working Group. Guidelines for investigating single cases of Legionnaires' disease. *Commun Dis Public Health* 2002; 5: 157–162.

4 Health and Safety Executive. *Water systems. Health Technical Memorandum 04-01: The control of Legionella, hygiene, 'safe' hot water, cold water and drinking water systems*. 2012. Available at http://www.hse.gov.uk/foi/internalops/sims/pub_serv/07-12-07/index.htm

5 Health and Safety Executive. *Legionnaires' disease: the control of legionella bacteria in water systems. Approved Code of Practice and Guidance* L8. HSE, 2000. HSE Books, PO Box 1999, Sudbury, Suffolk CO10 2WA.

6 Fraser DW, Tsai TR, Orenstein W et al. Legionnaires' disease: description of an epidemic of pneumonia. *N Engl J Med* 1977; 297: 1189.

7 Mulazimoglu L, Yu V. Can Legionnaires disease be diagnosed by clinical criteria? A critical review. *Chest* 2001; 120: 1049.

8 Wallensten A, Oliver I, Ricketts K, Kafatos G, Stuart JM, Joseph C. Windscreen wiper fluid without added screenwash in motor vehicles: a newly identified risk factor for Legionnaires' disease. *Eur J Epidemiol* 2010; 25: 661–665.

9 Sabrià M, Pedro-Botet ML, Gómez J et al. Fluoroquinolones vs macrolides in the treatment of Legionnaires disease. *Chest* 2005; 128: 1401–1405.

10 Blázquez Garrido RM, Espinosa Parra FJ, Alemany Francés L et al. Antimicrobial chemotherapy for Legionnaires disease: levofloxacin versus macrolides. *Clin Infect Dis* 2005; 40: 800.

11 Varner TR, Bookstaver PB, Rudisill CN, Albrecht H. Role of rifampin-based combination therapy for severe community-acquired Legionella pneumophila pneumonia. *Ann Pharmacother* 2011; 45: 967–976.

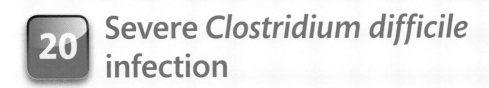

20 Severe *Clostridium difficile* infection

Jasmin Islam

ⓘ **Expert commentary** Martin Llewelyn

Case history

An 82-year-old man presented to the emergency department with a 4-day history of increased bowel frequency. He reported opening his bowels up to 20 times a day with no blood or mucus per rectum. There was no significant travel or dietary history but he had recently been discharged from hospital following suspected diverticulitis treated with co-amoxiclav. Past medical history included irritable bowel syndrome, peptic ulcer disease, and hypertension for which he took amlodipine and omeprazole. Examination revealed a soft abdomen with evidence of lower abdominal tenderness and normal bowel sounds. Blood test results showed a raised inflammatory response and deranged renal function (Table 20.1).

In view of the recent course of antibiotics, a diagnosis of *Clostridium difficile* infection (CDI) was suggested and oral vancomycin 125 mg four times a day was commenced due to the severity of his symptoms.

Table 20.1 Blood results and observations on admission

Haematology		Biochemistry		Observations	
Hb	16.0 g/dL	Na	134 mmol/L	Temperature	37.3°C
WCC	20.8 × 10⁹/L	K	4.8 mmol/L	BP	122/87 mmHg
Neutrophils	18.2 × 10⁹/L	Urea	14.2 mmol/L	Pulse	108 bpm
Leukocytes	4.2 × 10⁹/L	Creatinine	190 μmol/L	O₂ saturations	99%
Platelets	207 × 10⁹/L	CRP	180 g/dL	Glucose	7.3 mmol/L
INR	1.2	ALT	7 iu/L		
		Albumin	32 g/L		
		Lactate	1.6		

⊕ **Clinical tip** Risk factors associated with CDI

- Antibiotics*
- Increased age
- Nasogastric feeding
- PPIs
- Multiple co-morbidities
- Immunosuppression (HIV, BMT, SOT)

Risk factors for CDI recurrence

- Increased age
- Concomitant antibiotics (CA)
- Continued disruption to host microbiota
- Inadequate antibody response to *C. difficile* toxin a and toxin b
- Increased length of stay in hospital or long-term care facility

* Certain classes are strongly associated with increased risk. These include cephalosporins, fluoroquinolones, and broad-spectrum penicillins.

> ⭐ **Learning point** Epidemiology
>
> *Clostridium difficile* is a Gram-positive, spore-forming anaerobic organism that causes toxin-mediated intestinal inflammation ranging from mild diarrhoea to fulminant severe life-threatening disease. *C. difficile* remains the leading cause of nosocomial diarrhoea in the developed world, and predominately affects the older population. Several outbreaks were reported in the media that were later attributed to a previously inconspicuous strain known as ribotype 027. First identified in Canada, this strain was quinolone resistant and capable of producing more toxin, which resulted in a higher degree of mortality and morbidity [1]. In 2007, the Department of Health (DoH) implemented infection control measures and mandatory reporting of cases in patients aged 2 years and above to the HPA (now PHE). As a result reported rates have continued to fall from 36,095 in 2008 to 18,000 in 2011 [2, 3]. However, despite this success the epidemiology of CDI is changing. Cases have increased in previously low-risk groups including children, pregnant women, and patients in the community. Clinical isolates have been detected in food products introducing the possibility of an animal reservoir of disease. Finally, ribotype 027 has almost disappeared in the UK, recent data reports the emergence of new virulent strains such as 078 and 015.

> ⭐ **Learning point** Typing methods used in CDI
>
> *C. difficile* isolates are named based on the predominant molecular technique used for epidemiological typing. In the UK strains are classified by ribotype for example 'ribotype 027'. In 2007, the HPA established the *Clostridium difficile* Ribotyping Network (CDRN) to facilitate the investigation of outbreaks. A number of other techniques have been employed to characterize strains and are outlined below.
>
> **Ribotyping:** PCR is used to discriminate differences in spacer regions of 16s and 23s ribosomes. Amplification of DNA encoding these regions produces distinct bands and is viewed by gel electrophoresis. Each distinct pattern corresponds to an individual ribotype. Although this test can be performed easily and rapidly, it may have relatively less discriminatory power compared with other techniques.
>
> **Pulse field gel electrophoresis (PFGE):** Restriction enzymes are used to splice the bacterial genome into large fragments of DNA that are transferred to a polyacrylamide gel. An alternating current separates fragments based on their molecular size into multiple bands that represent the entire chromosome.
>
> **Restriction endonuclease analysis (REA):** This technique is similar to PFGE but involves more frequent cutting of the genome resulting in the generation of hundreds of fragments that can be difficult to interpret. This is further confounded by the presence of extra-chromosomal DNA.
>
> **Multilocus variable number tandem repeat analysis (MLVA):** PCR is used to detect variation in the number of tandem repeated DNA sequences that exist at different loci within a bacterial genome. This produces a unique MLVA profile that can easily be compared between laboratories via central databases. The CDRN has used this highly discriminatory technique to investigate outbreaks of CDI.

> ➕ **Clinical tip** Defining severity in CDI [3]
>
> **Mild CDI**
> - No associated rise in WCC
> - <3 stools/day, type 5–7 on Bristol Stool Chart
>
> **Moderate CDI**
> - Raised WCC <15×10^9/L
> - 3–5 stools/day
>
> **Severe CDI**
> - WCC >15×10^9/L
> - Acute rising serum creatinine (>50% increase above baseline)
> - Temperature >38.5°C
> - Evidence of severe colitis (abdominal or radiological signs)
> Note: Correlation between stool frequency and severe disease is less well established
>
> **Life-threatening CDI**
> - Hypotension
> - Partial or complete ileus (including vomiting and absent passage of stool)
> - Evidence of toxic megacolon seen on CT

> **ⓖ Expert comment** Choice of vancomycin as initial therapy
>
> Vancomycin is superior to metronidazole for the treatment of severe CDI, being associated with better response to treatment, lower mortality and lower relapse rate [4]. Although it has not been demonstrated specifically for CDI, the speed with which effective treatment is started is a major determinant of outcome in life-threatening infection. For these reasons, when a patient is treated empirically for CDI before a diagnostic test result is available, the choice of empiric therapy should be based on severity assessment, with vancomycin chosen if there are any markers of severe disease. In patients with an ileus in whom vancomycin given orally may not reach the colon, vancomycin enemas and dual therapy with IV metronidazole should be considered.

The diagnosis was confirmed the following day on stool testing and the patient was transferred for isolation to a cohort ward (Box 20.1).

✪ Learning point Diagnostic microbiology

C. difficile was named thus due to the difficulties associated with culturing this organism. Although culture remains the gold standard, this is laborious and time consuming. As a result, diagnostic testing became reliant on detection of toxin using commercial EIA kits. These were easy and quick to use; however, limited by poor sensitivity, they resulted in a large number of false-positives that contributed to an over-reporting of cases, which has implications for infection control. More recently, a two-stage testing approach has been adopted (Figure 20.1). This involves an initial sensitive test (GDH testing or NAAT), followed by a more specific test (EIA) as confirmation.

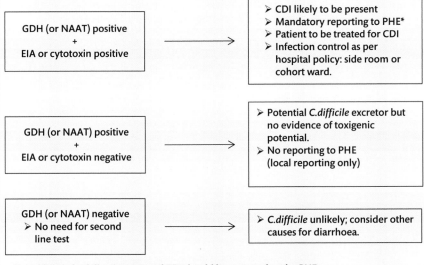

*In addition the following cases of CDI should be reported to the PHE:
- Pseudomembranous colitis diagnosed on colonoscopy or CT.
- Colonic histopathology characteristic of CDI (in the absence of diarrhoea or toxin detection) obtained during endoscopy or colectomy.
- *C. difficile* toxin positive faecal specimens at post-mortem with gross or microscopic evidence of -

Figure 20.1 *Clostridium difficile* diagnostic algorithm [5].
Source: Data from Department of Health, *Updated guidance on the diagnosis and reporting of Clostridium difficile.*
© Crown copyright 2012, available from http://www.dh.gov.uk/en/Publicationsandstatistics/Publications/PublicationsPolicyAndGuidance/DH_132927

(continued)

Glossary of diagnostic tests

EIA: Detects the presence of toxins A and B.

Cytotoxin: Reference test for the presence of toxins. Cell rounding occurs due to changes in the cell cytoskeletal structure.

GDH: This antigen is produced in large amounts by both toxin-producing and non-toxin-producing *C. difficile* strains and therefore only identifies the presence of the organism, not pathogenic potential.

Nucleic acid amplification technique: Detects the presence of toxin genes. PCR is a type of NAAT.

Culture: This is the gold standard but is limited by the time taken to grow the organism.

❝ Expert comment
Concomitant PPIs

PPIs and other drugs that suppress gastric acid secretion are considered to be risk factors for developing CDI. In reality the risk they confer appears to be relatively small, comparable to low-risk antibiotics such as parenteral vancomycin [7]. Doctors should ensure that PPIs are only prescribed to patients at risk of CDI when there is a clear indication; however, when a patient develops CDI the benefit of stopping PPIs is likely to be small.

Box 20.1 Infection control

Following outbreaks at Stoke Mandeville Hospital and Maidstone Hospital, the Healthcare Commission made several recommendations which are outlined in the DoH guidelines [1]. These include rapid isolation of patients in individual side rooms or transfer to a CDI-specific cohort isolation ward as an alternative. Suspected cases should be isolated as soon as possible and remain isolated until symptom-free for at least 48 hours when a formed stool has occurred. Movement of confirmed cases between wards and departments should be limited to avoid potential transmission of cases. It is well established that CDI spores are highly resistant and remain as fomites for several years. Several studies have shown that cleaning using detergent alone is insufficient; a chlorine-based agent should be used for environmental cleaning of bed spaces, commodes, and bathrooms.

Individual Hospital Trusts should have a designated infection control team with individual link practitioners for each clinical area whose role involves education, training, and conducting audits. They must provide regular feedback to staff on cleaning, isolation, and maintaining good hand hygiene as *C. difficile* spores are resistant to alcohol-based gels. In the future, novel molecular techniques such as whole genome sequencing (WGS) will help shape infection control in CDI. WGS provides an opportunity to establish the true genetic relatedness of strains and to accurately determine transmission events between patients. As the cost of sequencing falls it will allow the rapid and accurate identification of outbreaks at a local level, thereby informing infection control decisions [6].

❝ Expert comment Cohorting of patients with CDI

Shared time and space on a ward with a patient who has CDI is a major risk factor for developing CDI, at least when disease prevalence rates are high. Prompt isolation of patients has therefore been a cornerstone of efforts to reduce CDI rates in National Health Service settings. In many old hospitals a lack of side rooms has led to the establishment of cohort wards where patients with CDI are nursed together. This approach also has the advantage of allowing the development of medical and nursing expertise in the management of CDI. This in turn demonstrates that the hospital is focused on delivering best care to a patient who has developed CDI during their stay. Patients should not be transferred to a cohort ward unless they have laboratory-confirmed CDI. Patients on the cohort ward should be managed by a single medical team with multidisciplinary support to minimize the movement of medical staff between the ward and the wider hospital. Cohort wards will inevitably have lower bed occupancy rates than general wards and Hospital Trust managers will need to be advised of this. Higher nurse-to-patient ratios may be required, given the high dependency of patients with acute CDI and the need to maintain scrupulous infection control practice. Patients who have recently had CDI may remain infectious after diarrhoea has ceased. If patients continue to be nursed on a cohort ward after cessation of diarrhoea, contact with active cases of disease should be minimized to prevent the possibility of re-infection.

Omeprazole was discontinued and a plain abdominal film requested which revealed gas-filled loops of small bowel.

> **Clinical tip** Investigating CDI and differential diagnosis
>
> **Investigations**
> - **Stool microscopy and culture**
> - **Plain abdominal film ± CT:** Bowel dilatation, mural thickening, and thumb-printing can be seen due to thickening of haustral folds. In severe cases rapid bowel dilatation known as toxic megacolon can occur. This can progress to bowel perforation.
> - **Colonoscopy:** In fulminant cases a pseudomembranous colitis can be seen. This consists of yellow, polypoid lesions on a hyperaemic mucosa. Histology demonstrates a neutrophilic infiltration of the lamina propria and mucopurulent exudate eruption through the denuded surface epithelium.
>
> **Differential diagnosis**
>
> The main differential is antibiotic-associated diarrhoea (AAD), which occurs in up to 25% of individuals following a course of antibiotics. Other pathogens associated with AAD include *Klebsiella oxytoca*, *Staphyloccus aureus*, and norovirus. Antibiotics can directly affect the intestinal tract and increase transit time, resulting in diarrhoea. In the absence of an inflammatory response other causes of diarrhoea such as pancreatic insufficiency should be considered.

The patient responded well to initial treatment with a reduction in stool frequency. On day 5, he developed a productive cough and was commenced on tazocin for hospital-acquired pneumonia. CDI treatment was continued. Over the following 48 hours his respiratory symptoms settled and the patient reported feeling much improved. Unfortunately, on day 9 of his admission he developed diarrhoea and reported over 15 episodes in 24 hours.

> **Learning point** Pathophysiology and CA use in CDI
>
> CDI patients tend to be older, have prolonged hospitalization, and are often on antibiotics at the time of infection with CDI.
>
> Antibiotics disrupt the host intestinal microbiota, permitting overgrowth of indigenous *C. difficile* or allowing ingested environmental spores to colonize and germinate. The organism produces two main virulence factors, toxin A and toxin B, that belong to the large clostridial glucosylating toxins. These destroy the colonic epithelial integrity, resulting in epithelial detachment, fluid accumulation, and tissue destruction. Certain strains produce a third binary toxin whose function remains to be established. Mullane et al. evaluated the effects of CA in CDI patients [8]. The study found that 28% of patients were treated with CA at the same time as CDI treatment or during the 4-week follow-up period. Receipt of any CA was associated with a significant reduction in CDI cure rate from 96.2% to 84.4% (p <0.001) and prolonged the median time to resolution of diarrhoea by 43 hours. There was a trend towards CA use and increased recurrence with a 50% increased recurrence risk in patients receiving CA during the follow-up period (24.8% vs. 17.8%). Patients treated with 'high risk' CA, including carbapenems and fluoroquinolones, showed a tendency to increased recurrence rates although the effects did not reach statistical significance. Prescriptions of CA are often unavoidable; however, clinicians should aim to use low-risk antibiotics for the minimum duration to limit harmful effects.

Expert comment CA

Most patients diagnosed with CDI are receiving or will need to receive systemic antibiotics for other infections. This may reduce the efficacy of CDI treatment. One very useful lesson to come out of the fidaxomicin trials has been the data on efficacy of CDI treatment in the face of CA [11–13]. The results of the fidaxomicin trials should be interpreted with some caution since the patients were much younger than typical CDI patients in the UK and the protocol discouraged recruitment of patients likely to need CA. Nevertheless, it would appear that patients who need systemic antibiotic therapy do generally still respond well to CDI treatment, albeit more slowly and with a greater risk of recurrence. Clinicians should ensure optimal treatment of life-threatening infections such as nosocomial pneumonia in elderly patients even in the presence of active CDI.

Oral vancomycin therapy was therefore increased to 250 mg 4 times daily, and a colonoscopy was performed that showed an inflamed left colon but was otherwise grossly normal. By day 14 his symptoms had resolved and he was discharged. Unfortunately, 3 weeks after cessation of treatment he suffered a recurrence of his symptoms and was readmitted. The vancomycin was recommenced at 500 mg 4 times daily and symptom resolution was achieved after 72 hours. He was discharged on a tapering course of vancomycin and has remained in remission since.

Discussion

This case highlights the challenges associated with managing severe CDI which often requires multiple courses of antibiotics with frequent hospitalization and can cause great distress and morbidity to patients. Recurrence of CDI remains a significant problem in 20–30% of cases despite successful initial antimicrobial treatment and can be due to recrudescence of the same strain or re-infection following acquisition of a novel strain from an exogenous source.

CDI treatment is based on disease severity, with metronidazole reserved for mild cases and vancomycin for moderate to severe cases. Any unnecessary antibiotics should be discontinued at the earliest opportunity.

Evidence base Predicting severity in CDI

In 2009, the ESCMID released important guidelines that described factors associated with CDI severity and outlined different treatment options [9]. A combination of clinical observations, imaging, and laboratory parameters were identified and summarized by the HPA (now PHE) as possible markers of CDI severity (see Clinical tip: Defining severity in CDI) (3). Severe CDI defined as recurrence of disease or deterioration in clinical symptoms carries a higher risk of treatment failure. In a clinical setting, early identification of those patients most likely to experience severe CDI in order to guide treatment. Prognostic scores proposed have included different factors such as age, underlying co-morbidity, and CA use. However, the majority of scores tested used small derivation cohorts and failed to validate scores in a large prospective cohort. In a recent study, markers of severe CDI suggested in national guidelines (fever >38°C, leucocytosis >15 × 10^9, and renal failure defined as creatinine >133 μmol/L) were evaluated [10]. A database consisting of 1,105 patients recruited as part of the fidaxomicin phase III clinical trials was used (Evidence base: Fidaxomicin versus vancomycin for CDI). Both leucocytosis (RR 2.29, 95% CI 1.63–3.21) and renal failure (RR 2.52, 95% CI 1.82–3.50) were associated with treatment failure. Fever occurred too infrequently to be of use as a prognostic marker in severe CDI. Renal failure was also predictive of CDI recurrence. The group went on to show the importance of timing on the predictive value of laboratory parameters, reporting that a

(continued)

difference in timing of a single blood sample could lead to a difference in CDI severity classification. Creatinine is likely to be the most useful prognostic marker due to its inherent stability around the time of diagnosis. Future work should focus on identification and validation of biomarkers for severe CDI that can be used to develop clinical predictive tools.

Where ileus is suspected vancomycin can be given intra-colonically by enema with surgical colectomy reserved for life-threatening cases that includes toxic megacolon and colonic perforation.

CDI recurrence

An initial recurrence is treated with the same regime as the index episode; however, the evidence basis for managing multiple episodes is less well established. Vancomycin can be given tapered or pulsed, which involves alternating high-dose and treatment-free days. Rifaximin after a course of vancomycin as a 'rifaximin chaser' has been used in some cases but may be limited by emerging antibiotic resistance. An exciting development has been the introduction of fidaxomicin, the first new antimicrobial to be licensed for adult CDI in 25 years. This novel macrocyclic antibiotic inhibits RNA polymerase and has a narrow spectrum of activity. The drug is associated with lower recurrence rates and causes less perturbation to the host microbiota than vancomycin [11]. Of note, the clinical trials of fidaxomicin have not recruited patients with life-threatening disease and as such there is a lack of good evidence for the equivalence of fidaxomicin to vancomycin in this group. However, the limitation to widespread use of fidaxomicin is likely to be its cost, with a 10-day course priced at $2,800, almost 20 times the cost of vancomycin. Therefore, at present fidaxomicin will most likely be used on an individual basis in those with refractory disease.

⊘ Evidence base Fidaxomicin versus vancomycin for CDI [12,13]

Aim: To assess the safety and efficacy of fidaxomicin compared to vancomycin.

Study design: Two phase 3, multicentre, double-blind RCTs across 154 sites in North America, Canada, and Europe [12,13]. All adults with acute CDI symptoms and a positive stool toxin test were eligible for recruitment. Patients were randomized to 200 mg fidaxomicin twice daily or vancomycin 125 mg 4 times a day for 10 days and followed up for 28 days. The primary endpoint was clinical cure (resolution of symptoms with no further need for therapy). Secondary endpoints were recurrence of CDI (diarrhoea and a positive stool toxin test within 4 weeks of treatment) and global cure or sustained response (defined as cure with no recurrence). Outcomes were compared by treatment and subgroup analyses and included age, inpatient status, previous CDI, CA (infections other than CDI), severity, strain type, and region.

Results: A total of 1,164 patients were enrolled with similar results in both studies (Table 20.2). The main finding was an increase in global cure due to a significant reduction in recurrence rates. However, it is interesting that no difference was seen in patients infected with the BI/NAP1/027 strain. In the European study, a larger number of patients on CA achieved clinical cure when treated with fidaxomicin versus vancomycin (90.2% vs. 73.3%, p = 0.031). All other outcomes were similar between treatment groups on subgroup analyses, and adverse event rates were comparable between both treatments.

Conclusion: Fidaxomicin was non-inferior to vancomycin in terms of clinical cure. Patients treated with fidaxomicin experienced overall lower rates of recurrence and increased global cure.

(continued)

Table 20.2 Fidaxomicin RCT endpoints. Values shown are the modified intention-to-treat analysis. Results were consistent for the per-protocol analysis

| | Louie et al. [12] | | | Cornely et al. [13] | | |
| | 51 sites in N. America (n = 629) | | | 45 sites in Europe, 41 sites in N. America (n = 535) | | |
	Fidaxomicin	Vancomycin	p value	Fidaxomicin	Vancomycin	p value
Clinical cure	88.2	85.8	–	87.7	86.8	0.754
Recurrence rate	15.4	25.3	0.005	12.7	26.9	0.0002
Global cure	74.6	64.1	0.006	76.7	63.4	0.001

Direct replacement of the disrupted intestinal microbiota is an attractive option. Possibilities include faecal transplants (FTs), probiotics, and non-toxigenic *C. difficile* strains. In the healthy state the intestinal microbiota maintains a stable ecosystem by outcompeting pathogenic organisms for space, surface receptors, and nutrients through a process known as colonization resistance.

Faecal transplantation or faecal microbiota transplantation (FMT) was first described in 1950 and involves instillation of a liquid suspension of stool from a healthy donor into an infected patient's GI tract by nasogastric tube, colonoscopy, or rectal enema. The advantages of this treatment are its low cost and sustainable effects. FMT has been used to treat severe refractory disease and has resulted in resolution of symptoms in over 80% of cases that have previously been described in individual reports and case series [14]. The first RCT trial of FMT was recently conducted and compared infusion of donor faeces following standard vancomycin treatment and bowel lavage to vancomycin therapy with bowel lavage or vancomycin alone [15]. A total of 43 patients were recruited and a significantly higher cure rate was observed in patients treated with FMT compared to those that received vancomycin or vancomycin and bowel lavage (81% vs. 31% vs. 23%, p <0.001). However, the trial was terminated early after interim analysis because almost all patients in the control groups experienced CDI recurrence. The main limitations to FMT are the aesthetics involved with using donor faeces and the logistical challenges of harvesting and processing stool. This may be overcome in the future through the storage of pre-screened anonymous donor material.

Probiotics are live microorganisms that confer a health benefit to the host if given in adequate amounts. Several small studies have suggested they may play a role in preventing AAD including CDI; however, there is no evidence to support their use in the treatment of acute CDI. Only one study, using *Saccharomyces boulardii* as an adjunct to high-dose vancomycin, showed a significant reduction in CDI recurrence when compared to placebo and larger RCTs are needed [16].

A considerable body of evidence exists describing the role of the immune response in determining disease outcome in CDI. Antibodies to both toxin a and toxin b may be generated following transient colonization with the organism in infancy and over 60% of the adult population possess antitoxin antibodies. Lower antibody titres to toxin a levels have been shown to predispose individuals to CDI recurrence [17]. This has contributed to the scientific rationale for using intravenous pooled immunoglobulin to treat refractory disease. However, the grade of evidence is weak with a lack of RCTs and is not recommended in European or American guidelines [9, 18]. Human mAbs have shown promise in reducing recurrence rates and a toxoid vaccine is undergoing evaluation. The efficacy of such a vaccine may be limited in older patients who have an aged immune system characterized by reductions in B lymphocytes, antibody diversity, and antibody affinity.

A final word from the expert

The dramatic decline in C. *difficile* rates seen in the UK since 2006 and the waning of ribotype 027 should not be a reason for complacency about this disease. With the recognition of novel virulent strains of other ribotypes and an aging population, it is clear that CDI will remain a threat to elderly patients, particularly in hospital. This case illustrates the importance of early recognition, diagnosis, and assessment of severe CDI to ensure both optimal infection control and management. The advent of fidaxomicin represents a significant advance but important questions remain around selection of patients to receive this treatment. Faecal therapy is now supported by RCT evidence but more extensive clinical evaluation of this method, in particular the role of synthetic stool, is needed before this approach is likely to be widely adopted.

References

1 Pépin J, Valiquette L, Alary M-E et al. *Clostridium difficile*-associated diarrhea in a region of Quebec from 1991 to 2003: a changing pattern of disease severity. *CMAJ* 2004; 171: 466–472.

2 Health Protection Agency. *Summary points on Clostridium difficile infection(CDI)* [Internet]. 2011 Mar. Available from: http://www.hpa.org.uk

3 Health Protection Agency and Department of Health. *Clostridium difficile infection: how to deal with the problem* [Internet]. 2009 [cited 2012 Jul 20]. Available from: http://www.dh.gov.uk

4 Zar FA, Bakkanagari SR, Moorthi KM, Davis MB. A comparison of vancomycin and metronidazole for the treatment of *Clostridium difficile*-associated diarrhea, stratified by disease severity. *Clin Infect Dis* 2007; 45: 302–307.

5 Health Protection Agency and Department of Health. *Updated guidance on the diagnosis and reporting of Clostridium difficile* [Internet]. 2012 [cited 2012 Jul 19]. Available from: http://www.dh.gov.uk

6 Eyre DW, Golubchik T, Gordon NC et al. A pilot study of rapid benchtop sequencing of *Staphylococcus aureus* and *Clostridium difficile* for outbreak detection and surveillance. *BMJ Open* 2012; 2(3).

7 Dubberke ER, Reske KA, Yan Y, Olsen MA, McDonald LC, Fraser VJ. *Clostridium difficile*-associated disease in a setting of endemicity: identification of novel risk factors. *Clin Infect Dis* 2007; 45: 1543–1549.

8 Mullane KM, Miller MA, Weiss K et al. Efficacy of fidaxomicin versus vancomycin as therapy for *Clostridium difficile* infection in individuals taking concomitant antibiotics for other concurrent infections. *Clin Infect Dis* 2011; 53: 440–447.

9 Bauer MP, Kuijper EJ, Van Dissel JT. European Society of Clinical Microbiology and Infectious Diseases (ESCMID): treatment guidance document for *Clostridium difficile* infection (CDI). *Clin Microbiol Infect* 2009; 15: 1067–1079.

10 Bauer MP, Hensgens MPM, Miller MA et al. Renal failure and leukocytosis are predictors of a complicated course of *Clostridium difficile* infection if measured on day of diagnosis. *Clin Infect Dis* 2012; 55 Suppl 2: S149–153.

11 Louie TJ, Cannon K, Byrne B et al. Fidaxomicin preserves the intestinal microbiome during and after treatment of *Clostridium difficile* infection (CDI) and reduces both toxin reexpression and recurrence of CDI. *Clin Infect Dis* 2012; 55 Suppl 2: S132–142.

12 Louie TJ, Miller MA, Mullane KM et al. Fidaxomicin versus vancomycin for *Clostridium difficile* infection. *N Engl J Med* 2011; 364: 422–431.

13 Cornely OA, Crook DW, Esposito R et al. Fidaxomicin versus vancomycin for infection with *Clostridium difficile* in Europe, Canada, and the USA: a double-blind, non-inferiority, randomised controlled trial. *Lancet Infect Dis* 2012; 12: 281–289.

14 Bakken JS. Fecal bacteriotherapy for recurrent *Clostridium difficile* infection. *Anaerobe* 2009; 15: 285–289.

15 Van Nood E, Vrieze A, Nieuwdorp M et al. Duodenal infusion of donor feces for recurrent *Clostridium difficile*. *N Engl J Med* 2013; 368: 407–415.

16 Surawicz CM, McFarland LV, Greenberg RN et al. The search for a better treatment for recurrent *Clostridium difficile* disease: use of high-dose vancomycin combined with *Saccharomyces boulardii*. *Clin Infect Dis* 2000; 31: 1012–1017.

17 Kyne L, Warny M, Qamar A, Kelly CP. Association between antibody response to toxin A and protection against recurrent *Clostridium difficile* diarrhoea. *Lancet* 2001; 357: 189–193.

18 Cohen SH, Gerding DN, Johnson S et al. Clinical practice guidelines for *Clostridium difficile* infection in adults: 2010 update by the society for healthcare epidemiology of America (SHEA) and the infectious diseases society of America (IDSA). *Infect Control Hosp Epidemiol* 2010; 31(5): 431–455.

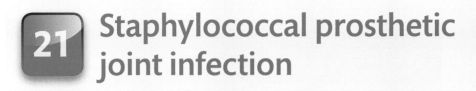

21 Staphylococcal prosthetic joint infection

Kate El Bouzidi

🎤 **Expert commentary** Matthew Laundy

Case history

A 72-year-old man presented to his general practitioner with a 10-day history of right hip pain which was limiting his mobility. He felt generally unwell and reported loss of appetite and lethargy. He had a history of type 2 diabetes mellitus and osteoarthritis for which he had undergone a right total hip replacement 3 years earlier. On examination, he had a temperature of 37.7°C, pulse 90 bpm and normal blood pressure. The right hip joint was tender on palpation with a reduced range of movement but there was no over-lying erythema or discharge. The GP suspected a prosthetic joint infection (PJI) and pre-scribed oral flucloxacillin before referring the patient for an urgent orthopaedic opinion.

The patient was admitted to hospital and an X-ray of the hip was consistent with prosthetic joint infection (Figure 21.1). On further questioning he had no history of recent skin breaks, trauma, or intravenous cannulation to suggest a source of infection, though he did have poor glycaemic control. There had been no wound complications following the total hip replacement.

> ➕ **Clinical tip** Radiological findings in bone and joint infection [1]
>
> **Plain radiography**
> - Periostitis, erosion, sclerosis, sequestra, soft tissue swelling, loose prosthesis
> - Remains normal for 10–14 days so not useful in acute osteomyelitis
>
> **Ultrasonography**
> - Effusions, synovial thickening, soft tissue collections
> - May be used to guide aspiration
>
> **CT**
> - Soft tissue/bone lesions, joint distention, fluid-filled bursae, hypoattenuation
> - Hardware artefact may interfere
>
> **MRI**
> - Standard modality for diagnosing native osteomyelitis
> - Less useful in PJI because of metal artefact
> - Cannot differentiate between marrow infection and reactive oedema
> - False-positive in postoperative phase and during non-infectious inflammation
>
> **Nuclear imaging**
> - Three-phase bone scan, white cell scan, PET
> - False-positive with recent surgery, degenerative disease, tumours

> 🎤 **Expert comment** GP referral
>
> The urgent referral by the GP, rather than awaiting outpatient investigations, was correct. Prosthetic joint infection is a serious complication which requires orthopaedic assessment and cannot be managed initially in the primary care setting. The prescribing of oral antibiotics was inappropriate, however, as they are unlikely to alter the course of infection and likely to hamper microbiological diagnosis, making treatment more difficult.

Initial investigations are summarized in Table 21.1. An ultrasound-guided joint aspi-ration yielded blood-stained purulent fluid which strongly suggested the diagnosis of

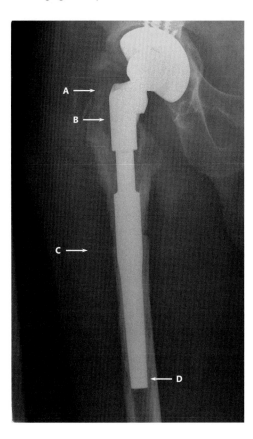

Figure 21.1 X-ray of the hip showing a) subcutaneous collection, b) periosteal reaction, c) small bony fragment in the adjacent soft tissues, and d) periprosthetic loosening.

prosthetic joint infection but fluid culture was negative despite prolonged incubation. Antibiotics were withheld as the patient remained haemodynamically stable and was closely monitored for signs of sepsis.

The surgical options were discussed with the patient and two-stage revision arthroplasty was agreed. The patient deteriorated following the joint aspiration, with a high-grade fever and tachycardia, and was taken urgently to theatre. The prosthesis was found to be loose and there were several tissue abscesses requiring drainage and irrigation. Intraoperative vancomycin and gentamicin were administered after periprosthetic tissue samples had been collected for microbiology and histology. The infected tissue was radically debrided and all prosthetic components were removed and replaced with a spacer loaded with vancomycin. Four of five tissue specimens cultured meticillin-sensitive *Staphylococcus aureus* (MSSA) and the infection was assumed to be the result of haematogenous seeding.

Table 21.1 Initial investigations

Haematology	Biochemistry	Microbiology
Hb: 13.4 g/dL	Urea: 10.6 mmol/L	Blood cultures: no growth
WCC: 11 × 10⁹/L	Creatinine: 210 µmol/L	MRSA screen: negative
Platelets: 460 × 10⁹/L	Albumin: 30 g/L	Hip aspirate: turbid fluid
ESR: 75 mm/hour	CRP: 132 mg/L	>95% neutrophils
		Gram: no organisms seen
		No growth at 5 days

> ✪ **Learning point** Prosthetic joint infection: classification and microbiology
>
> **Classification [4]**
>
> Early: <3 months after surgery
> - Often infected at time of surgery or by contiguous spread from wound
> - Virulent organisms, e.g. *Staphylococcus aureus* (*S. aureus*), GNB
>
> Delayed: 3–24 months after surgery
> - Usually occurs during prosthesis implantation, indolent presentation
> - Low virulence, e.g. coagulase-negative staphylococci, *Propionibacterium acnes*
>
> Late: >24 months after surgery
> - Haematogenous seeding during bacteraemia, acute presentation
> - Secondary infection from skin, respiratory, dental and urinary sources
>
> **Microbiology (see Table 21.2 [4])**
>
> Prosthetic joint infection may be caused by unusual pathogens such as fungi or *Mtb* in high-risk populations. [3]
>
> **Table 21.2 Relative frequency of organisms causing PJI**
>
> | Organism | Frequency |
> | --- | --- |
> | Coagulase-negative staphylococci | 30–43% |
> | *S. aureus* | 12–23% |
> | *Streptococcus* spp. | 9–10% |
> | Enterococci | 3–7% |
> | Gram-negative bacteria | 3–6% |
> | Anaerobes | 2–4% |
> | Polymicrobial infection | 10–11% |
> | Culture-negative infection | 11% |

Antibiotics were rationalized to intravenous flucloxacillin 2 g four times daily. After a period of inpatient rehabilitation the patient was referred to the outpatient parenteral antibiotic therapy (OPAT) team to allow ongoing administration at home. Teicoplanin was chosen for a convenient od regimen and therapeutic drug levels were achieved with a dose of 600 mg. In addition oral RIF was prescribed at a dose of 300 mg twice daily. Two weeks after discharge, blood samples sent from the OPAT clinic revealed a drop in the platelet count to 44×10^9/L. A glycopeptide-related thrombocytopenia was suspected and the antibiotic treatment was changed to ceftriaxone and the platelet count returned to normal. The CRP was <4 mg/L by the end of 6 weeks of treatment and the patient had a 2-week antibiotic-free period before the second stage operation. The spacer was removed and a new prosthesis was fixed with cement loaded with vancomycin and gentamicin. Prophylactic cefotaxime was given for 48 hours until negative tissue cultures of operative tissue confirmed eradication of the infection. The patient made an uneventful recovery and no further antibiotics were given. He remained well with good hip function and a normal CRP during 6 months of follow-up.

Discussion

This case highlights several challenges in the management of prosthetic joint infection (PJI). The organism was not confirmed until after the first operation and prior antibiotic treatment probably led to the negative aspirate culture. The patient opted for two-stage revision arthroplasty but there are several surgical strategies that can be used to manage prosthetic joint infection. There were also decisions to be made regarding inpatient and outpatient intravenous antibiotic therapy, use of a second antimicrobial agent, local antibiotics, and duration of therapy. Staphylococci account for the majority of prosthetic joint infections.

✪ **Learning point** Staphylococcal prosthetic joint infection: pathophysiology [4]

Pathogenesis

- Staphylococci can enter the joint at the time of prosthesis implantation, via contiguous spread from adjacent soft tissue infection, or from haematogenous seeding.
- The presence of a foreign body causes impaired granulocyte activity and a local immune response deficit which leaves the joint vulnerable to infection even with organisms of low virulence.
- *S. aureus* releases superantigens (enterotoxins A, B, C, D and toxic shock syndrome toxin 1; TSST-1) and cytolytic toxins (alpha, beta, and gamma toxin) which contribute to inflammation and tissue damage.
- *S. aureus* can evade the host immune response by invading osteoblasts and promotes osteolysis via cytokine release and osteoclast formation.
- *S. epidermidis* also releases virulence factors which allow it to attach to host matrix proteins and prosthetic surfaces.
- Raised intramedullary pressure causes bone ischaemia and the spread of abscesses into adjacent soft tissues.

Biofilm formation

- Microcolonies of bacteria coalesce to form a biofilm of cells embedded in an extracellular matrix of polysaccharide glycocalyx. This provides protection against bacterial clearance and prevents penetration of antibiotics.
- *S. aureus* binds to ligands on host proteins coating the implant via adhesins such as MSCRAMM (microbial surface components recognizing adhesive matrix molecules).
- *S. epidermidis* biofilm formation is mediated by specific adhesins such as the polysaccharide intercellular adhesin encoded by the intercellular adhesion (*ica*) operon.
- The sessile bacteria exhibit an altered phenotype with reduced metabolism and cell division and this stationary phase confers resistance to many antimicrobials.
- Cell-to-cell signalling molecules are used to communicate and coordinate gene expression between populations, which is known as quorum sensing.

Diagnosis

In this case there was high suspicion of infection based on the symptoms, radiological findings, and inflammatory markers, but indolent infections with organisms of low pathogenicity may be difficult to definitively diagnose. The patient had a diagnostic arthrocentesis in accordance with the IDSA guidelines on diagnosis and management of prosthetic joint infection [2]. Preoperative sampling is recommended to differentiate PJI from other conditions such as mechanical loosening or haemarthrosis, and to obtain microbiological diagnosis. Joint aspiration culture had a sensitivity of 73–80% and specificity of 94–95% for confirming infection in two studies including 239 knees [1]. Hip fluid culture identified the causative organism in 60% of infected hips (n = 291) [1].

The aspiration in this case revealed purulent fluid with polymorphic inflammation pattern which was sufficient evidence of PJI to proceed to immediate arthroplasty when the patient deteriorated. If the organism is not identified by aspiration, tissue may be obtained for culture by arthroscopy or during joint replacement surgery. Atkins et al. recommend collecting a minimum of five deep tissue specimens for culture using different sterile instruments before intraoperative antibiotics are administered [5]. They found that the isolation of indistinguishable organisms from three or more specimens was highly predictive of infection, with a sensitivity of 65% and specificity of 99.6% in a series of 41 prosthetic joint infections [5]. Gram stain, although highly specific for infection if positive, had a poor diagnostic yield of 12%. Histological examination of periprosthetic tissue for the presence of five or more polymorphonuclear leucocytes per high power field has 80% sensitivity and 91% specificity for diagnosing infection [1]. In practice this is limited by high interobserver variability [4].

An alternative method for microbiological diagnosis is sonication of the extracted prosthesis. Sonication uses sound waves to disrupt the biofilm coating on an explanted prosthesis and disperse the bacteria into a planktonic form in solution. The sonicate fluid is then cultured and the number of CFU is recorded. This technique preserves microbial viability and proponents argue that the results are more representative of the microorganisms involved in prosthesis infection than periprosthetic tissue culture. Trampuz et al. conducted a prospective trial of 331 patients undergoing revision arthroplasty to compare sonication to periprosthetic tissue culture [6]. This included 79 patients with PJI, as defined by visible purulence, neutrophilic tissue inflammation, or a communicating sinus tract. Tissue cultures were considered positive if two or more samples grew the same organism and the yield increased with the number of samples sent (50% with two samples and 72.7% with five or more). Optimal sensitivity and specificity for sonicate cultures were achieved if there were at least 5 CFU of the same organism. The overall sensitivity of tissue cultures was 60.8%, compared to 78.5% for sonicate fluid (p < 0.001). The specificity was similar, 99.2% and 98.8% respectively. In patients who had received antibiotics in the 14 days prior to surgery, the sensitivity fell to 45% for conventional cultures, but remained high at 75% for sonication (p < 0.001). Fourteen cases of infection were detected by sonication but missed by tissue sampling.

> **Expert comment** PCR
>
> Samples which are negative on culture may be investigated using established molecular techniques. Species-specific PCR assays are readily available for *S. aureus* and streptococcal species, among others. In cases where the organism is not detected using these techniques, a broad range 16S PCR followed by sequencing may be used to detect and identify bacteria. However, 16S PCR suffers from reduced sensitivity as compared to species-specific PCR, so should be used after specific PCR. At present limited information can be gained on antibiotic resistance patterns using these techniques, though this is likely to change in the future.

Surgery

This patient underwent two-stage revision arthroplasty, which is the most frequently performed surgery for prosthesis infection in the UK. This method accounted for 65% of hip and knee PJI surgery reported to the UK National Joint Registry in 2011. The patient must be fit enough to undergo two major operations and there is often poor function and limb instability between stages. There is no clear evidence regarding the optimum interval between stages, and in practice this is influenced by inflammatory markers, nutritional indices, wound healing, and patient factors.

A subset of patients may be managed with one-stage revision arthroplasty, a single operation in which the whole implant and all infected tissue are removed and a new prosthesis is implanted into the debrided cavity. This approach is often used for patients with a high anaesthetic risk and is also cheaper and preferred by patients as it permits earlier mobilization. However, potential candidates must fulfil strict criteria, as listed in Box 21.1 [3].

> **Box 21.1** Criteria for one-stage revision
> - No severe co-morbidities
> - No difficult-to-treat organisms
> - Uncomplicated anatomy
> - Satisfactory condition of soft tissue
> - No need for bone graft
> - Extensive debridement achieved

Bejon et al. reported the outcomes of 152 two-stage revisions for PJI managed at a tertiary bone infection unit [7]. All patients received a 6-week course of intravenous β-lactam or glycopeptide. Twenty-four patients (16%) underwent at least one additional debridement and a further course of antibiotics. Failure included revision of the prosthesis for any reason, amputation, and sinus recurrence. The overall success rate of two-stage revision surgery was 83%. Re-revisions did worse with only 73% retaining the prosthesis compared to 89% of first revisions.

An identical success rate of 83% was found in a review of 1,299 one-stage hip revisions with removal of all prosthetic components and reimplantation with antibiotic-impregnated cement. Factors associated with eradication were uncomplicated wound healing after the initial hip replacement, good general health of the patient, the use of an effective antibiotic in the cement, and MSSA and streptococcal infections [3].

There is a lack of randomized trials comparing the two methods and, as two-stage procedures tend to be performed on those with more complex infections, the literature is prone to selection bias demonstrating a favourable outcome with one-stage revision.

An alternative to one- or two-stage replacement surgery is debridement, antibiotics, and implant retention or 'DAIR'. This is a single operation which involves excision of the wound margins and open debridement of necrotic tissue. The prosthesis is retained if fixed and sound but all modular components are exchanged and any previous bone grafts are removed. Tissue cultures are used to guide targeted postoperative antibiotic therapy. Implant retention may be possible in early infection because the biofilm is not yet fully established. This approach may avoid the tissue destruction associated with resection arthroplasty in selected patients (Box 21.2) [3]. Reported success rates vary widely depending on the criteria and methods used.

⊘ Evidence base DAIR

Cobo et al. 2011: Prospective multicentre cohort study of 117 patients with early PJI [8]

- Time from implantation: mean 3–4 weeks
- Duration of antibiotics: ~10 weeks
- Follow-up: ~2 years
- *S. aureus* infection: 40%
- 67 (57%) were cured of infection
- 35 (30%) failed with DAIR and the prosthesis was removed
- 15 (13%) failed and were managed with chronic suppressive antibiotics
- Success rates similar with high- and low-virulence organisms

Westberg et al. 2012: Prospective study of 38 patients with early hip PJI [9]

- Time from implantation: <4 weeks
- *S. aureus* infection: 55%
- Duration of antibiotics: median 7 weeks
- Follow-up: median 4 years
- 27 (71%) were successfully treated including 5 that required a second debridement
- 11 failed: 6 then had a successful one- or two-stage revision
- DAIR appeared to be less effective in polymicrobial infection—8 of 15 patients cured

---

Box 21.2 Criteria for DAIR

- Early postoperative or acute haematogenous infection
- Short duration of symptoms, <3 weeks
- Stable prosthesis
- Intact soft tissues
- Known pathogen susceptible to antibiotics with surface-adhering bacterial activity

Antibiotics

The first antibiotic treatment decision was to rationalize the empirical regimen to intravenous flucloxacillin. The use of intravenous therapy rather than oral for bone and joint infections stems from early studies on the treatment of native osteomyelitis which showed poor outcomes using oral penicillins [4]. A number of agents have activity against staphylococci and the choice should take into account bioavailability, administration, adverse effects, and tolerability.

The next consideration was the antibiotic to use for OPAT. Ceftriaxone and teicoplanin were both suitable as od agents effective against MSSA. Teicoplanin is often used for PJI in Europe, particularly in penicillin-allergic patients, but is not yet licensed by the US FDA (Clinical tip: Teicoplanin). Dacquet reported 50 cases of bone and joint infection treated with teicoplanin in combination with either fusidic acid or an aminoglycoside; 25 patients (50%) had prosthetic joint infection and 43 (86%) were infected with staphylococci [10]. In all, 46 episodes (92%) were regarded as clinical successes including one patient who required a second course of teicoplanin. Adverse events were noted in 10% but did not require discontinuation of therapy. The patient in this case developed thrombocytopenia, an uncommon but well-described adverse reaction to glycopeptide therapy, which resolved upon changing to ceftriaxone.

✚ **Clinical tip** Teicoplanin

Teicoplanin is a glycopeptide antibiotic used to treat Gram-positive infections. Good penetration of bone and joint fluid has led to its use in staphylococcal PJI, particularly in the OPAT setting.

PK

Plasma level profile following IV administration:

- Rapid phase with a half-life of 0.3 hours
- More prolonged distribution phase with a half-life of 3 hours
- Slow clearance with a terminal elimination half-life of 150 hours
- Allows od dosing

Dose

Loading dose 400 mg 12-hourly for 3 doses then 400 mg od thereafter
Dose adjustment for renal impairment: normal dose for 3 days, then:

- Creatinine clearance 40–60 mL/min: half dose, e.g. 200 mg daily or 400 mg every 2 days
- Creatinine clearance <40 mL/min and haemodialysis patients: one-third normal dose or once every 3 days

Teicoplanin is not removed by dialysis

Therapeutic drug monitoring

- Levels should be taken after 5 days
- Target therapeutic range 20–60 mg/L
- Weekly monitoring of full blood count and renal function

Adverse drug reactions

Common (>1/100 to <1/10)

- Erythema, rash, itch
- Fever, pain

Uncommon (>1/1,000 to <1/100)
- Thrombocytopenia, leucopenia, eosinophilia
- Anaphylaxis, dizziness, headache, hearing loss, vestibular disorder
- Phlebitis, bronchospasm, GI upset

A controversial issue was the use of a second systemic antibiotic. The patient received RIF, which can eliminate stationary phase staphylococci and penetrate biofilms [3]. It is used in combination with other agents to avoid inducing drug resistance and clinical trials have demonstrated the efficacy of oral RIF-fluoroquinolone regimens in the treatment of osteomyelitis [3,11]. Senneville et al. reviewed the characteristics of 98 patients with *S. aureus* prosthetic joint infections, of whom 77 (79%) were in remission at a mean follow-up of 43.6 months [11]. Ten out of 68 (15%) patients treated with RIF combination therapy failed treatment compared with 11 of 30 (37%) patients who were not treated with RIF. Fusidic acid, co-trimoxazole, tetracyclines, and linezolid can also be used with RIF although there is scanty clinical evidence to support this [4].

> **⚖ Expert comment** Theoretical risk of reduced efficacy when RIF is used with vancomycin
>
> The use of RIF as a second agent divides opinion. Many experts hold that without it the treatment of retained implants is impossible. Others point to evidence that suggests that RIF drives vancomycin resistance when used together. My experience with patients on OPAT is that RIF is often associated with side effects which confuses treatment and make these patients more difficult to manage.
>
> The patient received 6 weeks of intravenous antibiotic therapy between stages but the optimal length of treatment is unknown. The IDSA guidelines suggest different durations depending on the surgical method used.

> **★ Learning point** Summary of Infectious Diseases Society of America Guidelines 2012 [2]
>
> See Tables 21.3 and 21.4.
>
> **Table 21.3 Staphylococcal prosthetic joint infection (antibiotics commonly used in Europe)**
>
> | Organism | Initial treatment | Continuation | Chronic suppression (if required) |
> |---|---|---|---|
> | Staphylococci: meticillin-susceptible | Preferred: IV flucloxacillin or ceftriaxone AND RIF
 Alternative: vancomycin or daptomycin or linezolid AND RIF | Preferred: RIF AND quinolone (e.g. ciprofloxacin, levofloxacin)
 Alternative: RIF AND other agent (e.g. co-trimoxazole, cephalexin, doxycycline, flucloxacillin) | Preferred: cephalexin
 Alternative: flucloxacillin or clindamycin or co-amoxiclav
 NB RIF is NOT recommended for chronic suppression |
> | Staphylococci: meticillin-resistant | Preferred: vancomycin AND RIF
 Alternative: daptomycin or linezolid AND RIF | Preferred: RIF AND quinolone (e.g. ciprofloxacin, levofloxacin)
 Alternative: RIF AND other agent (e.g. co-trimoxazole, doxycycline) | Preferred: co-trimoxazole or doxycycline |
>
> Source: Data from Osmon DR et al, Diagnosis and management of prosthetic joint infection: Clinical Practice Guidelines by the Infectious Diseases Society of America, *Clinical Infectious Diseases*, Volume 56, Issue 1, e1–25, Copyright © The Author 2012. Published by Oxford University Press on behalf of the Infectious Diseases Society of America.
>
> (continued)

Table 21.4 Postoperative treatment duration

Surgery	Organism	Initial treatment	Duration	Continuation	Total duration
DAIR	Staphylococci	IV antibiotics AND oral RIF	2–6 weeks (4–6 weeks if RIF not used)	RIF-containing oral combination therapy	3 months (6 months for TKA)
	Other	IV antibiotics OR highly bioavailable oral	4–6 weeks	± indefinite oral suppression (not unanimously recommended)	≥4–6 weeks
Resection arthroplasty ± reimplantation	Any	IV antibiotics OR highly bioavailable oral	4–6 weeks	No continuation therapy recommended	4–6 weeks
1-stage exchange	Staphylococci	IV antibiotics AND oral RIF	2–6 weeks (4–6 weeks if RIF not used)	RIF-containing oral combination therapy	3 months
	Other	IV antibiotics OR highly bioavailable oral	4–6 weeks	± indefinite oral suppression (not unanimously recommended)	≥4–6 weeks
Amputation	Any	Pathogen-specific antibiotics	24–48 hours	Stop if all infected bone and tissue removed and no sepsis syndrome or bacteraemia	≥24–48 hours

Source: Data from Osmon DR et al, Diagnosis and management of prosthetic joint infection: Clinical Practice Guidelines by the Infectious Diseases Society of America, *Clinical Infectious Diseases*, Volume 56, Issue 1, e1–25, Copyright © The Author 2012. Published by Oxford University Press on behalf of the Infectious Diseases Society of America.

> **❝ Expert comment**
>
> If you are considering using teicoplanin for coagulase-negative staphylococci (CNS) prosthetic joint infections, it is important that MICs are determined rather than relying on disc sensitivity testing. A proportion of CNS are resistant despite being sensitive to vancomycin and appearing sensitive to teicoplanin on disc testing.

Short courses of systemic antibiotics without oral continuation therapy have been used successfully for prosthesis-related infection. Hsieh et al. conducted a retrospective review of 99 patients with prosthetic hip infection managed by two-stage revision with antibiotic-loaded spacers and cement [12]. One group of 53 patients were managed with 1 week of intravenous antibiotics after the first stage and a comparator group of 46 patients received standard treatment of 4–6 weeks of IV therapy between stages. Each group received intravenous antibiotics for 3 days following the second stage operation. The overall success rate was 90% with no significant difference between the two groups. There is some evidence that thorough surgical debridement and local antibiotics are effective even with short courses of systemic antimicrobial therapy.

> **✓ Evidence base** Local antibiotics
>
> Local antibiotics can be used to target the infection while minimizing systemic effects. Antibiotic-loaded cement and spacers are commonly employed and need to be mechanically stable as well as pharmacologically effective. Therapeutic levels of antibiotic are maintained in periprosthetic tissue for several months after implantation, and adverse reactions including drug fevers have been reported.
>
> (continued)

An analysis of pooled data from 29 studies of hip prosthesis-associated infection managed with one-stage revision arthroplasty showed a cure rate of 86% with the use of antibiotic-impregnated bone cement, compared to 59% with plain cement [4]. This has led some to question whether prolonged systemic therapy is needed at all and several groups have published good outcomes with two-stage revisions and short courses of intravenous antibiotics.

Stockley et al. reported 114 patients with hip prosthesis infection [13]:

- 15 (13%) had *S. aureus* infection
- Local antibiotics: beads and cement (mainly vancomycin and gentamicin)
- Systemic antibiotics: 3 perioperative doses of IV cephalosporin at each stage
- Interval between stages: mean 6.4 months (range 2–22 months)
- Follow-up: mean 74 months
- Success rate: 88%
- No significant association found with respect to the infecting organism, positive second stage cultures, or co-morbidity
- A similar success rate of 89% was found in 53 infected knees managed with the same method

PJI is a serious complication which incurs higher investigation and treatment costs, and requires longer operating times and inpatient stays than aseptic revision. Some preventive measures are illustrated in Box 21.3. If initial management fails then postoperative recurrence may be managed with DAIR, if appropriate, or a further two-stage revision. If the infection cannot be controlled, amputation or a salvage procedure such as excision arthroplasty or arthrodesis may be offered. If the patient is not fit or willing for further surgery then long-term oral antibiotic therapy may be given with the aim of suppressing secondary bacteraemia rather than eradicating infection (Box 21.3).

Box 21.3 Infection control and prevention

Preoperative MRSA screening

- To guide perioperative prophylaxis and the need for decolonization

Perioperative antimicrobial prophylaxis

- Prophylaxis for primary arthroplasty reduces infection rates [4]
- Systemic antibiotics (e.g. cefotaxime or vancomycin) should be administered immediately before surgery to achieve adequate serum and tissue levels during the operation

Pre-operative *S. aureus* decolonization

- Bode et al. conducted a randomized placebo-controlled trial on the effect of screening surgical patients and decolonizing *S. aureus* carriers on surgical site infection [14]
- 917 *S. aureus* carriers: 504 treated with nasal mupirocin and chlorhexidine soap
- Rate of *S. aureus* infection was 3.4% (17/504) in the treatment group and 7.7% (32/413) after placebo (relative risk of infection, 0.42; 95% CI 0.23–0.75)

Theatre environment

- Ultra-clean air significantly reduces the rate of infection in orthopaedic implant surgery
- Laminar airflow systems are used with HEPA filters
- UK theatres should not exceed 180 CFU/m^3 of air for an average 5-minute period during periods of activity

❶ Expert comment The choice of oral agent for long-term suppression

The choice of oral agent for long-term suppression is not well defined and there is little evidence to support one regimen over the other. The ideal oral agent should have a high bioavailability, be able to penetrate well into bone, be active against the organism, be convenient to take, be well tolerated, and have low toxicity. Agents that fit these criteria to a greater or lesser extent that are regularly used include RIF, ciprofloxacin, moxifloxacin, doxycycline, trimethoprim, clindamycin, and fusidic acid. All variations and combinations are used and treatment choice is usually dependent on the sensitivities of the organism and the patient's ability to tolerate the medication.

A final word from the expert

Staphylococcal prosthetic joint infections present significant clinical challenges in diagnosis and management. Despite PJI being a condition that infection specialists and orthopaedic surgeons come across commonly, our knowledge of the optimum management is still limited. The type of surgery, selection of antibiotics, role of second agents, utility of local antibiotics, and duration of therapy is hotly debated and practice varies widely. The dearth of RCTs means that we are overly reliant on retrospective studies and expert opinion. This uncertainty and heterogeneity of opinion is reflected in the published guidelines. As a clinician, I gain some comfort that our practice falls broadly within these guidelines, but at the same time I am frustrated by the lack of knowledge.

In this case of a diabetic man with MSSA prosthetic hip infection, successful treatment was achieved with two-stage revision arthroplasty and a 6-week course of intravenous antibiotics. However, there is good evidence for one-stage revision and debridement with implant retention in a selected cohort. There is a continental divide in this with Europe more comfortable with the one-stage approach and the USA firmly in the two-stage camp, with Britain falling somewhere in between.

The use of short courses of intravenous antibiotics and local antibiotic delivery systems without prolonged systemic antibiotic therapy has also shown encouraging results.

The need for more well-designed studies is self-evident. One trial currently under way, the Oxford OVIVA trial, is comparing 6 weeks of IV antibiotics against 6 weeks of oral antibiotics. The results of trials like this may mean that our reliance on IV antibiotics and OPAT is greatly diminished. However, at present OPAT remains the mainstay of treatment in many centres. An effective well-managed OPAT service is essential to manage these patients appropriately.

The vagaries of guidelines and the complexity of the issues mean that an MDT approach is essential. I find an MDT meeting with orthopaedic surgeons, infection specialists (microbiologists and/or ID physicians), orthopaedic nurses, the OPAT team, and others allows us to manage the patients effectively from a surgical, antibiotic, social, and laboratory point of view.

A final point to be considered is the psychological effects that prosthetic joint infections have on patients. The loss of independence, loss of mobility, pain, and the extended periods of treatment all have an impact on the patient. Patients often become over-dependent on caregivers. In my experience depression is common and suicide does occur. These psychological factors must be considered in any patient management programme treating these infections.

References

1 Della Valle C, Parvizi J, Bauer TW et al. Diagnosis of periprosthetic joint infections of the hip and knee. *J Am Acad Orthop Surg* 2010; 18: 760–770.

2 Osmon DR, Berbari EF, Berendt AR et al. Diagnosis and management of prosthetic joint infection: Clinical Practice Guidelines by the Infectious Diseases Society of America. *Clin Infect Dis* 2013; 56: e1–e25.

3 Leone S, Borre S, Monforte A et al. Consensus document on controversial issues in the diagnosis and treatment of prosthetic joint infections. *Int J Infect Dis* 2010; suppl 4: S67–S77.

4 Zimmerli W, Trampuz A, Ochsner PE. Prosthetic-joint infections. *N Engl J Med* 2004; 351: 1645–1654.

5 Atkins BL, Athanasou N, Deeks JJ et al. Prospective evaluation of criteria for microbiological diagnosis of prosthetic-joint infection at revision arthroplasty. The OSIRIS Collaborative Study Group. *J Clin Microbiol* 1998; 36: 2932–2939.

6 Trampuz A, Piper KE, Jacobson MJ et al. Sonication of removed hip and knee prostheses for diagnosis of infection. *N Engl J Med* 2007; 357: 654–663.

7 Bejon P, Berendt A, Atkins BL et al. Two-stage revision for prosthetic joint infection: predictors of outcome and the role of reimplantation microbiology. *J Antimicrob Chemother* 2010; 65: 569–575.

8 Cobo J, Miguel LG, Euba G et al. Early prosthetic joint infection: outcomes with debridement and implant retention followed by antibiotic therapy. *Clin Microbiol Infect* 2011; 17: 1632–1637.

9 Westberg M, Grogaard B, Snorrason F. Early prosthetic joint infections treated with debridement and implant retention: 38 primary hip arthroplasties prospectively recorded and followed for median 4 years. *Acta Orthop* 2012; 83: 227–232.

10 Dacquet V. Treatment of bone and joint infection with teicoplanin: a retrospective analysis of 50 cases. *Int J Antimicrob Agents* 1996; 7: 49–51.

11 Senneville E, Joulie D, Leqout L et al. Outcome and predictors of treatment failure in total hip/knee prosthetic joint infections due to *Staphylococcus aureus*. *Clin Infect Dis* 2011; 53: 334–340.

12 Hsieh PH, Huang KC, Lee PC, Lee MS. Two-stage revision of infected hip arthroplasty using an antibiotic-loaded spacer: retrospective comparison between short-term and prolonged antibiotic therapy. *J Antimicrob Chemother* 2009; 64: 392–397.

13 Stockley I, Mockford BJ, Hoad-Reddick A, Norman P. The use of two-stage exchange arthroplasty with depot antibiotics in the absence of long-term antibiotic therapy in infected total hip replacement. *J Bone Joint Surg Br* 2008; 90: 145–148.

14 Bode LG, Kluytmans JA, Wertheim HF et al. Preventing surgical-site infections in nasal carriers of *Staphylococcus aureus*. *N Engl J Med* 2010; 362: 9–17.

22 Meticillin-resistant *Staphylococcus aureus* bacteraemia

James Price

ⓘ **Expert commentary** Martin Llewelyn

Case history

A 20-year-old intravenous drug user (IVDU) was admitted to hospital with a 1-week history of fevers, rigors, dyspnoea, and productive cough. On further questioning he described progressive lethargy and coryzal symptoms over the preceding month. He had no significant past medical history and was not taking any prescribed medications. He had no recent weight loss and had never travelled outside the United Kingdom. He was a smoker and denied heavy alcohol consumption. On initial examination he was febrile (38.9°C) and haemodynamically stable. There was evidence of injection drug use in both groins but no associated cellulitis. His oxygen saturation was 92% on room air. Auscultation of his chest revealed coarse crepitations throughout both lung fields. He had no peripherial stigmata of infective endocarditis (IE) and precordial examination revealed no audible murmurs. Initial biochemical investigations revealed a marked inflammatory response (WCC 18.2×10^9/L, CRP 253 mg/L). Blood cultures were taken.

➕ **Clinical tip** Secondary-site infections in *Staphylococcus aureus* bacteraemia (SAB)

Metastatic infection complicates up to one-third of SAB cases and can lead to considerable disability and even death. Several risk factors have been associated with the development of secondary-site infections including:

- Prosthetic devices *in situ*
- Community acquisition
- IVDU
- Failure or delay in removing a focus
- Unidentifiable source of bacteraemia. Up to 40% of patients will not have an identifiable focus of infection despite detailed investigation; intriguingly, these patients are particularly at risk of secondary-site infections, principally IE [5].

A CXR revealed multiple areas of opacification and possible cavitating lesions (Figure 22.1). He was treated for community-acquired pneumonia with intravenous (IV) co-amoxiclav and clarithromycin. The patient was reviewed by the ID physician. Concerns were raised of invasive *S. aureus* disease. Reflecting high local prevalence of MRSA colonizing IVDUs, IV vancomycin was added as empirical treatment. An unenhanced CT scan of the thorax confirmed multiple cavitating nodules consistent with lung abscesses (Figure 22.2). Right-sided IE was suspected and urgent transthoracic echocardiogram (TTE) revealed a large mobile vegetation on the native tricuspid valve (Figure 22.3).

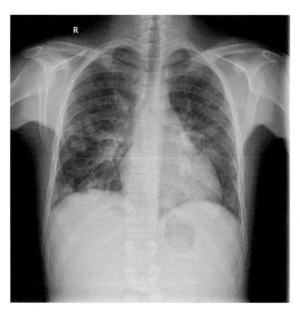

Figure 22.1 CXR showing multiple lesions throughout both lung fields consistent with pulmonary abscesses.

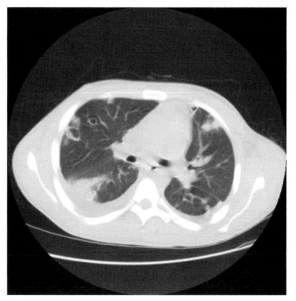

Figure 22.2 Transverse image of mid-thorax taken from a non-contrast-enhanced CT scan highlighting multiple cavitating pulmonary abscesses.

> **❝ Expert comment**
>
> When a patient presents with suspected *S. aureus* bacteraemia the choice of antibiotic treatment pending blood culture isolate sensitivities is crucially important. There is now a wealth of evidence that glycopeptides are inferior to β-lactams for treatment of MSSA bacteraemia. The finding by Lodise et al. [2] that mortality is greater even if glycopeptide treatment is switched to a β-lactam once sensitivities are known underscores the importance of including a β-lactam in the initial regimen if possible. At the current time only around 20% of *S. aureus* bacteraemias in the UK are caused by MRSA, but where there is a significant risk of MRSA infection, empiric treatment should cover this possibility. In addition to traditional risk factors for MRSA (previous documented MRSA, recent hospital contact, exposure
>
> (continued)

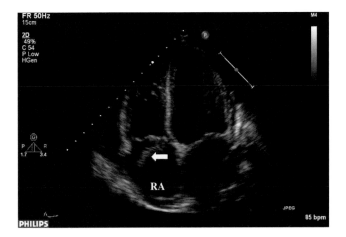

Figure 22.3 TTE. Apical four-chamber view depicting a triscupid valve vegetation (arrow) extending into the right atrium (RA).

to broad-spectrum antibiotics) there have been reports from several urban centres in the UK of high MRSA rates among drug users particularly in association with prison contact and the sex industry. Such MRSA strains are usually community-associated strain types (e.g. sequence type (ST) 1) and not typically PVL-producing.

Admission blood cultures grew MRSA. Antimicrobial therapy was rationalized to IV vancomycin and oral RIF. The MIC to vancomycin was tested and found to be 0.75 mg/L. The sample was sent to the reference laboratory for bacterial genotyping. Panton–Valentine Leukocidin (PVL) toxin genes were not detected and the strain was reported as EMRSA-15 (see Learning point: Epidemiology of MRSA infections). Repeat blood cultures were negative at 48 hours after starting treatment. The patient received 6 weeks of antimicrobial therapy and is being considered for triscuspid valve repair.

⊕ **Clinical tip** Consider the following infective causes of cavitating lung lesions

Bacteria
- Oral anaerobes
- *S. aureus, Streptococcus pyogenes, Streptococcus pneumoniae, Klebsiella pneumoniae, Haemophilus influenzae*
- Enteric GNB
- *Nocardia* spp, *Actinomyces* spp

Mycobacteria
- *Mtb*
- Atypical mycobacteria

Fungi
- Opportunistic pathogens (*Aspergillus* spp, *Cryptococcus* spp)
- Endemic mycoses (Histoplasma, Coccidioides, Blastomyces)

Parasites
- *Paragonimus* spp, *Entamoeba* spp, *Echinococcus* spp

- Ensure appropriate empirical antimicrobial therapy by assessing risk of MRSA
- Rationalize treatment with culture results
- Early removal of infective foci (if possible)
- Regular examinations for evidence of metastatic spread
- Define treatment duration; a minimum of 2 weeks IV treatment in uncomplicated disease, prolonged to 4–6 weeks in deep-seated infections or with unremovable foci
- Repeat blood cultures at 48–96 hours
- Echocardiography in patients with persistent bacteraemia or a cardiac prosthesis.

⭐ **Learning point** PVL toxin

Recent interest in PVL reflects its reputed importance as a virulence factor in community infections, yet its precise role in disease pathogenesis remains unclear. PVL is encoded by two genes (*lukS-PV* and *lukF-PV*) which are present on a mobile phage in both meticillin-susceptible *S. aureus* (MSSA) and MRSA strains. Expression results in formation of a cytotoxin which creates pores in host cell membranes causing tissue necrosis and neutrophilic destruction. In contrast to other highly prevalent leukocidins, the epidemiology of PVL is variable. Universally present among community-acquired MRSA (CA-MRSA), two PVL-expressing clones (USA300/400) have successfully spread through North American communities. Commonly associated with aggressive skin and soft tissue infections in young healthy individuals, CA-MRSA also causes severe bone and joint infections, necrotizing pneumonia, and sepsis. Surprisingly, bacteraemia caused by PVL-expressing strains is associated with better treatment outcomes [3]. In Europe PVL-related disease is uncommon and more frequently associated with MSSA. The reason for geographical variation remains unclear.

In suspected PVL-associated isolates, antibiotic susceptibility profiles have been used as a screening tool. While MSSA expressing PVL have variable antibiotic susceptibility patterns, PVL-positive MRSA strains are typically susceptible to most anti-staphylococcal agents [4]. Consequently ciprofloxacin susceptibility has been used as a surrogate marker [4]. Most microbiology laboratories do not have the facilities to routinely genotype strains and currently suspected PVL-expressing strains are sent to reference centres for PCR-based identification. Due to its retrospective nature, genotyping is used most effectively in surveillance, prevention, and management of recurrent skin infections.

⭐ **Learning point** Epidemiology of MRSA infections

In healthcare settings in endemic countries (UK, USA) ~5% of patients and healthcare workers carry MRSA as well as various environmental fomites. Infection control policies aim to reduce the burden of MRSA as carriage precedes infection. Nosocomial MRSA infections are caused by few circulating epidemic clones. Varying between countries these clones naturally wax and wane, being replaced by novel strains over time. In the UK 95% of MRSA infections are currently caused by two clones: EMRSA-15 (CC22, ST22) and EMRSA-16 (CC30, ST36, USA200). Stain nomenclature varies according to the typing method used and country of origin. Clonal complex (CC) refers to the lineage assigned by any appropriate typing method whereas ST represents multi-locus sequence typing characterization. The prefix USA- denotes dominant American strains whereas EMRSA- signifies UK epidemic MRSA clones. Such variations have led to confusion.

Traditionally associated with healthcare facilities, MRSA typically causes infections in the elderly and in patients with chronic diseases, indwelling devices, and receiving long-term antibiotics. However, the epidemiology of MRSA disease is changing. In the UK it is not uncommon for patients to present to hospital with MRSA bacteraemia which is technically of community onset but has in fact been acquired through previous hospital contact. These strains are phenotypically similar to nosocomial strains. In contrast, CA-MRSA infections have been increasingly described in some parts of the world where the clinical phenotype is remarkably different (see Learning point: PVL toxin). Such newly emerging strains have caused outbreaks in hospitals, prisons, military units, and sports facilities.

⭐ **Learning point** Infective endocarditis and when to perform cardiac surgery

IE commonly complicates SAB. Rates are highest when associated with prosthetic heart valves and cardiac rhythm management devices (CRMD) (20–55%) compared to native heart valves (14–25%). Clinical findings can be non-specific or absent. Subsequently international guidelines recommend echocardiography in all patients with SAB. A common scenario is deciding which imaging modality to use. TTE is a portable and non-invasive screening tool but has limited sensitivity (50–82%). Transoesophageal echocardiography (TOE) has a sensitivity approaching 100% and is superior for detecting small vegetations on both native and prosthetic valves and CRMD. TOE is an invasive procedure requiring a skilled user and has associated operative risks. With improving sensitivity TTE continues to be a valuable first-line screening tool, with TOE preferred in patients with high suspicion.

(continued)

Although successful medical management is achieved in many cases of native valve IE, surgery may be required. Prosthetic valves and CRMD infections commonly require a combination of surgical removal and antimicrobial therapy as definitive treatment. International guidelines recommend early surgical intervention in those patients with life-threatening congestive heart failure or cardiogenic shock. Surgical indications in haemodynamically stable patients remain less clear. Many advocate surgery in uncontrolled infections, emboli prevention, structural abnormalities, abscesses or infections caused by MDR organisms (such as MRSA). The treatment of IVDUs with triscuspid valve IE with associated regurgitation or large vegetations (as in the clinical case) can include triscuspid valve repair, valvectomy, or vegectomy. Optimal timing for surgery remains unclear and early consultation with cardiac surgeons is essential.

Discussion

The clinical vignette describes a case of MRSA bacteraemia complicated by pulmonary and cardiac secondary-site infections. The patient presented with signs and symptoms of community-acquired pneumonia which made the diagnosis of invasive *S. aureus* disease challenging. Evidence to support *S. aureus* as the causative organism comes from: (i) risk factors (IVDU); (ii) clinical features (sepsis); (iii) microbiological information (sputum Gram stain); and (iv) radiological features (pulmonary abscesses). Appropriate antimicrobial therapy is vital to improve outcomes in SAB so while awaiting identification and antibiotic susceptibility testing effective empirical therapy is essential. When *S. aureus* disease is suspected an assessment of MRSA risk should be performed based on: (i) local endemnicity (see Box 22.1), (ii) previous carriage, and (iii) risk factors of MRSA colonization including previous hospital admission, recent antibiotic use, skin lesions, and underlying chronic disease (diabetes, haemodialysis, HIV). In this case the patient was deemed at high risk due to locally high prevalence of MRSA in IVDUs, and vancomycin was added to the β-lactam regimen. Glycopeptides are commonly used as empirical treatment in *S. aureus* infections pending antibiotic susceptibility testing. Interestingly there is data to suggest that glycopeptides are inferior to β-lactams in the treatment of SAB (MRSA or MSSA) with excess infection-related mortality observed in glycopeptides regimens even when rationalization to β-lactam therapy with sensitivity results (see Evidence base). It is postulated that glycopeptides do not sterilize the blood as quickly as β-lactams, leading to persistent bacteraemia. As in this case, some clinicians recommend β-lactam and glycopeptide combinations as empirical treatment. Rationalization should be performed with susceptibility results.

Box 22.1 How the NHS in England and Wales responded to rising MRSA bacteraemia rates

During the 1990s there was a dramatic rise in the rate of MRSA bacteraemia in the UK, becoming one of the highest in Europe. In 2001 the Department of Health in England responded by introducing a surveillance programme requiring mandatory reporting of all cases of MRSA bacteraemia in acute hospital trusts [1]. In contrast to other national surveillance programmes, rates of MRSA bacteraemia were determined for individual trusts and made available in the public domain. In the following years (2001–2004) UK MRSA bacteraemia rates remained high at over 7,000 cases per year. This strengthened growing public concerns regarding hospital hygiene and received significant media attention. In response further measures were instigated. First, mandatory surveillance was enhanced to obtain detailed clinical and epidemiological information on each case to determine the proportion acquired in each hospital trust. Second, a national target was set for trusts to decrease MRSA bacteraemia rates by 50% over a 4-year period. Third, strategies to promote and improve infection control practices were introduced including enhanced hand hygiene, contact precautions, intravascular line care bundles, restricted antibiotic prescribing policies, deep-cleaning of clinical areas, and decolonizing MRSA carriers. Between 2004 and 2008 a reduction of 56% was made in MRSA bacteraemia rates in England [1]. It remains unclear which measures, if any, contributed to the fall in rates or whether this was the natural waning of the dominant MRSA clones in UK hospitals. Interestingly, during the same period rates of bacteraemia caused by MSSA remained high.

> **⊘ Evidence base** Impact of empirical-therapy selection on outcomes of IVDUs with infective endocarditis caused by meticillin-susceptible *S. aureus* [2]
>
> **Study design:** A retrospective single-centred population-based cohort analysis comparing infection-related mortality for empirical β-lactam and vancomycin therapy among IVDU with MSSA IE.
>
> **Methods:** Between 1 January 1997 and 31 July 2001 all hospitalized IVDUs diagnosed with IE caused by *S. aureus* were identified. Study inclusion criteria included: (i) the diagnosis of MSSA bacteraemia satisfying the modified Dukes Criteria for IE; (ii) recent use of IV drugs prior to admission; and (iii) empirical treatment with either vancomycin or a β-lactam. Data was collected on patient demographics and co-morbidities, IE diagnostic features, treatment regimens given, and clinical outcomes.
>
> **Definitions:** Empirical treatment was defined as the antibiotic regime administered before the identification and determination of susceptibility of the infecting organism. Outcome was assessed as death related to MSSA IE defined as (i) MSSA-positive blood cultures at time of death; (ii) death occurring prior to resolution of IE symptoms; (iii) death in hospital without an unrelated, alternative cause; and (iv) *S. aureus* confirmed as cause of death by post-mortem.
>
> **Results:** During the study period 84 cases of MSSA IE were identified, 12 of which were excluded as they did not receive either vancomycin or β-lactam regimens. Of the 72 cases included, 28 received vancomycin and 44 received β-lactam regimens (36 semi-synthetic penicillins and 8 ceftriaxone). There were no statistical differences in baseline clinical features between the two treatment groups. A total of 16/72 (22.2%) patients died. In the outcome analysis a significantly higher infection-related mortality was identified in patients who received empirical vancomycin therapy compared to those who were empirically treated with β-lactam agents (39.4% vs. 11.4%; $p = 0.005$). Following logistical regression analysis, vancomycin use remained highly predictive of infection-related mortality (adjusted OR 6.5; 95% CI 1.4–29.4). Of the 28 patients who received vancomycin empirically, 21 were changed to a semi-synthetic penicillin regimen following susceptibility results. There was no difference in infection-related mortalities between patients who received vancomycin as the primary regimen and patients who had vancomycin switched to β-lactam therapy (33.3% vs. 40.9%; $p = 0.7$).
>
> **Conclusion:** These findings suggest that the use of vancomycin is inferior to β-lactams in the treatment of SAB.

The patient in the case was reviewed by an IDs physician who directed investigation and management according to best evidence. There is evidence that input from an infection specialist consultation significantly improves outcome in patients with SAB (see Evidence base box). This is felt to be through improved adherence to best practice. There remains a paucity of evidence available to guide the management of SAB, particularly relating to MRSA. Current practice is mostly based on clinical experience and observational studies [5]. The optimum treatment for MSSA bacteraemia remains penicillinase-stable penicillins. Despite no RCTs, prospective observational studies suggest that most cephalosporins are as effective as penicillins in the treatment of SAB [5]. This does not include cefonicid or ceftazidime, which have been associated with treatment failures. The management of MRSA bacteraemia, or those patients with anaphylactic penicillin allergy, remains less clearly defined. Glycopeptides, such as vancomycin and teicoplanin, probably remain the treatment of choice.

> **⊘ Evidence base** The value of ID consultation in SAB [6]
>
> **Study design:** A prospective single-centre cohort study conducted in an American tertiary referral centre evaluating the impact of infection specialist input on the mortality of SAB.
>
> **Methods:** Between July 2005 and July 2007 all adult patients diagnosed with SAB, as defined by *S. aureus* in at least one blood culture and evidence of clinical infection, were prospectively evaluated. Exclusion criteria included: (i) patients less than 18 years old; (ii) patients previously diagnosed with SAB or *S. aureus* IE in preceding 12 months; or (iii) death within first 2 days of positive blood culture. Demographic and clinical data was collected including bacteraemia duration, metastatic complications, antimicrobial therapy regimens, and removal of infected foci. Medical records were reviewed to determine whether patients received consultation by an infectious diseases (ID) specialist. All-cause mortality at 28 and 365 days after first positive blood culture was evaluated by reviewing both medical records and the US Social Security Death Index.
>
> **Results:** A total of 341 patients with SAB were evaluated; 111 (33%) had an ID consultation, of which 87 (78%) took place within 5 days of first positive blood culture. Those patients receiving an ID consult were more likely to have congestive heart failure, cardiac or orthopaedic prostheses *in situ*, HIV, community-associated infection, metastatic infection, and prolonged bacteraemia. Patients receiving chronic haemodialysis, central venous catheter *in situ*, history of smoking, or current diagnosis of malignancy were less likely to receive an ID consult. Patients who had an ID consult were more likely to receive appropriate antimicrobial agents, undergo TOE investigation, and have an appropriately planned duration of therapy.
>
> The overall all-cause 28-day mortality rate for patients with SAB was 16% (54/341; 95% CI 12–20); 9 with ID consultation and 45 without specialist input. ID consultation was associated with a 56% reduction in 28-day mortality (AHR 0.44; 95% CI 0.22–0.89, p = 0.022). A total of 287 patients survived the first 28 days following first positive blood culture. The overall 1-year all-cause mortality was 41% (140/341; 95% CI 36–46). There was no statistical difference in 1-year mortality between patients who did and did not receive an ID consultation (crude HR 0.88; 95% CI 0.56–1.38, p = 0.579).
>
> **Conclusion:** ID consultation in patients with SAB is independently associated with reduced short-term mortality.

In the case the decision to add a second agent, RIF, was made following diagnosis of organism and secondary-site infection. Adjunctive therapies are commonly used in the treatment of SAB [7], although the benefits remain unclear. Synergistic gentamicin has been used in *S. aureus* endocarditis but due to high levels of renal toxicity it is no longer recommended. Combination therapy with fluoroquinolones, RIF, and fusidic acid are frequently used in *S. aureus* disease associated with deep infective foci and bone and joint infections. Rationale for their use is limited and comes from studies evaluating patients with persistent bacteraemia despite removal of infective foci and commencing effective antimicrobial agents with good bactericidal activity *in vitro*. This is concerning as positive blood cultures 48–96 hours after starting effective antimicrobial therapy is the most important predictor of complicated disease and death [8]. A proposed reason for persistence is intracellular survival of *S. aureus*. Traditionally regarded as an extracellular pathogen, it has become clear that *S. aureus* can invade and survive within viable and dead human cells. As β-lactam and glycopeptide agents have poor intracellular activity, intracellular organisms can evade the effects of these antibiotics promoting persistence, dissemination, and subsequent infective seeding.

The use of adjunctive agents with good intracellular penetration, such as RIF, has shown promising results in animal models. To date the best clinical evidence for adjunct RIF therapy comes from a study primarily designed to evaluate levofloxacin combination therapy in SAB [9]. Although the addition of levofloxacin to standard therapy did not reduce mortality, the study found that patients with deep-seated infections given combination RIF treatment had lower mortality rates than those receiving standard therapy alone. Adjunctive RIF is currently used in 38% of MRSA and 17% of MSSA bacteraemia treatment regimens [7]. At the time of writing (February 2014) a large multi-centre study which will determine the efficacy of adjunctive RIF has started in the UK.

The patient in the clinical scenario was treated for 6 weeks with IV therapy. The length of antimicrobial therapy for SAB remains subject to debate as, to date, no RCTs have examined effective treatment duration. Recommendations are based on case series and clinical experience [5,10]. In cases with identifiable and removable foci, with no evidence of secondary-site infections, current guidance suggests a minimum of 14 days. In complicated infections, such as deep-seated infections or unremovable sources, a prolonged course of antibiotics (>4 weeks) is advised as retained foci are associated with recurrence. Traditionally it has been recommended to complete all treatment regimens with IV therapy. This is usually given on an inpatient basis although some centres operate an OPAT service for clinically stable patients. The basis for recommending parenteral therapy has been from observational studies and expert opinion. The administration of IV antibiotics is a rapid and reliable route to establish therapeutically effective antibiotic concentrations, avoid uncertainties of absorption, and ensure medication compliance. However, prolonged IV therapy is expensive, inconvenient for patients, and holds associated risks from long-term cannula placement. The effective use of oral antibiotics in the treatment of SAB is yet to be established but the oral route is felt to be less effective than parenteral therapy, especially for severe or metastatic disease. Few randomized controlled studies have directly compared IV and oral therapy and, while some have found comparable cure rates, these studies contained small patient numbers with varying selection criteria. The use of oral antibiotics following an initial course of IV treatment has been proposed. Case series evaluating clinical outcome following IV to oral switch within 2 weeks of commencing treatment have shown no excess of complications. Of note, patient numbers were small, the timing of switching antibiotic administration route was inconsistent, and total duration of antibiotics was variable. Large randomized controlled studies are needed to address these issues.

In this clinical case the microbiology laboratory assessed vancomycin susceptibility by determined the MIC. PHE (formerly the HPA) currently recommends that MIC evaluation should be used to determine vancomycin (or teicoplanin) susceptibility as disc diffusion testing is not accurate at detecting low-level resistance and is unreliable at determining high-level resistance. PHE suggests that MIC testing may be confined to those *S. aureus* isolates causing invasive or clinically severe infections (as in this case) or treatment failures. Accurate determination of susceptibility is becoming particularly important as there are now reports of clinically-relevant MRSA isolates with reduced susceptibility to vancomycin. This is worrying as there is an association between higher vancomycin MICs and poor clinical outcome. A number of studies have found that despite remaining within the susceptibility range (<2 mg/L) the vancomycin MICs of clinically-relevant MRSA isolates have increased over time, termed the vancomycin 'MIC creep' [11]. Furthermore, a range of clinical isolates have also been identified with vancomycin MICs >2mg/L, including (i) vancomycin-resistant *S. aureus* (VRSA; MIC ≥16 mg/L), (ii) vancomycin-intermediate *S. aureus* (VISA; MIC 4–8 mg/L), and (iii) heterogenous vancomycin-intermediate *S. aureus* (hVISA; MIC <4 mg/L with subpopulations

⓺ Expert comment
Importance of finding a focus

It is widely understood that all foci of infection in *S. aureus* bacteraemia should be identified and where possible controlled by drainage or removal of infected material. Non-infection specialists may find it counterintuitive that even with modern medical management, including easy availability of TOE, patients in whom no focus of infection is found still do worse than patients with known foci of infection [7]. New, high-sensitivity technologies such as FDG-PET have the potential to identify foci which are difficult to find using conventional techniques (e.g. endovascular infections) and improve outcome.

growing at higher MICs). Unsurprisingly these have been associated with treatment failures. Currently the prevalence of these isolates is low, but with increasing MRSA burden and subsequent vancomycin use this is expected to change. The BSAC recommends that all isolates with an MIC > 8 mg/L should be referred to a reference laboratory for confirmation. As vancomycin susceptibility diminishes and resistance follows, alternative therapeutic agents are urgently needed. Daptomycin has now been approved by the US FDA for the treatment of SAB and right-sided IE. A number of other alternative antimicrobial agents are currently being evaluated including linezolid, tigecycline, and telavancin [5,12]. Furthermore, novel agents including dalbavancin, oritavancin, ceftobiprole, and ceftaroline are undergoing clinical trials [12].

ⓕ Expert comment MIC creep

There has been considerable concern about the phenomenon of MIC creep. This refers to a situation in which *S. aureus* isolates with higher vancomycin MICs become more common over time, although the MICs still remain within the susceptible range of the drug. Studies which have reported this effect have generally been from single centres or single geographical regions. Several recent studies have challenged whether this effect exists. Most notably Reynolds et al. [13] used an archive of *S. aureus* isolates from across the UK held by the HPA to look for changes in MIC over time, and found a small but statistically significant downward trend in MIC with time. This may be because MIC creep occurs in some settings and not others, depending for example on local use, or may be because the findings of small single-centre studies are skewed by, for example, changes in testing methodology. There is good evidence that a broth dilution MIC >1 is associated with poor outcome on vancomycin treatment, and in this situation other agents such as daptomycin may be preferable.

In the clinical vignette the MRSA isolate was sent for genotyping due to disease severity and the possibility of PVL-related necrotizing pneumonia. In the UK, the Staphylococcal Reference Unit (part of PHE) performs PCR-based toxin gene profiling on isolates from suspected toxin-mediated disease, including enteric (*S. aureus*-related food poisoning) and non-enteric (toxic shock syndrome, impetigo, scalded skin syndrome) infections. At the current time, as part of a national surveillance scheme, PHE requests isolates (MSSA and MRSA) from patients with clinical features suggestive of PVL-related diseases including (i) recurrent boils and abscesses, (ii) necrotizing skin and soft tissue infections, and (iii) necrotizing pneumonia, purpura fulminans, or necrotizing fasciitis.

A final word from the expert

Although rates of MRSA bacteraemia have fallen markedly in the UK, *S. aureus* bacteraemia remains a common clinical entity associated with substantial morbidity and mortality. This case illustrates the key elements of optimal management. Early diagnosis and prompt initiation of treatment are crucial. Unless the infection is known to be caused by MRSA, treatment should include a β-lactam drug where possible. It is not established whether using combination antibiotic therapy improves outcome. Foci of infection must be identified promptly by thorough and repeated clinical examination and radiological investigation and removed as soon as possible. Patients with persisting fever and bacteraemia 48–96 hours after starting treatment are at highest risk of complications. Current best evidence indicates that patients with *S. aureus* bacteraemia should receive intravenous treatment for a minimum of 2 weeks, with this duration increasing to 4–6 weeks in patients with endocarditis or unremovable foci of infection.

References

1 Johnson A, Davies J, Guy R, Abernathy J, Sheridan E, Pearson A, Duckworth G. Mandatory surveillance of methicillin-resistant *Staphylococcus aureus* (MRSA) bacteraemia in England: the first 10 years. *J Antimicrob Chemother* 2012; 67: 802–809.

2 Lodise TP, McKinnon PS, Levine DP, Rybak MJ. Impact of empirical-therapy selection on outcomes of intravenous drug users with infective endocarditis caused by methicillin-susceptible *Staphylococcus aureus*. *Antimicrob Agents Chemother* 2007; 51: 3731–3733.

3 Lalani T, Federspiel JJ, Boucher HW, et al. Associations between the genotypes of *Staphylococcus aureus* bloodstream isolates and clinical characteristics and outcomes of bacteremic patients. *J Clin Microbiol* 2008; 46: 2890–2896.

4 Nathwani D, Morgan M, Masterton RG et al. Guidelines for UK practice for the diagnosis and management of methicillin-resistant *Staphylococcus aureus* (MRSA) infections presenting in the community. *J Antimicrob Chemother* 2008; 61: 976–994.

5 Thwaites GE, Edgeworth JD, Gkrania-Klotsas E et al. Clinical management of *Staphylococcus aureus* bacteraemia. *Lancet Infect Dis* 2011; 11: 208–222.

6 Honda H, Krauss MJ, Jones JC, Olsen MA, Warren DK. The value of infectious diseases consultation in *Staphylococcus aureus* bacteremia. *Am J Med* 2010; 123: 631–637.

7 Thwaites GE, and United Kingdom Clinical Infection Research Group (UKCIRG). The management of *Staphylococcus aureus* bacteremia in the United Kingdom and Vietnam: a multi-centre evaluation. *PLoS One* 2010; 5: e14170.

8 Fowler VG, Olsen MK, Corey GR et al. Clinical identifiers of complicated *Staphylococcus aureus* bacteremia. *Arch Intern Med* 2003; 163: 2066–2072.

9 Ruotsalainen E, Järvinen A, Koivula I et al. Levofloxacin does not decrease mortality in *Staphylococcus aureus* bacteraemia when added to the standard treatment: a prospective and randomized clinical trial of 381 patients. *J Intern Med* 2006; 259: 179–190.

10 Liu C, Bayer A, Cosgrove SE et al. Clinical practice guidelines by the infectious diseases society of america for the treatment of methicillin-resistant *Staphylococcus aureus* infections in adults and children. *Clin Infect Dis* 2011; 52: e18–e55.

11 Steinkraus G, White R, Friedrich L. Vancomycin MIC creep in non-vancomycin-intermediate *Staphylococcus aureus* (VISA), vancomycin-susceptible clinical methicillin-resistant *S. aureus* (MRSA) blood isolates from 2001–05. *J Antimicrob Chemother* 2007; 60: 788–794.

12 Rasmussen RV, Fowler VG, Skov R, Bruun NE. Future challenges and treatment of *Staphylococcus aureus* bacteremia with emphasis on MRSA. *Future Microbiol* 2011; 6: 43–56.

13 Reynolds R, Hope R, Warner M, MacGowan AP, Livermore DM, Ellington MJ; BSAC Extended Working Party on Resistance Surveillance. Lack of upward creep of glycopeptide MICs for methicillin-resistant Staphylococcus aureus (MRSA) isolated in the UK and Ireland 2001–07. *J Antimicrob Chemother.* 2012; 67: 2912–2918.

23 Pneumococcal meningitis: antibiotic options for resistant organisms

Sathyavani Subbarao

Expert commentary Claire P. Thomas

Case history

A 55-year-old current smoker presented to his local emergency department with a 16-hour history of neck stiffness, fever, and confusion. Prior to this admission, he had received various courses of antibiotics for presumed exacerbations of chronic obstructive pulmonary disease (COPD) and sinusitis within the last 6 months. He had one admission 1 week previously for a community-acquired pneumonia, which was treated with 2 days of intravenous co-amoxiclav and he was discharged on the oral equivalent. His COPD was managed by his general practitioner with a regular Seretide inhaler and Salbutamol as required. He had no other medical problems and he was up-to-date with influenza and pneumococcal vaccinations.

> **Expert comment**
>
> Acute infective exacerbations of COPD are often viral in cause. However, BI can follow viral infections (RSV, rhinovirus, influenza, para-influenzae, meta-pneumovirus), leading causes being *S. aureus*, *Streptococcus pneumoniae*, and *Streptococcus pyogenes*. One of the most well-known viral–bacterial interactions is the synergism between influenza virus and *S. pneumoniae*. *S. pneumoniae* binds strongly to fibronectin, which is exposed at the epithelial basement membrane after viral infection leading to increased bacterial adherence, and invasion. In a co-infection model with influenza virus and *S. pneumoniae* in mice, excess IL-10 production following co-infection resulted in enhanced bacterial colonization and increased mortality [1]. Yearly 'flu' vaccination of vulnerable groups and healthcare workers is a key public health focus, with 5-yearly pneumococcal vaccination [2].

> **Clinical tip** The 23-valent pneumococcal polysaccharide vaccine [2]
>
> *Streptococcus pneumoniae* is classified into serotypes based on their polysaccharide capsule antigens. There are more than 90 distinct serotypes, which are grouped according to similarities in structure. Pneumococcal polysaccharide vaccine (PPV) includes polysaccharide antigens from the 23 serotypes that cause 96% of invasive pneumococcal disease in adults in in the United Kingdom. Studies suggest that PPV protects against invasive disease (including meningitis) but there is still controversy as to whether it protects or reduces mortality in non-bacteraemic pneumonia. Additionally, it has no effect in prevention of otitis media or exacerbations of COPD and, although recommended, may not have full effect in the immunosuppressed. Current UK 'Green Book' guidelines suggest re-immunization with PPV every 5 years in the following groups:
>
> - Adults >65 years
> - Adults aged 19–64 with COPD, cardiovascular disease, diabetes, chronic liver disease, smokers
> - Sickle cell disease/other haemoglobinopathies or acquired/congenital asplenia
>
> (continued)

- Patients with cochlear implants
- Patients with CSF leaks following trauma or major skull surgery
- Immunocompromised patients

In comparison the pneumococcal conjugate vaccine (PCV) contains capsular antigens from 13 common capsular types, conjugated to a protein (CRM197) to make it more immunogenic particularly in young children. It is now given routinely as part of the universal infant immunization programme.

He lived at home with his wife and 8-year-old child who were all well. His younger brother and 3-year-old niece (from Spain) also lived with them and had returned 10 days ago from a holiday in Spain. The older child was attending school and the 3-year-old had previously attended nursery and daycare in Spain. The 3-year-old child had missed a considerable number of his vaccinations due to travel.

> ✪ **Learning point** Pneumococcal carriage and pneumococcal conjugate vaccination
>
> *Streptococcus pneumoniae* acquisition is via respiratory droplets, and colonization of the nasopharynx is required before the development of disease. Asymptomatic colonization occurs in 20–40% of children (usually after 6 months of age) and may continue to be present in 5–10% of adults. Daycare attendance is a significant risk factor for pneumococcal carriage and children often act as the reservoir for adult disease [3].
>
> In the UK, the seven-valent pneumococcal conjugate vaccine (PCV-7) was introduced into the routine childhood vaccination schedule in 2006 and converted to the 13-valent vaccine in 2010. Reported cases of invasive disease in England and Wales have reduced by 34% from an adjusted average annual incidence of 16.1/100,000 before to 10.6/100,000 after introduction of the vaccine. The total reduction encompassed a reduction in vaccine type (VT) disease plus an increase in non-vaccine type (NVT) disease (vaccine replacement) [4].
>
> The introduction of the vaccine has led to reduction of pneumococcal disease in both those who had received the vaccine and in adults who had not, stressing the importance of children as a reservoir for adult disease and the importance of herd immunity [4]. Similar results have been seen in other countries including the USA.

On arrival in the emergency department he was pyrexial with a temperature of 38.5°C and had one generalized tonic clonic seizure, which lasted 1 minute. Following the seizure he was minimally confused but did not have any focal neurological deficit. He had marked neck stiffness that was associated with a positive Kernig's and Brudzinski's sign. Routine blood samples were taken including for blood cultures, intravenous ceftriaxone (1 g dose) was commenced for presumed meningitis, and the patient was transferred for a CT scan of his brain.

> ❖ **Expert comment**
>
> The history and examination findings are highly suggestive of meningitis and 2–4 g of Ceftriaxone should have been started straight away. Many would also have started dexamethasone at this stage. Had the history of the link to Spain been known, the addition of vancomycin should have been considered. There should be readily available local guidelines for meningitis based on best practice, with mention made of likely aetiology, associated with age and pre-morbidities. Causes of bacterial meningitis in adults are *Neisseria meningitidis, Streptococcus pneumoniae*, and *Listeria*, particularly in individuals older than 60, or those who are immunocompromised.

> ➕ **Clinical tip** The need for CT of the head before LP in meningitis
>
> There is often a debate about whether CT of the head is required prior to LP for suspected meningitis. The concern is that in patients with a space-occupying lesion, a LP could cause cerebral herniation due to a downward displacement of the cerebrum following a relative pressure gradient.
>
> The risk of serious complications following LP has been calculated as being low; however, risks are likely to be increased in certain settings. One study involving 301 patients demonstrated that the clinical features at baseline that were associated with abnormal findings on CT scan of the head were: age ≥60 years; immunocompromised; previous history of central nervous system disease; a history of a seizure ≤1 week previously; inability to follow two consecutive commands; or the
>
> (continued)

presence of focal neurological findings [5]. While these findings have not been formally validated, the current IDSA [6] and the BIA guidelines [7] recommend that in the clinical setting of bacterial meningitis, an immediate CT scan prior to an LP should be performed only in those meeting at least one of the following criteria:

- Immunocompromise
- History of CNS disease
- New-onset seizure
- Papilloedema
- Altered level of consciousness
- Focal neurological deficit
- Or any event that might delay in the performance of an LP.

Blood results revealed a raised white blood cell count at 18.9 × 10^9 cells/L (neutrophil count 16.3 × 10^9 cells/L) and raised CRP at 99 mg/dL. The remainder of his full blood count, renal function, and LFTs were in normal range. A chest radiograph showed early changes in keeping with COPD but did not demonstrate any focal abnormality.

The CT scan of the brain was normal and an LP was performed 3 hours after receiving the initial antibiotics. The initial tap appeared purulent and a dose of dexamethasone was given immediately.

> **⊗ Learning point** Steroids and meningitis
>
> The question of adjuvant steroids in suspected bacterial meningitis has rarely been met with a uniform answer, largely because of discrepancies among trial data. The current IDSA and BIA guidelines recommend the use of dexamethasone with CA [6,7]. Initial support came from clinical studies showing benefit of dexamethasone in infants with *Haemophilus influenzae* type b (Hib) meningitis. In 2000, five large RCTs were performed. A trial in Europe demonstrated a reduction in mortality and fewer other unfavourable outcomes, with the greatest effect on pneumococcal meningitis (**Evidence base: Do steroids improve mortality and morbidity in meningitis?**) [8]. Another large Vietnamese trial showed a beneficial effect only in those with proven bacterial meningitis while the other three trials did not confer additional benefit [6]. A meta-analysis in 2010 combined all these trials. Dexamethasone was not associated with a significant reduction in death (270 of 1,019 [26.5%] on dexamethasone versus 275 of 1,010 [27.2%] on placebo; OR 0.97, 95% CI 0.79–1.19). Additionally, dexamethasone had no effect on outcomes from meningitis caused by pneumococcus, suggesting that the overall benefit of steroids remains unproven [9]. The Cochrane review and meta-analysis in 2010 also did not show any benefit to mortality rates with the use of steroids; however, it did show that in pneumococcal meningitis there was a significantly reduced rate of hearing loss and short-term neurological sequelae. Additionally, sub-analyses for timing of corticosteroids (before or with the first dose of antibiotic versus after the first dose of antibiotic) showed no differences in the efficacy of corticosteroids with regard to timing [10].
>
> One interpretation of the current data would be to give dexamethasone once there is evidence of true meningitis (e.g. cloudy CSF, definite meningism) and evidence of a pneumococcal source (e.g. Gram-positive cocci seen on the CSF Gram stain, chest radiography findings, or positive pneumococcal urinary antigen test).

> **✔ Evidence base** Do steroids improve mortality and morbidity in meningitis?
> Dexamethasone in adults with bacterial meningitis [8]
>
> **Study design:** A prospective randomized double-blind placebo-controlled multi-centre trial conducted in the Netherlands.
>
> **Method:** 301 adults (≥17 years of age) with suspected bacterial meningitis in association with either cloudy CSF, bacteria seen on Gram stain of CSF, or CSF WCC of over 1,000 were randomly assigned to
>
> (continued)

either dexamethasone (157 patients) or placebo treatment (144 patients). Dexamethasone 10 mg was given intravenously 15–20 minutes before the first dose of antibiotic and every 6 hours for the next 4 days.

The primary outcome was the level of disability at 8 weeks after randomization as measured on the Glasgow outcome score. A score of 1–4 is unsatisfactory (1, death; 2, vegetative state; 3, severe disability and unable to live alone; 4, moderate disability and unable to go back to work but can live alone; 5, mild disability or no disability) and a score of 5 is satisfactory. Secondary outcomes were death, focal neurological abnormalities, hearing loss, GI bleeding (clinically relevant bleeding with a decreased serum haemoglobin level), fungal infection, herpes zoster, and hyperglycaemia (a blood glucose level higher than 144 mg/dL [8.0 mmol/L]). Sub-group analysis for both *Streptococcus pneumoniae* and *Neisseria meningitidis* was performed.

Results: Both groups had similar rates of *Streptococcus pneumoniae* (35%) and *Neisseria meningitidis* (33%) as causes of the meningitis. Treatment with dexamethasone was associated with a reduction in the risk of unfavourable outcome (relative risk, 0.59; 95% CI 0.37–0.94; p = 0.03) and death (relative risk 0.48; 95% CI, 0.24–0.96; p = 0.04). The beneficial effect of dexamethasone was most obvious in patients with pneumococcal meningitis (relative risk, 0.50; 95% CI 0.30–0.83; p = 0.006). GI bleeding occurred in two patients in the dexamethasone group and five patients in the placebo group. No difference in hearing loss or neurological deficit was found.

Conclusion: The conclusion from this study was that steroids were beneficial especially in pneumococcal meningitis.

The initial Gram stain on the cerebral spinal fluid (CSF) demonstrated scanty Gram-positive cocci in pains, 26 polymorphs/mL, protein 0.61 g/L, and CSF glucose 1.3 mmol/L (paired serum glucose 4.5 mmol/L), suggesting an initial diagnosis of pneumococcal meningitis. The patient was transferred to a side room in the acute assessment unit and was started on ceftriaxone 1 g twice a day. The case was notified to the local health protection unit.

Cultures from both anaerobic and aerobic blood culture bottles and the CSF grew *Streptococcus pneumoniae* the next day; the CSF grew 10^3 CFU/mL.

⊕ Clinical tip Diagnosis vs. speed of antibiotic administration

There is often a debate between the emergency department and the medical or IDs team with regard to the timing of the LP and antibiotic administration. The BIA guidelines suggested that antibiotics should be withheld until after an LP if the LP can be performed and antibiotics given within 30 minutes [7]. The current IDSA guideline for meningitis recommends immediate LP followed by antibiotics unless there is a delay while CT is performed [6]. However, many UK emergency departments will have guidelines for administering antibiotics to patients with possible sepsis within a specific time frame as part of 'Surviving Sepsis' care bundles and will ask the medical team to perform the LP later. There is a rationale for early administration of antibiotics in meningitis from retrospective studies and CSF analysis studies but no randomized controlled studies have been performed, for ethical reasons. One retrospective study of 305 patients found that the death rates were lower in those who had received antibiotics prior to admission (1 death in 53; 1.9%) compared to those who had not (30 deaths out of 252; 12%) [7].

While the rate at which antibiotics clear bacteria from the CSF has not been established in humans, animal studies of pneumococcal meningitis show that penicillin produces a 2-log drop in CSF bacterial concentration every hour, so that sterilization is achieved by 8 hours [11]. In the presence of prior antibiotic administrations the sensitivity of CSF Gram stain and culture drops to 40–60% and less than 50%, respectively [12]. Blood cultures should ideally be sent before antibiotic administration, where possible, and have been reported to be positive in 50–90% of adults with bacterial meningitis.

CSF and serum can also be sent for PCR. A sensitivity of 92–100% and specificity of 100% has been reported for pneumococcal meningitis [13].

Antibiotic susceptibility plates including E-tests for penicillin G and ceftriaxone were set up on day 2 and read on day 3. By day 3, the patient was still febrile and not improving; disc diffusion showed a diameter of 17 mm around the oxacillin disc and E-test results confirmed reduced susceptibility to both penicillin and ceftriaxone. The results of susceptibility testing were:

- Penicillin G: MIC 0.16 microgram/L — BSAC intermediate susceptibility
- Ceftriaxone: MIC 1 microgram/L — BSAC intermediate susceptibility

> ⭐ **Learning point** Resistance testing and pneumococcus
>
> Currently three methods are used by hospital-based microbiology laboratories to determine antibiotic susceptibilities. Disc diffusion is the most common and usually sufficient. However, in certain instances correlation between disc diameter and resistance profile is not accurate and a more precise method is required. The antibiotic gradient method (E-test) is used as a simple method to obtain a formal MIC (Figure 23.1). Molecular techniques are likely to play a larger role in the future but currently are only used to identify a few resistance markers, e.g. Mec A detection in MRSA screening.
>
> The standardization of inhibition diameters, MIC, and breakpoints is regulated by the BSAC in the UK and the CLSI in the US. The BSAC disc diffusion method for *S. pneumoniae* currently uses a 1-microgram oxacillin disc as a screening tool to detect penicillin-resistant pneumococci. A zone size ≥20 mm is required for an organism to be reported as susceptible to the β-lactams (penicillin, cephalosporins, and carbapenems). Zone sizes ≤19 mm require further testing for MIC via an E-test to interpret [14].
>
> BSAC categorizes *S. pneumoniae* isolates into three groups according to susceptibility patterns. Penicillin definitions are as follows: susceptible (MIC ≤0.06 mg/L); intermediate (MIC 0.12–2 mg/L); and resistant (MIC >2 mg/L).
>
> It is recommended that for infections involving the CNS, penicillin should be avoided if the MIC in the intermediate range. In non CNS infections, high doses of penicillins may be adequate to overcome the MIC.
>
> Susceptibility to third-generation cephalosporins (cefotaxime and ceftazidime) is also divided into three categories: susceptible (MIC ≤0.5 mg/L); intermediate (MIC 1–2 mg/L); and resistant (MIC >2 mg/L).

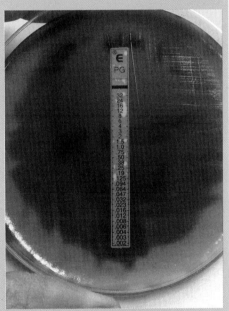

> **Figure 23.1** E-test strip. A penicillin gradient strip sits on an agar plate inoculated with *Streptococcus pneumoniae*. An elliptical zone is seen around the strip and the point of interception (0.023 microgram/mL) corresponds to the MIC.
> With thanks to Ms. Amita Patel and Dr. Pasco Hearn (Guys and St Thomas's NHS Foundation Trust) for developing the penicillin E-test for the chapter.

➕ **Clinical tip** Summary of IDSA guideline on choice of antimicrobial agents for β-lactam resistant pneumococci causing CNS infection [6]

See Table 23.1.

Table 23.1 IDSA guidelines for the management of pneumococcal meningitis

Pen MIC ≤0.06 mg/L	Penicillin G, amoxicillin or third-generation cephalosporin
Pen MIC >0.06 mg/L plus ceftriaxone MIC <1.0 mg/L	Third-generation cephalosporin
Pen MIC >0.06 mg/L plus ceftriaxone MIC ≥1.0 mg/L	Third-generation cephalosporin plus vancomycin (some would add RIF as well if dexamethasone has been given) or carbapenem if sensitive or fluroquinolone is listed as an alternative agent

Source: Data from Tunkel AR et al, Practice guidelines for the management of bacterial meningitis, *Clinical Infectious Diseases*, Volume 39, Issue 9, pp. 1267–84, Copyright © 2004 by the Infectious Diseases Society of America. All rights reserved.

The ceftriaxone dose was increased to 2 g twice daily and vancomycin 60 mg/kg per day was also added.

✔ **Evidence base** Attaining adequate levels of CSF vancomycin

Levels of vancomycin in CSF of adult patients receiving adjunctive corticosteroids to treat pneumococcal meningitis [15]

Vancomycin is a large molecule with poor CSF penetration. Further reduction in penetration in the CSF with concomitant dexamethasone was postulated and confirmed in the rabbit meningitis model.

Study design: A prospective observational study was performed in four intensive care units in France to look at CSF vancomycin levels during treatment for pneumococcal meningitis with dexamethasone as well as antimicrobials.

Method: Thirteen adult patients with suspected pneumococcal meningitis were treated with high doses of intravenous vancomycin (15 mg/kg loading dose followed by 60 mg/kg/day) along with intravenous dexamethasone and cefotaxime. All participants had a second LP performed on day 2 or 3 to assess the evolution of the meningitis and to check vancomycin levels. Matched serum levels were taken at the same time.

Results: The mean concentration of serum vancomycin was 25.2 mg/L (range 14.2–39.0 mg/L) and the mean concomitant concentration of CSF vancomycin was 7.9 mg/L (range 3.1–22.3 mg/L) and there was positive correlation between the two. The concentration of vancomycin in CSF was at least 10-fold the MIC in 8 patients, 8-fold the MIC in 2 patients, and 4-fold the MIC in 1 patient.

Conclusion: This study showed that therapeutic concentrations of vancomycin can be attained in the CSF by administrating high intravenous doses.

The patient improved significantly and the treatment was continued for 14 days, after which he was discharged without any neurological complications.

✖ **Learning point** Outcomes in pneumococcal meningitis

Prior to the advent of antibiotics, pneumococcal meningitis was uniformly fatal. However, even in the era of antimicrobials and treatment, in high-income countries mortality is still in the range of 20–30% in adults and around 10% in children. Rates of neurological complications are as high as 50% even with

(continued)

optimum care. Complications include seizures, intellectual impairment, cranial nerve palsies, loss of cognitive function, and hearing impairment. Outcomes in the era of cephalosporin resistance have not so far been shown to be worse; however, most of the studies have been performed in countries where it is routine to give vancomycin as well as cephalosporins.

Discussion

This case highlights the many challenges in the management of acute pneumococcal meningitis, made more complicated by intermediate penicillin and cephalosporin resistance. The patient was lucky to survive without any neurological consequences considering the nature of the organism, his clinical presentation, resistance profile, and the initial sub-therapeutic dose of cephalosporin that he was given at the outset. Although in this case the patient was treated with cefotaxime rapidly by the emergency department, it was not given at the meningitis dose of 2 g twice a day and his condition did not improve. On day 3 of admission the infecting organism was found to have intermediate resistance to cefalosporins which led to the addition of vancomycin and the increase of the cefotaxime dose to 2 g. Any adult presenting with meningitis should be treated empirically with a CNS dose of cefotaxime or ceftriaxone. If they have recently had multiple courses of antibacterials or traveled to an area when penicillin or cephalosporin resistant pneumococci are prevalent in the last 3 months, empirical vancomycin should also be given.

In parts of the world where resistance rates are high, empirical choice of antibiotics for bacterial meningitis includes a third-generation cephalosporin and vancomycin (see IDSA guidelines). In the UK rates of pneumococcal resistance currently remains relatively low, with rates of cephalosporin resistance even lower. Current UK guidelines do not recommend the routine addition of empirical vancomycin except in high-risk groups (see Box 23.1), so a blanket policy for all of adding vancomycin is not recommended. However, rates of resistance are higher in certain areas of the country (e.g. London) and in certain at-risk groups (Box 23.1).

Risk factors for invasive disease with resistant organisms have been identified in retrospective analyses, suggesting that patients can be stratified according to risk [17]. Risk factors include travel to area with high resistance, previous antibiotic use, residence in long-term care facility, recent hospitalization, chronic pulmonary disease, and community or household contact with resistant strains. Our patient had three risk factors for resistance: prolonged household contact with a child who had recently come from Spain and was unvaccinated, COPD, and recent antibiotic use. Although there is no evidence yet that a risk assessment approach leads to better outcomes, many authorities are advocating this approach. For example, the current UK paediatric NICE guidance suggests that patients with recent travel overseas and multiple or prolonged courses of antibiotics in the previous 3 months should receive vancomycin as well as third-generation cephalosporin [18]. Many clinicians will also follow this guidance for adult patients, de-escalating to narrow-spectrum antibiotics when susceptibility data is available.

Could this patient have been treated with cefotaxime alone, considering that the isolate was only just at the intermediate resistance breakpoint of 1 mg/L. Multiple case reports from the 1990s have shown that treatment with cefotaxime/ceftriaxone when the isolate has a MIC $\geq$2 mg/L consistently results in clinical failure [19]. Due to the high rates of adverse outcomes from pneumococcal meningitis it is difficult to interpret case reports of failure without repeat LP data, which was included in some of the reports. Sterilization for sensitive isolates usually occurs within hours [11]. Further evidence

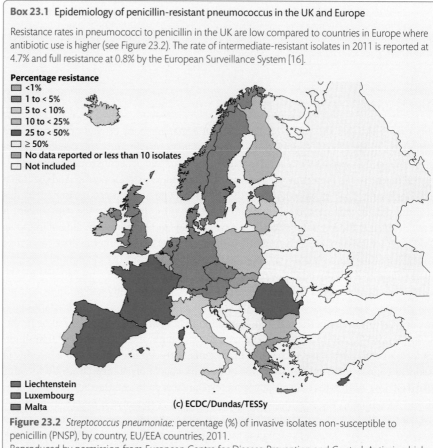

Box 23.1 Epidemiology of penicillin-resistant pneumococcus in the UK and Europe

Resistance rates in pneumococci to penicillin in the UK are low compared to countries in Europe where antibiotic use is higher (see Figure 23.2). The rate of intermediate-resistant isolates in 2011 is reported at 4.7% and full resistance at 0.8% by the European Surveillance System [16].

Percentage resistance
- <1%
- 1 to < 5%
- 5 to < 10%
- 10 to < 25%
- 25 to < 50%
- ≥ 50%
- No data reported or less than 10 isolates
- Not included

- Liechtenstein
- Luxembourg
- Malta

(c) ECDC/Dundas/TESSy

Figure 23.2 *Streptococcus pneumoniae*: percentage (%) of invasive isolates non-susceptible to penicillin (PNSP), by country, EU/EEA countries, 2011.
Reproduced by permission from European Centre for Disease Prevention and Control, Antimicrobial resistance surveillance in Europe 2011, Annual Report of the European Antimicrobial Resistance Surveillance Network (EARS-Net), ECEC, Stockholm, Sweden, Copyright © European Centre for Disease Prevention and Control, 2012.

Malta and Spain harbour some of the highest rates of penicillin resistance in Europe with non-susceptibility rates (resistant and intermediate-resistant) reported at 50% and 30% respectively. High rates are also high in many Asian countries and the USA [16].

Introduction of PCV-13 vaccination has led to a reduction in carriage and disease from resistant strains in the USA. This is due in part to including serotypes with high levels of resistance in the vaccine and is also thought to be due to reduced use of antibiotics in vaccinated recipients.

that an MIC ≥2 mg/L is likely to fail came from the rabbit pneumococcal meningitis model where ceftriaxone did not reach levels required to sterilize the CSF when the MIC was in the 2–4 mg/L range [19]. In the rabbit model, vancomycin in addition to ceftri-axone led to synergy between the two antibiotics and good sterilization. In the presence of dexamethasone, CSF levels of both antibiotics were reduced and the addition of RIF (not affected by dexamethasone in the rabbit model) is therefore advocated by some authorities for resistant isolates treated with adjunctive dexamethasone. The majority of reports for isolates with an MIC of 1 mg/L (intermediate range) tend to show effective treatment with cefotaxime alone. However, failure at 1 mg/L has been reported and this tends to be the cut-off at which vancomycin is added [19].

⑥ Expert comment

There are unfortunately few alternatives to penicillin and cephalosporins for *S. pneumoniae* meningitis. Vancomycin is active against β-lactam resistant pneumococcus, but is not particularly bactericidal, and CSF penetration is limited and possibly further reduced by dexamethasone. RIF could be considered as adjunctive treatment, as studies with vancomycin and/or ceftriaxone show additional clearance of the CSF and bactericidal killing. RIF also demonstrates a non-antibiotic effect of lowering proinflammatory bacterial products. In low-resource settings, chloramphenicol continues to be used to treat bacterial meningitis, but toxicity and increasing resistance rates reduce its usefulness. Chloramphenicol could be considered where severe penicillin allergy is an issue. Another older drug is co-trimoxazole which has good penetration through inflamed meninges, and has been used to treat pneumococcal meningitis. Among the β-lactams the carbapenem, meropenem, is licensed for use in meningitis; however, cross-resistance in penicillin-resistant and cephalosporin-resistant isolates can occur and MIC assessment is required. Linezolid has good CSF penetration, but little data is available, apart from an animal model, where it was found to be inferior to ceftriaxone. Therefore linezolid is very much used as a last resort, often in combination. The new fluoroquinolones, levofloxacin and moxifloxacin, have good CNS penetration and activity against *S. pneumoniae*, but clinical experience in severe sepsis and meningeal pneumococcal disease is limited.

A final word from the expert

Bacterial meningitis is a leading cause of morbidity and mortality worldwide. Advances such as vaccination, introduced routinely for children and at-risk adults, has reduced the risk of invasive pneumococcal infections (including the reduction of some resistant strains) for both children and adults. However, antibiotic choices for resistant isolates continue to pose a challenge.

Solutions for better management in the case described include easily accessible hospital prescribing guidelines (e.g. on the hospital intranet) and early referral to an infection team. Many centres have developed an MDT of pharmacists, ID physicians, and clinical microbiologists, who offer a rapid response consult service. Daily infection-focused ward rounds on the medical admissions unit would also have picked up this case early.

References

1 Bosch AA, Biesbroek G, Trzcinski K, Sanders EA, Bogaert D. Viral and bacterial interactions in the upper respiratory tract. *PLoS Pathog* 2013; 9: e1003057.

2 Department of Health. *Immunisation against infectious disease – 'The Green Book'.* Pneumococcal: Chapter 25. https://www.gov.uk/government/uploads/system/uploads/attachment_data/file/147977/Green-Book-Chapter-25-v4_0.pdf.pdf (accessed 10 April 2013).

3 Dudley S, Ashe K, Winther B, Wendley JO. Bacterial pathogens of otitis media and sinusitis: detection in the nasopharynx with selective agar media. *J Lab Clin Med* 2001; 138: 338–342.

4 Miller E, Andrews NJ, Waight PA, Slack MP, George RC. Herd immunity and serotype replacement 4 years after seven-valent pneumococcal conjugate vaccination in England and Wales: an observational cohort study. *Lancet Infect Dis* 2011; 11: 760–768.

5 Hasbun R, Abrahams J, Jekel J, Quagliarello VJ. Computed tomography of the head before lumbar puncture in adults with suspected meningitis. *N Engl J Med* 2001; 345: 1727–1733.

6 Tunkel AR. Practice guidelines for the management of bacterial meningitis. *Clin Infect Dis* 2004; 39: 1267–1284.

7 Heyderman RS, Lambert HP, O'Sullivan I, Stuart JM, Taylor BL, Wall RA. Early management of suspected bacterial meningitis and meningiococcal septicaemia in adults. *J Infect* 2003; 46: 75–77.

8 de Gans J, van de Beek D; European Dexamethasone in Adulthood Bacterial Meningitis Study Investigators. Dexamethasone in adults with bacterial meningitis. *N Engl J Med* 2002; 347: 1549–1556.

9 van de Beek D, Farrar JJ, de Gans J et al. Adjunctive dexamethasone in bacterial meningitis: a meta-analysis of individual patient data. *Lancet Neurol* 2010; 9: 254–263.

10 Brouwer MC, McIntyre P, de Gans J, Prasad K, van de Beek D. Corticosteroids for acute bacterial meningitis (review). *Cochrane Database Syst Rev* 2010; (9): CD004405.

11 Sande MA, Korzeniowski OM, Allegro GM, Brennan RO, Zak O, Scheld WM. Intermittant or continuous therapy of experimental meningitis due to *Streptococcus pneumoniae* in rabbits: preliminary observations on the postantibiotic effect *in vivo*. *Rev Infect Dis* 1981; 3: 98–109.

12 Blazer S, Berant M, Alon U. Bacterial meningitis. Effect of antibiotic treatment on cerebrospinal fluid. *Am J Clin Pathol* 1983; 80: 386–387.

13 Werno AM, Murdoch DR. Medical microbiology: laboratory diagnosis of invasive pneumococcal disease. *Clin Infect Dis* 2008; 46: 926.

14 British Association for Antimicrobial Chemotherapy (BSAC). Methods for Antimicrobial Susceptibility Testing 2013. http://bsac.org.uk/wp-content/uploads/2012/02/Version-12-december-2012_final.pdf (accessed 10 April 2013).

15 Ricard JD, Wolff M, Lacherade JC et al. Levels of vancomycin in cerebrospinal fluid of adult patients receiving adjunctive corticosteroids to treat pneumococcal meningitis: a prospective multicenter observational study. *Clin Infect Dis* 2007; 44: 250–255.

16 Susceptibility of *Streptococcus pneumoniae* isolates to penicillins in Europe in 2011. http://ecdc.europa.eu/en/activities/surveillance/EARS-Net/database/Pages/tables_report.aspx (accessed 10 April 2013).

17 Vanderkooi OG, Low DE, Green K, Powis JE McGeer A. Predicting antimicrobial resistance in invasive pneumococcal infections. Clin Infect Dis 2005; 40: 1288–1297.

18 Pollard AJ (GDG chair), Cloke A et al. *Bacterial meningitis and meningococcal septicaemia: Management of bacterial meningitis and meningococcal septicaemia in children and young people younger than 16 years in primary and secondary care.* Issue date: June 2010, revised September 2010. http://guidance.nice.org.uk/CG102/Guidance/pdf/English (accessed 13 April 2013).

19 Kaplan SL, Mason EO Jr. Management of infections due to antibiotic resistant *Streptococcus pneumoniae. Clin Microbiol Rev* 1998; 11: 628–644.

Urinary sepsis: vancomycin-resistant enterococci

Julia Howard

ⓒ **Expert commentary** Sorrush Soleimanian

Case history

A 76-year-old gentleman presented to the emergency department with a 2-hour history of rigors and difficulty in passing urine. He had a past medical history of a radical perineal prostatectomy for carcinoma of the prostate 9 years previously, hypertension, and a recent transurethral resection of bladder tumour (TURBT) for transitional cell carcinoma (TCC).

At presentation he was tachycardic, hypertensive, and pyrexial. On abdominal examination he was found to have suprapubic and left-sided loin tenderness. Systems examination was otherwise unremarkable. He was found to have urethral clot retention and a three-way catheter was inserted under gentamicin cover. Urine and blood cultures were taken at this time. Blood tests revealed an increased WCC (WCC 13.4×10^9/L) and CRP 157 mg/L. In view of these findings and his pyrexia, he was started on intravenous piperacillin/tazobactam for presumed urinary sepsis. Renal function was normal. He was admitted under the care of the urology team. He remained clinically stable and became apyrexial after 36 hours. Blood results were negative and urine culture was reported as no significant growth.

> ➕ **Clinical tip** Urine culture in the microbiology laboratory and reporting of results
>
> The initial urine sample in this case was reported as no significant growth. Bacteriuria is considered significant when a pure growth of an organism is identified at over 10^5 CFU/mL [1]. Growth below this concentration is most likely to be due to contamination. However, significant results can occur with concentrations that are lower in certain populations and clinical situations. For example, counts as low as 10^3 CFU/mL have been shown to be significant in young men and counts of 10^2 CFU/mL in acutely symptomatic young women [1]. Conversely, counts over 10^5 CFU may not always require treatment or be significant. For example, elderly patients may develop asymptomatic bacteriuria with significant counts on culture but they may not require antibiotic treatment. Looking at the WCC in the urine and whether antibacterial activity is detected (reported by some laboratories) in the sample can help interpret a urine result. Significant pyuria is defined as 10^4 WBC/mL, although a level of 10^5 WBC/mL is a more useful indicator of clinical infection because high white cell counts can exist in healthy women [1]. Repeat urine microbiological examination is necessary if the laboratory result is not consistent with the clinical situation.
>
> In this case the patient's symptoms, the fact that the urine was collected after the initiation of antibiotics, and the presence of white cells in the urine all suggested urinary infection despite the 'no significant growth' result of the urine culture.

On day 5 of his admission he underwent a CT scan of his abdomen and pelvis which showed left hydronephrosis secondary to a bladder tumour. On day 6 a cystoscopy was performed with a failed attempt to pass a ureteric stent. He underwent left nephrostomy insertion a day later and, although pus was drained, unfortunately none was sent for microscopy and culture.

The patient received 10 days of treatment with piperacillin/tazobactam for presumed pyonephrosis with good response. However, 24 hours after stopping antibiotics he became pyrexial and haemodynamically unstable. Blood cultures and a sample from the nephrostomy drain were taken, and he was commenced on meropenem. On day 11, two days after he had become pyrexial again, blood cultures grew *Escherichia coli* (*E. coli*) which showed intermediate susceptibility to piperacillin/tazobactam by direct disc susceptibility testing and susceptibility to meropenem.

The sample from the nephrostomy drain grew *E. coli* with identical sensitivities to that found in the blood culture and a vancomycin-resistant *Enterococcus faecium* (VRE) (Table 24.1).

> **⊕ Clinical tip**
>
> Ensure that samples are sent for microscopy, Gram stain, and culture to guide appropriate microbiological and clinical management.
>
> A valuable opportunity (sending the pus from the drainage at nephrostomy insertion) was missed. An analysis of the sample from the sterile site would have been more helpful to guide antimicrobial therapy than the drain fluid that the laboratory eventually received.

> **⊕ Clinical tip** Ensure you distinguish between colonization and infection
>
> Enterococci are low-virulence organisms that may colonize rather than cause infection [2].
>
> Make sure you consider the result in the clinical context of the patient. Consider whether the patient clinically has an infection or not and remember to look back through previous microbiological results to see if they have been colonized or infected with the organisms previously. Consider risk factors for invasive infection. For VRE the risk factors for invasive infection are malignancy, immunosuppression, intensive care unit (ICU) care, being a patient on a renal unit, haematology or liver unit, repeated or prolonged hospital admissions, indwelling medical devices, and multiple courses of antibiotics [2].
>
> Look carefully at results of fluid samples and compare with cultures from other sites. Has the sample been taken from a sterile site? If the site is not sterile there is a high likelihood that the organism may not be significant. If there is no indication of the source on the form, chase it up with the clinical team.

Table 24.1 Microscopy and culture of fluid from left-sided nephrostomy drain

Microscopy and Gram stain	Culture	Antimicrobial sensitivities
Turbid, WCC seen +++		
Gram-positive cocci seen +	Moderate growth of *Enterococcus faecium* isolated	Penicillin R Ampicillin R Erythromycin R Vancomycin R (MIC 256 microgram/mL) Teicoplanin R (MIC 256 microgram/mL) RIF R Gentamicin R Linezolid S
Gram-negative rods seen ++	Heavy growth of *Escherichia coli* isolated	Ampicillin R Cephalexin R Ciprofloxacin R Nitrofurantoin S Trimethoprim R Gentamicin R Piperacillin/tazobactam I Meropenem S

I, intermediate; MIC, minimum inhibitory concentration; R, resistant, S, sensitive.

> **☼ Learning point** Epidemiology
>
> VRE is a major cause of nosocomial infection worldwide. The use of the glycopeptide avoparcin in animals is thought to have encouraged the development of VRE [3,4,5,6] and it was withdrawn from the market in 2000. The first clinical report of an outbreak of VRE was published in 1988 and this described a VRE outbreak in a cohort of end-stage renal failure patients in Europe. Subsequently outbreaks were reported in some hospitals in the United States [2,6,7]. The clinical incidence varies from country to country. Across Europe, the prevalence of vancomycin resistance in enterococcal clinical isolates varies widely from very low prevalence rates in some countries (e.g. the Netherlands) to over 40% in others (such as Greece and Portugal) [4]. For 2010 (latest data) in England, Wales, and Northern Ireland, the prevalence of vancomycin resistance was 1% for *E. faecalis* and 17% for *E. faecium* [8]. The success seen in the Netherlands has been attributed to various factors including good antimicrobial stewardship and national search-and-destroy policies for MDR organisms [8]. VRE isolates are most frequently *E. faecium* [2]. Patients with VRE infection have worse clinical outcomes and a higher mortality than those with vancomycin-susceptible enterococci infections [2].
>
> **Surveillance:** In England there is voluntary reporting of enterococcal bacteraemias. Clinically significant VRE bacteraemias (blood culture isolates) have been part of mandatory reporting in England since 2003 under a joint Department of Health (DH) and PHE (formerly HPA) scheme. Currently there are just over 500 reports a year and these are reported on a National Health Service (NHS) Trust basis.
>
> In England, there is no mandatory reporting for isolates from other sites (wounds, urine, other sterile fluids, etc.). There are schemes for screening patients for faecal colonization with VRE in some parts of the world using selective media and NAATs, but this type of screening is not routinely carried out in England.

In this case, culture of the nephrostomy drain fluid grew an identical *E. coli* to that found in the blood cultures. Therefore the VRE was felt to be simply colonizing the drain fluid and specific antibiotic therapy for VRE was not instituted.

> **☼ Learning point** Isolation, identification, and antimicrobial susceptibility testing of enterococci from clinical samples
>
> **Appearance on culture, Lancefield grouping, and speciation**
>
> Enterococci are Gram-positive cocci usually seen in short chains. They belong to the Lancefield group D streptococci, are aesculin-positive, and may be beta-haemolytic. They are facultative anaerobes and are catalase and oxidase-negative. They will grow on MacConkey, CLED (cystine-lysine-electrolyte deficient agar) and bile-containing media. In clinical practice in England, Wales, and Northern Ireland, the most commonly identified enterococci in blood cultures are *E. faecalis* (44.5%) and *E. faecium* (28.7%). However, 22.4% of enterococcal bacteraemia reports to the HPA in 2010 did not record the species [8]. Speciation is usually carried out using a commercially available biochemical identification test kit (e.g. API) but they can also be identified by MALDITOF.
>
> **Vancomycin-resistant enterococci:** VRE are glycopeptide-resistant enterococci. A large antimicrobial surveillance programme of all VRE clinical isolates carried out in 2003, covering 839 sites in the US and Canada and 56 sites in Europe, found that 91% of VRE were *E. faecium* and 7.8% were *E. faecalis* [9]. However, other species such as *Enteroccocus gallinarium*, *Enterococcus casseliflavus*, and *Enterococcus flavescens* may be found.
>
> **Antimicrobial resistance testing**
>
> First-line disc testing for enterococci usually includes penicillin, amoxicillin, vancomycin, teicoplanin and, where relevant, gentamicin 200 micrograms. Further sensitivity testing to linezolid, daptomycin, and tigecycline should be requested if vancomycin resistance is detected. Testing for sensitivity to quinupristin-dalfopristin is appropriate for *E. faecium* only [2]. Testing for sensitivity to nitrofurantoin may be appropriate for uncomplicated urinary tract infection (UTI) [2].
>
> Resistance to teicoplanin and/or vancomycin seen on disc testing should be confirmed with a commercially available epsilometer test (E-test) to establish MICs. The Clinical and Laboratories Standards Institute (CLSI) breakpoints define vancomycin susceptibility for enterococci as having a MIC ≤4 microgram/mL and resistance as ≥32 microgram/mL [2].

> ❝ **Expert comment**
>
> *Enterococcus* spp grow on non-selective media and the majority of selective media including media containing NaCl 6.5%. Their colonies on blood agar can appear as α, γ, or β-haemolytic. Their ability to grow on media containing NaCl 6.5% is an important characteristic of the organism as this distinguishes it from *Streptococcus bovis*. *S. bovis* is also catalase-negative, aesculin-positive, and also reacts with Lancefield group D. It is also important to distinguish between *Leuconostoc* spp and VRE as the former appear as Gram-positive cocci in chains or pairs, are aesculin-positive, are inherently resistant to vancomycin and teicoplanin, and grow on NaCl 6.5%. However, *Leuconostoc* spp do not react with Lancefield group D.

> ❝ **Expert comment**
>
> Remember that trimethoprim *in vitro* susceptibility does not correlate with *in vivo* clinical response seen in the patient due to the ability of enterococci to utilize preformed folic acid. Therefore, trimethoprim is not recommended as a treatment option, even for urinary tract infections. Doxycycline and chloramphenicol have been used in different clinical settings in the past with some success if the isolate appears to be sensitive to these antibiotics. *Enterococcus* spp including VRE are resistant to low concentrations of gentamicin disc (10 micrograms). If clinically the isolate is felt to be related to infective endocarditis, a high concentration gentamicin disc (200 micrograms) should be tested to determine if the isolate is sensitive to it.

On discussion with the microbiology team the patient was moved to a side room for barrier nursing (Box 24.1).

Box 24.1 Infection control

Reservoir of carriage

The main site of carriage in humans is the lower GI tract and colonization may persist for months or even years [3]. There is no evidence of effectiveness for decolonization with non-absorbable antibiotics and this is not recommended. Healthcare staff have been found to be carriers of VRE; however, no evidence of transfer to patients has been found and so screening of staff is not recommended [3].

Transmission

Key routes of transmission of the organism include hands, fomites, as well as the potential long-term presence of enterococci in the environment [3].

Guidelines available

Guidelines on the control of glycopeptide-resistant enterococci in healthcare settings were published in 2003 in the United States by the Society for Healthcare Epidemiology of America (SHEA) [10] and in 2006 in the United Kingdom by a working party of the Hospital Infection Society (HIS), Infection Control Nurses Association, and the BSAC [3].

Both the SHEA [10] and the UK guidelines [3] make recommendations about limiting the use of vancomycin to improve control. The UK guidelines recommend that all hospitals try to avoid using glycopeptides when possible [3], and the American guidelines recommended restricting vancomycin use [10]. However, a systematic review [11] which reviewed 13 studies published from January 1987 to March 2006 concluded that the role of strategies that aim to restrict the use of vancomycin in the control of VRE colonization and infection in hospitals located in the USA is uncertain.

What to do in everyday practice
- Consult local guidelines.
- Tell your infection control team and the clinical team looking after the patient.
- Ensure that the patient is nursed in a side room with ensuite toilet facilities. If there are not enough side rooms, discuss with infection control and prioritize VRE patients with diarrhoea as these are most likely to spread the infection. In an outbreak consider cohorting patients.

(continued)

- Ensure that the nursing staff and clinical teams use barrier precautions when attending the patient. Hand washing is the most important precaution. Alcohol gel is effective on the physically clean hand.
- Use dedicated equipment such as commodes.
- When the patient is discharged the room will need deep cleaning with a chlorine-based agent.
- Ensure surveillance is carried out to detect an outbreak if it occurs.
- If an outbreak occurs, ensure screening is carried out to detect colonization and enable isolation. Screening of stool samples should be carried out by use of specific selective media such as agar containing bile salts and an indicator such as aesculin and containing 6 microgram/L of vancomycin [3]. Other methods such as using specific chromogenic agar or specific PCRs that detect the *vanA* and *vanB* genes are currently undergoing scientific evaluation.

It was considered that the *E. coli* was the clinically significant pathogen and that the VRE was colonizing his drain, so he remained solely on meropenem.

The patient made good clinical progress and the meropenem was stopped on day 10 of treatment. He was sent home with a left-sided nephrostomy *in situ* with a plan for palliative chemotherapy and tumour debulking surgery in the future.

Four weeks later he returned to hospital complaining of fevers and reduced output from the nephrostomy. He complained that the output from the drain had changed from clear urine to thick pus. On admission he was found to be pyrexial and tender over the left loin. Blood cultures and samples from the left-sided nephrostomy drain were taken. He was commenced on meropenem in view of his previous *E. coli* infection. A CT scan of the abdomen showed that the tumour had progressed, partially blocking the nephrostomy drain, and there was a collection behind the drain. Both the blood cultures and the drain fluid cultured VRE but no *E. coli*. After a discussion with the microbiology team, linezolid was added to the meropenem; however, it was felt that surgical drainage of the collection was the most important intervention and the patient was taken to theatre the next day for drainage of the collection and insertion of a new nephrostomy tube. On day 10 he developed thrombocytopenia and the linezolid was switched to daptomycin. Repeat blood cultures were negative at day 3 and he finished a 2-week course of antibiotic therapy before undergoing definitive surgery.

Discussion

This case presented two major challenges. The first challenge was when to consider the VRE as causing invasive infection. When the patient first presented, correlation with the blood culture findings and the evidence that the VRE was grown from drain bag fluid rather than a sterile sample suggested that the VRE was only colonizing the site and this growth was of doubtful significance. Unfortunately, a key opportunity was missed; sending a sample for microscopy and culture from the procedure when the pyonephrosis was drained and the nephrostomy tube was inserted. When he re-presented, finding the VRE in the blood culture suggested that it had become a pathogen and required treatment both with antibiotics and with surgical drainage to remove the collection of pus. Many patients who present with invasive VRE disease may be colonized in the bowel; however, there is no evidence for the effectiveness of decolonization currently [3,6], so it is unlikely that screening would have influenced the outcome as decolonization would not have been undertaken.

The second challenge was the choice of antibiotics for the treatment of the VRE bacteraemia. Limited high-quality evidence exists to inform the optimal treatment of VRE bacteraemia. This case highlights a patient with a VRE of the *E. faecium* variety

Expert comment

One of the risk factors for VRE is previous vancomycin therapy either intravenous or oral. For example, there is an association between VRE bacteraemia and CDI thought to be due to vancomycin treatment. In this case there was no other patient known to be colonized or infected with VRE on the ward. This is always worth checking to ensure that the possibility of cross-transmission is not missed.

Expert comment

Among carbapenems only imipenem demonstrates good activity against penicillin-susceptible enterococcal spp (e.g. *Enterococcus faecalis* including VRE). Isolates of *Enterococcus faecium* including VRE should be resistant to carbapenems. Meropenem generally has poor activity against *Enterococcus faecalis* and ertapenem is considered as having no activity against such isolates.

Expert comment

Please note that some studies have demonstrated that addition of an antibiotic with activity against enterococcal spp (this includes VRE) to empirical therapy of intra-abdominal sepsis did not have effect on the outcome and subsequent complications of patients. On the other hand, some other studies showed a degree of benefit.

which are normally resistant to ampicillin and aminoglycosides. *E. faecalis* VRE are much rarer and are often sensitive to ampicillin.

⊗ **Learning point** Resistance in enterococci

Enterococci are intrinsically more resistant than other streptococci, with *E. faecium* displaying more resistance than *E. faecalis*. Resistance to cephalosporins, low concentrations of aminoglycosides, clindamycin, and trimethoprim-sulfamethoxazole (*in vivo* by using exogenous folate) are all intrinsic to enterococci. Resistance to amoxicillin, glycopeptides, and vancomycin are all commonly acquired [6]. Glycopeptides inhibit cell wall production by binding to the D-alanyl-D-alanine (D-Ala-D-Ala) terminus of the peptidoglycan precursor leading to chain termination. The replacement of alanine with lactate leads to resistance through reduced affinity for glycopeptides. Acquired resistance is encoded by five main gene clusters (VanA, VanB, VanD, VanE, and VanG), VanA and VanB being the most common. VanC is intrinsic to *Enterococcus gallinarium* and *Enterococcus casseliflavus/Enterococcus flavescens*. All types display resistance to vancomycin (to varying degrees) but they differ in whether they lead to teicoplanin resistance and whether teicoplanin resistance can be induced. VanA leads to high-dose vancomycin and teicoplanin resistance, and resistance can be induced by either antibiotic, whereas VanB are resistant to a range of vancomycin concentrations and are sensitive to teicoplanin [7]. The clinical significance is that VRE can be treated with teicoplanin if resistance testing suggests the isolate is sensitive. However, resistance to teicoplanin may be induced [7] (Table 24.2).

Table 24.2 Rates of antimicrobial resistance in *E. faecalis* and *E. faecium*

	E. faecalis	E. faecium
Amoxicillin	R in 5% of isolates [8]	R in 90% of isolates [8]
	If R mechanism is via a penicillinase	If R mechanism is via reduced affinity of penicillin binding protein PBP5
High-level gentamicin	R in 32% of isolates [8] Aminoglycoside modifying enzymes	R in 54% of isolates [8]
Vancomycin	R in 1% of isolates [8] VanB > VanA	R in 17% of isolates [8] VanA > VanB

Source: Data from Health Protection Agency, *Enterococcus* spp. bacteraemia reports for England, Wales and Northern Ireland: 2006–2010, Copyright © 2010, available from http://www.hpa.org.uk/Topics/InfectiousDiseases/InfectionsAZ/EnterococciSpeciesAndGRE/EpidemiologicalData/VoluntarySurveillanceData/EnterococcusSpp/

A few VRE are still sensitive to teicoplanin (if they contain VanB or VanC) and can be treated with this glycopeptide, although this may induce teicoplanin resistance [7]. (Note: teicoplanin is not available in the USA.) However, as in this case, most VRE are not sensitive to teicoplanin. Most consensus opinion suggests linezolid or daptomycin should be first-line agents with quinupristin-dalfopristin as an alternative option for *E. faecium* only [2]. Tigecycline is licensed for the treatment of complicated skin and soft tissue infection and intra-abdominal infections; however, due to its PK, tigecycline is not suitable for the treatment of VRE bacteraemia [2].

Linezolid, an oxazolidinone antimicrobial that interferes with bacterial protein synthesis at the ribosomal level, is another option for treatment. Linezolid is bacteriostatic and has good absorption orally (100% bioavailability [5]). The main side effect is bone marrow suppression, as was seen in this case when the patient became thrombocytopenic. In England the licensed duration of treatment is limited to a maximum of 2 weeks in view of potential bone marrow suppression. When recommending treatment with linezolid it is therefore important to ask the clinician to perform regular monitoring of the full blood count. VRE may develop resistance to linezolid via a ribosomal mutation;

however, this is rare and is more likely to be seen when linezolid is used for long periods of time or when a focus of infection is left *in situ* or undrained [5].

Daptomycin is a lipopeptide which interferes with bacterial cell membranes. It is only active against Gram-positive bacteria and is bactericidal [12]. When using daptomycin it is important to ask the clinician to monitor serial CK and check for muscular aches and pains in case the patient develops myopathy [2].

Daptomycin is currently only licensed by the EMA for complicated skin and soft-tissue infections, staphylococcal bacteraemia, and right-sided staphylococcal endocarditis in adults, hence its use for the treatment of VRE bacteraemia is off-licence. Controversy remains about the optimal dosing for complex infection; however, it can be given in a once-a-day dosing regimen [12].

> **🕦 Expert comment**
>
> Baseline CK should be obtained at the beginning of daptomycin therapy, and weekly monitoring is recommended if the CK level remains normal. More frequent monitoring is indicated if CK starts to rise during therapy.

✔ Evidence base Comparison of outcomes from daptomycin or linezolid treatment for vancomycin-resistant enterococcal bloodstream infection: a retrospective, multicenter, cohort study [13]

Study design: A retrospective, multicentre cohort study (three US hospitals) performed via notes review. The hospitals included in the study all used either linezolid or daptomycin in the treatment of VRE bacteraemia.

Inclusion criteria: Patients aged 18 and over with VRE as sole cause of bacteraemia were included from 2003 to 2007 (n = 101); 67 patients were treated with daptomycin and 34 with linezolid. The two groups were similar in that the most common source of the bacteraemia was intravascular line (51% daptomycin vs. 38% linezolid, p = NS) followed by an abdominal source (10% daptomycin vs. 12% linezolid). There was one case of infective endocarditis in the daptomycin group only. The groups differed significantly in that those treated with daptomycin were more likely to be shocked (31.3% vs. 11.8%; p = 0.049) and to have received previous linezolid treatment (31.8% vs. 0%; p <0.001).

Outcomes: The outcomes assessed were mortality and duration of bacteraemia defined by time of initial positive blood culture to time of first negative blood culture.

Results: No significant difference in inpatient mortality was seen in patients receiving daptomycin (31/67, 46.3%) versus linezolid (10/34, 29.4%). However there was a trend towards worse outcomes in the daptomycin group. It must be remembered that the daptomycin group were more likely to be shocked and to have had prior antibiotic treatment, suggesting more prolonged infection. Antibiotic selection did not affect the mean duration of positive cultures (daptomycin, 2.9 days vs. linezolid, 1.6 days; p = 0.12).

Results: The study found that increased mortality among participants was related to shock (OR 14.24, p = 0.008), *E. faecium* infection (OR 53.10, p = 0.024), previous treatment with linezolid (OR 6.63, p = 0.031), and a source of infection which was not line-related (OR 6.67, p = 0.019).

Quinupristin-dalfopristin inhibits protein synthesis and has various side effects including arthralgia, myalgia, and various GI effects. It is recommended for use in the treatment of *E. faecium* infections only as it is only poorly active against *E. faecalis* [2].

It has been acknowledged in national guidelines that there is limited high-quality evidence to guide therapy of VRE infective endocarditis (IE). The latest BSAC guidelines published in 2012 did not make specific recommendations for the treatment of VRE IE in light of this [14].

> **Evidence base** Treatment of VRE infective endocarditis
>
> The latest BSAC guidelines for the antibiotic treatment of infective endocarditis (IE) published in 2012 did not make specific recommendations for the treatment of VRE IE as there is limited data available. The evidence that is available suggests treatment with linezolid or daptomycin and this is based on case reports and animal models. However, the development of resistance to daptomycin has been seen [14].
>
> Vouillamoz et al. [15] carried out a study evaluating daptomycin use at doses simulating kinetics in humans at 6 mg/kg od in rats with experimental infective endocarditis due to *E. faecalis* or *E. faecium*. They showed that daptomycin is effective against both susceptible and MDR strains of *E. faecalis* and *E. faecium in vitro* and in experimental endocarditis in rats.

> **Expert comment**
>
> Generally, for treatment of IE, a bactericidal antibiotic needs to be deployed to reduce treatment failure rate. In order to achieve the bactericidal effect, dual therapy with gentamicin or streptomycin (in the case of gentamicin resistance), if the isolate appears to be sensitive to the particular aminoglycoside, is advocated. Although daptomycin has demonstrated *in vitro* bactericidal effect, it has been used in a limited number of cases of IE caused by enterococci spp [12]. In some of these cases a higher dose of daptomycin (8–10 mg/kg rather than the licensed dose of 6 mg/kg which is used for MSSA or MRSA infective endocarditis) has been used with a second agent such as an aminoglycoside or amoxicillin where the organism's sensitivity pattern shows susceptibility [16].

The guidelines do, however, make reference to animal models which have shown that there is a benefit in using daptomycin or linezolid over glycopeptides [14]. Patel et al. [17] demonstrated that linezolid treatment was more active ($p < 0.05$) than vancomycin or no treatment in a rat model of vanA vancomycin-resistant *E. faecium* experimental endocarditis.

The IDSA guidelines published in 2009 for the treatment of intravascular catheter-related bacteraemia [18] recommend linezolid or daptomycin as a first-line agent, with quinupristin-dalfopristin as an alternative. However, as previously discussed, quinupristin-dalfopristin is only suitable for infection caused by *E. faecium*.

A final word from the expert

In comparison with some virulent Gram-positive bacteria such as Group A streptococcus, Group B streptococcus and *Streptococcus pneumoniae*, *Enterococcus* spp including VRE are low-virulence organisms. VREs are not considered more virulent than vancomycin-sensitive enterococci. The reason why VRE are considered a problem is that treatment options are limited.

VRE are commonly associated with urinary tract and intra-abdominal infections. However, this does not necessarily mean that empirical antibiotic therapy chosen for these conditions should have activity against *Enterococcus* spp. For example, the use of empirical therapy with antibiotics active against *Enterococcus* spp in intra-abdominal infection still remains controversial.

Appropriate β–lactam agents (e.g. amoxicillin or penicillin), glycopeptides, quinupristin-dalfopristin, linezolid, tigecycline, nitrofurantoin, and fosfomycin are all bacteriostatic for treatment of *Enterococcus* spp including VRE. Daptomycin has shown bactericidal activity *in vitro* against isolates of *Enterococcus* spp including VRE. Among the antibiotics mentioned above, nitrofurantoin and fosfomycin only play a role in treatment of uncomplicated UTI if the isolate displays an appropriate sensitivity pattern.

Linezolid is only licensed for 2 weeks of therapy and manufacturers advise that linezolid should not be used for more than 4 weeks. Along with bone marrow suppression, prolonged linezolid therapy is also associated with optic neuritis.

Tigecycline is generally active against VRE and is currently also licensed for intra-abdominal sepsis due to the broad spectrum of its activity against many facultative Gram-negatives and anaerobes. However, its level in blood may not reach the therapeutic level and there are concerns about its usage in bloodstream infection.

Treatment of infections such as UTI, intra-abdominal infections, and bacteraemias in the absence of IE may not require dual therapy with an aminoglycoside agent.

In summary, this case highlighted a case of VRE bacteraemia associated with pyonephrosis. Removal of the source (drainage of pus) was the most important intervention in management of the patient. There are limited choices of antibiotics in treatment of VRE infection. This is more challenging where bactericidal effect is essential (e.g. infective endocarditis and osteomyelitis) as there is no strong evidence to influence the optimal choice of antibiotics.

References

1 Health Protection Agency. *UK Standards for Microbiology Investigations: Investigation of Urine* (August 2012). Available from: http://www.hpa.org.uk/ProductsServices/ MicrobiologyPathology/UKStandardsForMicrobiologyInvestigations/TermsOfUseForSMIs/ AccessToUKSMIs/SMIBacteriology/smiB41InvestigationofUrine/

2 Rivera AM and Boucher HW. Current concepts in antimicrobial therapy against select Gram-positive organisms: Methicillin-resistant *Staphylococcus aureus*, penicillin-resistant pneumococci, and vancomycin-resistant enterococci. *Mayo Clin Proc* 2011; 86: 1230–1242.

3 Cookson BD, Macrae MB, Barrett SP et al. *HIS Guidelines for the control of glycopeptide-resistant enterococci in hospitals*. Available from: http://www.his.org.uk/ files/4113/7338/2928/GRE_guidelines.pdf

4 Werner G, Coque TM, Hammerun AM et al. Emergence and spread of vancomycin resistance among enterococci in Europe. *Eurosurveillance* 2008; 13(47); 1–11.

5 Greenwood D, Finch A, Davey D and Wilcox M. *Antimicrobial Chemotherapy*, 5th edition 2008. Oxford University Press.

6 Gold HS. Vancomycin-resistant enterococci: mechanisms and clinical observations. *Clin Infect Dis* 2001; 33: 210–219.

7 Courvalin, P. Vancomycin resistance in Gram-positive cocci. *Clin Infect Dis* 2006; 42: S25–S34 (Suppl 1).

8 Health Protection Agency. *Enterococcus* spp. bacteraemia reports for England, Wales and Northern Ireland: 2006–2010 Available from: http://www.hpa.org.uk/Topics/ InfectiousDiseases/InfectionsAZ/EnterococciSpeciesAndGRE/EpidemiologicalData/ VoluntarySurveillanceData/EnterococcusSpp/

9 Deshpande LM, Fritsche TR, Moet GJ et al. Antimicrobial resistance and molecular epidemiology of vancomycin-resistant enterococci from North America and Europe: a report from the SENTRY antimicrobial surveillance program. *Diagn Microbiol Infect Dis* 2007; 58: 163–170.

10 Muto CA, Jernigan JA, Ostrowsky BE et al. SHEA guideline for Preventing Noscomial Transmission of Multidrug-Resistant Strains of *Staphylococcus aureus* and *Enterococcus*. Available from: http://www.shea-online.org/View/ArticleId/7/Guideline-for-Preventing-Nosocomial-Transmission-of-Multidrug-Resistant-Strains-of-Staphylococcus-au.aspx

11 de Bruin MA, Riley LW. Does vancomycin prescribing intervention affect vancomycin-resistant enterococcus infection and colonization in hospitals? A systematic review. *BMC Infect Dis* 2007; 7: 24.

12 Livermore D. Future directions with daptomycin. *J Antimicrob Chemother* 2008; 62: S3, iii41–iii49.

13 Crank CW, Scheetz MH, Brielmaier B et al. Comparison of outcomes from daptomycin or linezolid treatment for vancomycin-resistant enterococcal bloodstream infection: A retrospective, multicenter, cohort study. *Clin Ther* 2010; 32: 1713–1719.

14 Gould FK, Denning DW, Elliott TSJ et al. Guidelines for the diagnosis and antibiotic treatment of endocarditis in adults: a report of the Working Party of the British Society for Antimicrobial Chemotherapy. *J Antimicrob Chemother* 2012; 67: 269–289.

15 Vouillamoz J, Moreillon P, Giddey M, Entenza JM. Efficacy of daptomycin in the treatment of experimental endocarditis due to susceptible and multidrug-resistant enterococci. *J Antimicrob Chemother* 2006; 58: 1208–1214.

16 Mandell GL, Bennett JE, Dolin R. *Principles and Practice of Infectious Diseases*, 7th edition, 2010. Churchill Livingstone Elsevier.

17 Patel R, Rouse MS, Piper KE, Steckelberg JM. Linezolid therapy of vancomycin-resistant *Enterococcus faecium* experimental endocarditis. *Antimicrob Agents Chemother* 2001; 45: 621–623.

18 Infectious Diseases Society of America. *IDSA Clinical Practice Guidelines for the Diagnosis and Management of Intravascular Catheter-Related Infection*. 2009 updates by the IDSA. Available from: http://www.idsociety.org/uploadedFiles/IDSA/Guidelines-Patient_Care/PDF_Library/Prevention%20IV%20Cath.pdf

Disseminated nocardiosis

Amber Arnold and Jayne Ellis

ⓘ **Expert commentary** Robert Hill

Case history

A 79-year-old retired mechanic presented to his general practitioner with a 5-week history of a lump in the posterior triangle of his neck.

> ⊕ **Clinical tip** Infective causes of a neck mass
>
> - Mycobacteria: *Mtb*, atypical mycobacteria
> - Bacterial: *Streptococcus pyogenes*, *S. aureus*, *Bartonella henselae* (cat scratch), *Actinomyces* spp, *Nocardia* spp, *Francisella tularensis*, *Brucella* spp
> - Viral: respiratory viruses (e.g. adenovirus, rhinovirus), EBV, CMV, HIV, HSV
> - Fungal: *Histoplasma capsulatum*, *Cryptococcus neoformans*, *Coccidioides* spp
> - Parasite: *Toxoplasma gondii*
> - Spirochaete: *Leptospira* spp, *Treponema pallidum* (syphilis)

The GP referred him to his local hospital for a lymph node aspirate, being concerned about malignancy or TB. The history given to the IDs team was as follows.

The patient had first noticed the lump towards the end of a holiday in Sri Lanka from which he had returned 3 weeks ago. He had been in Sri Lanka visiting relatives for 2 months; while there he had noticed a small laceration on his right foot after walking barefoot. The laceration had been covered in mud on first detection and he was surprised that it was not painful considering its size. He cleaned it and it healed slowly over the next few weeks. He reported reduced mobility over the last 6 months. He had also suffered with weight loss and night sweats for a month and intermittent rigors, fevers, and cough for a week.

The patient had a history of hypertension requiring medication and COPD for which he regularly used inhalers. The COPD was not limiting and he had not required antibiotics or hospital admission in the past. He had been diagnosed with temporal arteritis 3 years ago when he had presented with headaches. He underwent a temporal artery biopsy which confirmed the diagnosis, and had been taking varying doses of prednisolone ever since. Currently he was taking prednisolone 15 mg a day, a dose he had been on for several months and was asymptomatic with regard to the arteritis. He had been diagnosed with glaucoma a year ago which was thought to be secondary to the prolonged use of steroids.

Table 25.1 Blood results

Test	On admission
Hb	11.1 g/dL
Mean corpuscular volume (MCV)	98 fL
WCC	16×10^9/L
Neutrophils	14.7×10^9/L
Lymphocytes	0.8×10^9/L
Platelets	296×10^9/L
Urea	6 mmol/L
Creatinine	90 µmol/L
Sodium	140 mmol/L
Potassium	3.5 mm/L
ALT	32 IU/mL
ALP	120 IU/mL
Bilirubin	10 µmol/L
Albumin	30 g/L
CRP	290 mg/L
Fasting glucose	4.4 mmol/L
T4	110 mmol/L
TSH	4 mU/L

On examination he was apyrexial, with oxygen saturations of 98% and a blood pressure of 145/85 mmHg. He was tachycardic at 110 bpm. He was noted to have oral candida. In the right posterior triangle of his neck was a solitary non-tender and non-erythematous nodule 2 cm in diameter. He had no other lesions or other palpable lymphadenopathy. Cardiovascular, respiratory, and abdominal examinations were unremarkable. A scar suggestive of a healed ulcer was noted on the right metatarsophalangeal joint. Neurological examination revealed that he had reduced sensation to pinprick and vibration testing in a glove-and-stocking distribution up to his elbows in his arms and to his mid-calves in the legs. He also had distal weakness in the arms and legs. The rest of the power in his limbs was normal. He had no ankle reflexes, equivocal plantars, and the rest of the reflexes were normal.

Blood tests were sent from the emergency department and revealed a raised CRP and a neutrophilia (Table 25.1). He was slightly lymphopaenic. Otherwise blood tests were unremarkable, as was a chest radiograph. Urine dip and culture were clear as were three sets of blood cultures. ECG was unremarkable. He was admitted to a side room on the infection ward.

On the ward the neck nodule was aspirated and sent for histological and microbiological investigation. An induced sputum specimen was sent for AFB analysis. That evening his temperature rose to 39°C and he became increasingly tachycardic despite fluids. He was treated for sepsis of unknown source with co-amoxiclav plus gentamicin according to hospital guidelines.

The next day a staging CT scan of the chest, abdomen, and pelvis revealed scattered bilateral pulmonary nodules and no other masses or enlarged lymph nodes. The microbiological report of the aspirate showed neutrophils and AFB analysis was negative. The microbiological report revealed no malignancy and confirmed the presence of neutrophils.

After 3 days the aspirate sample plated on aerobic blood agar grew scanty white chalky colonies. Gram staining revealed Gram-positive branching bacilli which were modified acid-fast. They were presumptively identified as *Nocardia* species and a slope specimen was sent to the reference laboratory for confirmation.

⊗ **Learning point** Identification of Gram-positive branching bacilli [1,2]

Nocardia spp will grow on a wide range of non-selective media (blood agar, chocolate, Sabouraud dextrose agar, Löwenstein-Jensen [LJ] slopes) and can take up to 3 weeks to grow. Colony morphology, Gram staining appearance, and demonstration of modified acid-fast staining are the main investigations in the local laboratory. After presumptive identification samples should be sent to the reference laboratory for confirmative 16S PCR and susceptibility testing. The organisms are hazard group 2 organisms.

The differential of Gram-positive branching bacilli (Figure 25.1)

Aerobic

- *Nocardia* **spp:** wrinkled chalky white or cream to pink-coloured colonies, filamentous branching bacilli with fragmentation, aerial hyphae, modified acid-fast
- *Streptomyces* **spp**: waxy heaped colonies, extensive branching with no fragmentation, aerial hyphae, modified acid-fast negative
- *Rhodococcus* **spp,** *Gordonia* **spp,** *Tsukamurella* **spp**: indistinguishable on colony and Gram stains. Pink, or cream to orange, sometimes slimy colonies of cocci that grow in zigzag pattern and can rarely germinate into branching bacilli, no aerial hyphae, may be modified acid-fast
- *Actinomadura* **spp**: white to red, often mucoid, molar tooth-like colonies, branching filamentous bacilli, variable aerial hyphae, modified acid-fast negative

Anaerobic

- *Actinomyces* **spp:** anaerobic media (without neomycin), anaerobic conditions. White gritty molar tooth-like colonies, thin filamentous bacilli and modified acid-fast negative. Metronidazole resistant, spot indole negative.

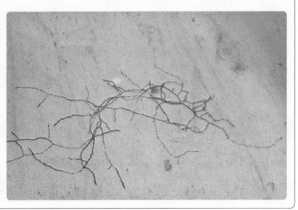

Figure 25.1 Smear preparation of *Nocardia asteroides* showing Gram-positive branching bacilli. Reproduced from Nick Mansell and Ann Millar, *Oxford Desk Reference Respiratory Medicine*, Figure 8.5.1, p. 182, Copyright © 2009, with permission from Oxford University Press.

❝ **Expert comment**

The key to the diagnosis of nocardiosis is the isolation of the infecting organism by culture. However, it is advisable to submit multiple clinical specimens because of the low rate of positivity. Histological features of *Nocardia* lesions show an abundance of neutrophils, lymphocytes, and macrophages consistent with the development of cell-mediated immunity.

⊕ **Clinical tip** Modified Ziehl-Neelsen (ZN) stain [1]

The modified ZN stain is used for the identification of certain branching Gram-positive bacilli (especially *Nocardia*). A heat-fixed slide is flooded with 3% carbol fuchsin and left to stain. Unlike the classical ZN stain, further heating is not required. The slide is then decolorized with 1% sulphuric acid (instead of 3% v/v acid-alcohol solution in the classical ZN stain) and counterstained with methylene blue or malachite green. *Nocardia* species will appear red/purple (Figure 25.2).

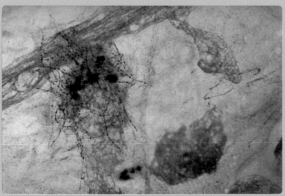

Figure 25.2 *Nocardia asteroides* (modified acid-fast stain, ×450), showing classical filamentous branching. Reproduced with permission from Abinash Virk, Specific Microorganisms. In Amit Ghosh (Ed), *Mayo Clinic Internal Medicine Board Review*, ninth edition, Oxford University Press, New York, USA, Copyright © 2010 Mayo Foundation for Medical Education and Research.

On day 3 the patient continued to suffer with fevers and his CRP had risen to 400 mg/L. He was switched to imipenem and intravenous co-trimoxazole for presumed disseminated *Nocardia* (lymphatic and possible pulmonary) infection.

⊕ Clinical tip Co-trimoxazole dosing for nocardiosis

Co-trimoxazole remains the most commonly used drug in nocardiosis. Treatment should consist of 3–6 weeks of intravenous therapy followed by a prolonged oral phase to prevent relapse. There are no controlled trials and data is at best from previous cases series. See Table 25.2.

Table 25.2 Co-trimoxazole treatment for nocardiosis

Dose	• 5–15 mg/kg/day of the trimethoprim component (30–90 mg/kg/day of co-trimoxazole) in 2–4 divided doses, with higher doses for disseminated infection
	• Sulfonamide levels should be monitored in severe disease, when high doses are used and in those with renal impairment. A serum concentration between 100 and 150 microgram/mL is considered to be therapeutic [4]
Treatment duration	Depends on sites of infection and immune status of host [4]
	• Immunocompetent host with isolated cutaneous disease: 3 months
	• Immunocompromised host with cutaneous disease: 6 months
	• Immunocompetent host with pulmonary or disseminated disease: 6 –12 months
	• Immunocompromised host with pulmonary, disseminated, or central nervous system (CNS) disease and immunocompetent host with CNS disease: 12 months

Source: Data from *Mayo Clinic Proceedings*, Volume 87, Number 4, John W. Wilson, Nocardiosis: Updates and Clinical Overview, pp. 403–407, Copyright © 2012 Mayo Foundation for Medical Education and Research. Published by Elsevier Inc. All rights reserved.

The reference laboratory confirmed a diagnosis of *Nocardia farcinica*. It was postulated that bacteria had gained entry through the laceration on the foot which the patient was not aware of due to the peripheral neuropathy.

★ Learning point *Nocardia* epidemiology and link with immunosuppression

Nocardia species are environmental saprophytes found in soil and water and are part of the aerobic actinomycetes group. Human infection occurs through inhalation or direct skin and soft tissue penetration, as is presumed to have occurred in our patient. Over 30 species of *Nocardia* have

(continued)

been associated with human disease. The most commonly isolated species in one US-based study were: *N. asteroides* complex (including *N. asteroides sensu stricto*, *N. farcinica*, and *N. nova*), *N. braziliensis*, and *N. cyriacigeorgica* [5]. Infection with *Nocardia* spp is rare with 53 isolates sent to the UK HPA between November 2004 and March 2007 (~23 per year) [6].

Nocardia spp are opportunistic pathogens more common in immunosuppressed populations. Cohort reviews show about 60% of cases associated with a form of immunosuppression including alcoholism, diabetes, chronic corticosteroid use, chemotherapy, and organ transplantation [4]. Both neutrophil activity (CGD is a risk factor) and cell-mediated immune activity are required for an effective immune response.

In a study of over 5,000 organ transplantation patients 35 were diagnosed with *Nocardia* infection (0.6%) and high-dose glucocorticoid use in the preceding 6 months was found to be an independent risk factor for *Nocardia* infection. *N. nova* and *N. farcinica* were found to account for 77% of infections [7].

❝ Expert comment

Nocardiae are not readily communicable. Routinely patients with Nocarida infections are not a priority for a side room to prevent infection to others, (they may warrant a side room due to immunosuppression) and regular hand hygiene should prevent spread. Some older reports have suggested nosocomial spread between patients via healthcare workers. However these reports are often based on susceptibility patterns of organisms and temporal relationships. Furthermore, the observation that a small number of patients have been affected in a given ward area over a period of time is more likely to point to a common source, such as dust (e.g. due to building works), rather than cross-infection. Molecular methods using random amplified polymorphic DNA analysis (RAPD) or ribotyping offer varying degrees of strain differentiation. It is likely that next generation WGS will be required to increase the sensitivity of the detection of strain differences to refine epidemiology.

★ Learning point

Pulmonary, cutaneous/lymphocutaneous, and disseminated nocardiosis (predominantly affecting the central nervous system) are the most common manifestations of *Nocardia* infection.

Pulmonary disease following inhalation of the bacteria is the commonest manifestation. Most pulmonary infections are primary but secondary spread from other sites may occur. Pulmonary nocardiosis presents with non-specific respiratory symptoms: dry or productive cough, dyspnoea, pleuritic chest pain, haemoptysis with systemic upset including fever, night sweat, fatigue, and weight loss. Onset of symptoms may be acute, subacute, or chronic.

Radiological features of pulmonary nocardiosis are variable and non-specific, often leading to diagnostic confusion. Disease may be focal or multifocal with evidence of nodular disease, cavitation, interstitial infiltrates, or consolidation. Pulmonary TB, malignant disease, and invasive fungal infections are important differentials.

Approximately 50% of pulmonary infections disseminate to sites outside the lungs. Local spread resulting in pleural effusions, empyema formation, mediastinitis, and/or pericarditis may occur. Haematogenous spread is common, especially to the CNS, occurring in 4–50% of disseminated cases [4].

CNS disease is characterized by parenchymal abscess formation and patients present with headache, fevers, and seizures with or without neurological deficits related to the site of the lesion. Neurological symptoms usually present gradually and are usually seen in conjunction with pulmonary disease.

Primary cutaneous nocardiosis results from traumatic inoculation of bacteria and may present as cellulitis, superficial abscess formation, or ulceration. The lesions are non-specific and may be clinically

(continued)

indistinguishable from other soft tissue infections [4]. Lymphocutaneous nocardiosis occurs when primary nocardial skin infection spreads to involve the local lymph nodes, resulting in a single or linear chain of nodular lesions. Lymphocutaneous nocardiosis is often called sporotrichoid nocardiosis, given the similar presentation of sporotrichosis [4].

In advanced cutaneous nocardiosis a mycetoma may occur. Mycetoma is a chronic cutaneous infection most commonly affecting the foot ('madura' foot) characterized by painless swelling, induration, and eventual sinus tract formation over several years.

Table 25.3 Blood results day 7

Biochemistry	Day 7 blood tests
Urea	10 mmol/L
Creatinine	150 µmol/L
Sodium	29 mmol/L
Potassium	6 mmol/L
CRP	100 mg/L
Cortisol (early morning)	700 mg/L

Over the next few days he clinically improved. His fevers resolved and his inflammatory markers in the blood settled. However, his renal function deteriorated and he became hyponatraemic and hyperkalaemic (Table 25.3).

Although no crystals, white cells, nor casts were found in the urine, making a crystal nephropathy or interstitial nephritis unlikely, the team were concerned that the renal impairment and hyperkalaemia were due to the high dose of co-trimoxazole.

Clinical tip Side effects of co-trimoxazole

Co-trimoxazole is composed of two synergistic anti-folate drugs, trimethoprim and sulfamethoxazole, in the ratio of 1:5. Side effects at regular doses are uncommon at around 8%, with rash and GI effects occurring most commonly.

The patient in the case suffered renal impairment and hyperkalaemia. Renal complications are more common when co-trimoxazole is used at higher doses, in the elderly, and in those with baseline renal impairment. Renal impairment may occur due to crystal formation and interstitial nephritis but may also occur for other reasons.

One retrospective cohort study found that acute renal impairment occurred in 5.8% (33/573) of patients treated with co-trimoxazole [8]. The majority of patients were given regular doses (960 mg twice a day) for skin and soft tissue and urinary infections. Diabetes and hypertension were identified as risk factors.

Table 25.4 Side effects of co-trimoxazole

Renal	Crystaluria, renal calculi, interstitial nephritis, hyperkalaemia, hyponataemia
Metabolic	hypoglycaemia
Gastro-intestinal	Nausea/vomiting, diarrhoea, glossitis, stomatitis, anorexia, hepatotoxicity (jaundice, hepatic necrosis), pancreatitis, antibiotic-associated colitis
Cutaneous/ musculoskeletal	Rash (including rarely Stevens-Johnson syndrome, toxic epidermal necrolysis, photosensitivity), myalgia, rhabdomyolysis (reported in HIV+ patients), arthralgia
Neurological	Aseptic meningitis, depression, seizures, peripheral neuropathy, ataxia, tinnitus, vertigo, hallucinations
Haematological	Megaloblastic anaemia, leucopenia, thrombocytopenia, eosinophilia
Cardio-respiratory	Myocarditis, cough, pulmonary infiltrates
Other	Systemic lupus erythematosis (SLE)-like syndrome, vasculitis, uveitis

(continued)

In none of the cases was the renal impairment thought to be due to crystal formation or interstitial nephritis.

Trimethoprim is excreted unchanged in the urine and can cause reversible hyperkalaemia by blocking the sodium channels in the collecting tubules, a similar mechanism to the diuretic amilioride. Hyperkalaemia over 6.0 mmol/L has been reported at a rate of 12% (3/25) in one case study in HIV-positive patients treated with high-dose co-trimoxazole [9]. Although more common at higher doses, hyperkalaemia has also been reported at low doses and in most cases co-trimoxazole has to be stopped. See Table 25.4.

He was switched to oral co-trimoxazole and the dose was reduced. He was restarted on intravenous fluid rehydration. His creatinine improved a little but he continued to suffer with intractable hyponatraemia and a decision was made to stop co-trimoxazole. By this time he had received 3 weeks of intravenous antibiotics, his fevers had resolved the previous week, and his CRP was down to 10 mg/L. The susceptibility results were available from the reference laboratory (Table 25.5) and a decision was made to change the patient's medication to co-amoxiclav and moxifloxacin. The aim was to continue the dual regimen for 12 months as an outpatient.

Table 25.5 Susceptibility data

Antibacterial	MIC	Breakpoint	Interpretation
Meropenem	4	Not available	Probably resistant
Imipenem	0.25	4	S
Co-amoxiclav	1	8	S
Moxifloxacin	0.0032	Not recorded	S
Ciprofloxacin	0.125	Not recorded	S
Linezolid	2	4	S
Amikacin	0.5	8	S
Co-trimoxazole	0.5	2	S

S, sensitive.

❻ Expert comment

Susceptibility testing is a major difficulty and MIC accuracy is not readily achievable. One significant problem is that isolates often do not grow well during testing (regardless of the method), leading to difficulties with the uniformity of inoculum size and length of incubation to achieve readable growth. Results are also not readily available as one-off readings and staff require regular experience of culturing and testing to obtain consistent results.

Due to the problems with susceptibility testing, speciation is important as this can help antibiotic choice based on knowledge of pathogenicity and previous phenotypic sensitivity data as well as genotypic data.

N. farcinica used to be classified as *N. asteroides* but findings of cefotaxime resistance in this species led to its differentiation. *N. farcinica* is potentially life-threatening because of its preponderance for dissemination and its common association with antibiotic resistance. A complete genome sequence of *N. farcinica* strain IFM 10152 [10] found resistance genes for all aminoglycosides except amikacin; three β-lactamases; ribosomal RNA methyltransferases conferring resistance to erythromycin, clindamycin, and clarithromycin; an efflux pump conferring resistance to chloramphenicol; a MurA mutation conferring resistance to fosfomycin; and RpoB2 conferring resistance to RIF. Remaining susceptibilities for isolate IFM were to trimethoprim, ofloxacin, imipenem, and possibly minocycline. There was no information concerning linezolid, which is the first new antimicrobial to be active against all clinically significant species of *Nocardia*.

During his stay he was reviewed by the neurologist and his steroids were reduced to 5 mg per day. He underwent EMG and nerve conduction studies which showed a mixed motor and sensory demyelinating peripheral neuropathy and he was given the provisional diagnosis of chronic inflammatory demyelinating polyneuropathy (CIDP).

Discussion

Diagnosing infections due to *Nocardia* spp can prove to be a challenge due to the need for biopsy or FNA and the slow growth of the organism. However, in this case diagnosis was achieved relatively quickly and antibiotic choice proved to be the main challenge.

Treatment for nocardiasis is problematic for several reasons. First, the organism has a propensity to relapse unless treatment is prolonged, often requiring a year of therapy in disseminated disease. Second, the infection is rare and the clinical manifestations and patient population diverse, so randomized trials of treatment are impossible. Third, the degree to which *in vitro* susceptibilities correlate with *in vivo* response is not fully elucidated.

Most experience in treatment is with co-trimoxazole and it remains the current drug of choice for susceptible isolates.

Co-trimoxazole has excellent tissue and CSF penetration both in the intravenous and oral form. However, successful outcomes with co-trimoxazole monotherapy in disseminated disease can be as low as 50% [12]. Furthermore, as in our patient, side effects are common when co-trimoxazole is used at high dose for prolonged periods. Therefore, finding alternative agents with better success rates, fewer side effects, and less resistance is an imperative.

Information regarding the use of alternative antimicrobial agents comes from *in vitro* susceptibility data, animal models, and retrospective analysis of case series and case reports. Antimicrobials with *in vitro* activity against *Nocardia* spp include the carbapenems (imipenem, meropenem, not ertapenem), cephalosporins (cefotaxime, ceftriaxone), aminoglycoside (amikacin), extended fluoroquinolones (moxifloxacin and levofloxacin), minocycline, tigecycline, and linezolid. Co-amoxiclav only has limited activity and so should only be used for stepdown treatment and in combination.

In the case, the patient was treated with intravenous imipenem and co-trimoxazole initially. *In vitro* and animal model studies show that imipenem is an effective antimicrobial against *Nocardia* (**Evidence base: *In vitro* models and Evidence base: Animal models**). There is some evidence from these data that these antimicrobials in combination work synergistically and therefore might produce better outcomes than co-trimoxazole alone. Interestingly, *in vitro* data and animal models suggest imipenem alone is more effective than co-trimoxazole alone. Co-trimoxazole-free combinations include cefotaxime plus imipenem or imipenem plus amikacin.

🕕 **Expert comment**

In the UK approximately 95% of isolates are susceptible to co-trimoxazole *in vitro*. There have been various alarming reports of resistance to co-trimoxazole ranging from 16.1% to 42% of isolates. However, in a survey aimed at verifying these results, careful susceptibility testing of 552 isolates of *Nocardia* species revealed only 2% resistance [11]. Difficulties in interpreting susceptibility results in the laboratory are thought to play an important role in overestimating resistance.

✓ **Evidence base** *In vitro* models for effective antimicrobial therapy

Synergism of imipenem and amikacin in combination with other antibiotics against *Nocardia asteroides* [13]

A total of 26 isolates of *N. asteroides* were collected and the agar dilution method was used to establish the MIC for amikacin, imipenem, co-trimoxazole and cefotaxime alone and in combination to these

(continued)

isolates. The MIC was defined as the lowest antibiotic concentration suppressing all growth at 48 h of incubation at 37°C. Synergy between the antimicrobials was defined as a fourfold or greater reduction in the MIC of both antimicrobials.

Results: Amikacin and imipenem had the lowest MICs. Synergy was observed in 83% of samples treated with amikacin plus co-trimoxazole, 80% of samples treated with imipenem plus co-trimoxazole, and 92% of samples treated with imipenem plus cefotaxime. An additive effect was observed with amikacin + imipenem and amikacin + cefotaxime. No antagonism was observed.

Conclusions: This study confirmed other studies showing low MICs for amikacin and imipenem and that synergy between certain antibiotics is observed. Importantly, no evidence of inhibition is observed *in vitro*, suggesting that dual treatment *in vivo* may be effective.

✔ **Evidence base** Animal models for effective antimicrobial therapy

Mouse model of cerebral nocardiasis (*N. asteroides*)

The effectiveness of antibiotics against cerebral nocardiasis was assessed in the mouse model. Brain tissue was harvested from the mice after 72 hours of antibiotic or saline (control) treatment and cultured. A comparison was made of the number of CFU per gram of brain tissue that grew in culture.

Amikacin and imipenem were the most effective of the agents tested and both were significantly better than co-trimoxazole. However, co-trimoxazole was significantly better than saline control. Minocycline was no better than saline control [14].

In a follow-up study that looked for synergy, a trend towards a better outcome with imipenem plus co-trimoxazole and imipenem plus cefotaxime was seen, but results were not significantly different from treatment with imipenem alone [15].

Conclusions: Amikacin, imipenem, and cefotaxime are all superior choices of antibiotic than co-trimoxazole in the mouse cerebral model, suggesting there may be a role for these antibiotics in combination with co-trimoxazole human nocardiasis.

In our patient, at the point where the side effects of co-trimoxazole forced the team to switch medications the patient was ready for an oral switch. Oral options that did not include co-trimoxazole included co-amoxclav, the fluoroquinolones, minocycline, and linezolid.

Linezolid is expensive and due to side effects is not routinely recommended for treatment beyond 2 weeks. However, a case series of 6 patients from one institution in the USA reported successful treatment with linezolid (600 mg twice daily) alone or in combination [16]. Two of the patients were receiving ongoing treatment with corticosteroids, as was our patient. The study confirmed a high rate of side effects; these occurred in 50% of patients with three patients becoming anaemic and one also suffering from thrombocytopenia, lactic acidosis, and peripheral neuropathy.

The patient in the case had improved significantly and already had multiple co-morbidities including peripheral neuropathy, so the team preferred a regimen that did not include linezolid. Moxifloxacin was chosen based on the *in vitro* susceptibility data as well as evidence from a few case reports of treatment success with this agent in the treatment of *Nocardia* brain abscesses [17]. Co-amoxiclav was also chosen based on the *in vitro* data and case reports [18].

A final word from the expert

Nocardiosis is uncommon in the UK. *N. farcinica* is even rarer and is only responsible for a minority of cases of nocardiosis. Infected individuals usually have a predisposing immunosuppression, including any condition that requires long-term corticosteroid usage as exemplified here. Although the majority of infections due to *N. farcinica* have pulmonary involvement, there are reports of foot trauma leading to infection. Infection often disseminates to the lymphatic system leading to the neck lump in this case; dissemination to the brain, kidneys, joints, bones, and eyes is also common.

Nocardia are soil-borne aerobic actinomycetes. They are often referred to as 'higher bacteria', because they have a propensity to form filamentous growth with true branching, reproduction being achieved by fragmentation of filaments into bacillary or coccoid elements. In the past, classification difficulties resulted in errors of diagnostic and therapeutic significance, but molecular methods have resolved these issues.

When isolated as a pure culture, growth is often achieved after 48 hours on Sabouraud glucose or blood agars but may take up to 4 weeks to develop from mixed cultures. *Nocardia* may not grow well on selective media for pathogenic fungi. Although the cell wall of *Nocardia* is composed of a peptidoglycan formed from meso-diaminopimelic acid, arabinose, and galactose, isolates are weakly Gram-positive but can be acid-fast. This odd staining profile is probably due to the presence of tuberculostearic acids and short-chain mycolic acids which are characteristic of *Nocardia*.

Susceptibility testing is difficult and MIC accuracy a major problem; speciation is recommended to help guide antibiotic choice. Sulfonamides are the antimicrobials of choice for nocardial infection and can usefully be prescribed before having the results of susceptibility testing due to low rates of resistance. In the case of sulfonamide allergy or a sulfonamide-resistant organism, minocycline, amikacin, cefotaxime, ceftriaxone, and imipenem can be used, but the choice should always be guided by testing results and speciation. In the case presented, moxifloxicin was a good choice based on susceptibility data and speciation.

The diagnosis and successful choice of antibiotics to treat nocardiosis remain a source of clinical complexity.

References

1 Health Protection Agency. *UK Standards for Microbiology Investigations: Identification of Aerobic Actimonycetes*. Available at http://www.hpa.org.uk/webc/hpawebfile/hpaweb_c/1317131061186

2 Health Protection Agency. UK Standards for Microbiology Investigations: Identification of Anaerobic *Actinomyces* species. Available at http://www.hpa.org.uk/webc/hpawebfile/hpaweb_c/1313155004718

3 Verroken A, Janssens M, Berhin C, Bogaerts P, Huang T-D, Wauters G, Glupezynski Y. Evaluation of Matrix-Assisted laser desorption ionization-time of flight mass spectrometry for identification of Nocardia species. *J Clin Microbiol* 2010; 48: 4015–4021.

4 Wilson J W. Nocardiosis: Updates and Clinical Overview. *Mayo Clin Proc* 2012; 87: 403–407.

5 Fraser TN, Avellaneda AA, Graviss EA, Musher DM. Acute kidney injury associated with trimethoprim/sulfamethoxazole. *J Antimicrob Chemother* 2012; 67: 1271–1277.

6 Trimethoprim is a potassium-sparing diuretic like amiloride and causes hyperkalemia in high-risk patients. Perazella MA. *Am J Ther* 1997; 4: 343–348.

7 Ishikawa J, Yamashita A, Mikami Y, Hoshino Y, Kurita H, Hotta K, Shiba T, Hattori M. The complete genomic sequence of Nocardia farcinica IFM 10152. *PNAS* 2004; 101: 14925–14930.

8 Uhde KB, Pathak S, McCullum I Jr, et al. Antimicrobial-resistant nocardia isolates, United States, 1995–2004. *Clin Infect Dis* 2010; 51: 1445.

9 Hill RLR, Pike R, Warner M. Antimicrobial susceptibility of *Nocardia* spp. – experience in England and Wales. Available at http://www.hpa.org.uk/webc/HPAwebFile/ HPAweb_C/1194947364282 (accessed 12 March 2012).

10 Peleg AY, Husain S, Qureshi ZA, et al. Risk factors, clinical characteristics, and outcome of Nocardia infection in organ transplant recipients: a matched case–control study. *Clin Infect Dis* 2007; 44: 1307.

11 Brown-Elliot B, Biehle J, Conville PS et al. Sulfonamide resistance in isolates of Nocardia spp. from a U.S. multicenter survey. *J Clin Microbiol* 2012; 50: 670–672.

12 Sorrell TC, Iredell JR, Mitchell DH. *Nocardia* species. In: *Mandell, Douglas, and Bennett's Principles and Practice of Infectious Diseases*, 5th edition, 2010; Churchill Livingstone.

13 Gombert ME, Aulicino TM. Synergism of imipenem and amikacin in combination with other antibiotics against *Nocardia asteroides*. *Antimicrob Agents Chemother* 1983; 24: 810–811.

14 Gombert ME, Aulicino TM, duBouchet L, Silverman GE, Sheinbaum WM. Therapy of experimental cerebral nocardiosis with imipenem, amikacin, trimethoprim-sulfamethoxazole, and minocycline. *Antimicrob Agents Chemother* 1986; 30: 270–273.

15 Gombert, M. E., L. duBouchet, T. M. Aufldno, and L. B. Berkowitz. 1989. Antimicrobial synergism in the therapy of experimental cerebral nocardiosis. J. Antimicrob. Chemother. 23:3943.

16 Moylett EH, Pacheco SE, Brown-Elliott BA et al. Clinical experience with linezolid for the treatment of *Nocardia* infection. *Clin Infect Dis* 2003; 36: 313–318.

17 Fihman V, Berçot B, Mateo J et al. First successful treatment of *Nocardia farcinica* brain abscess with moxifloxacin. *J Infect* 2006; 52: e99–102.

18 Nolt D, Wadowsky RM, Green M. Lymphocutaneous *Nocardia brasiliensis* infection: a pediatric case cured with amoxicilin/clavulanate. *Pediatr Infect Dis J* 2000; 19: 1023–1025.

26 Urinary sepsis: extended spectrum β-lactamase-producing *E. coli*

Rishi Dhillon and Amber Arnold

⑥ Expert commentary Hugo Donaldson

Case history

A 72-year-old woman presented to the emergency department with a 48-hour history of fever, vomiting, and abdominal pain. She complained of dysuria, but no other symptoms. Prior to the acute symptoms, she had been feeling generally unwell for over a week, with increasing lethargy and general malaise. She had had well-controlled diabetes for many years, with no known clinical complications. She had recently been suffering from recurrent UTIs, which were managed in the community by her general practitioner. She had received a variety of antibiotics but no mid-stream urine (MSU) specimen had been sent.

On examination, she was alert and orientated but appeared flushed. Her blood pressure was low (110/70 mmHg compared to her normal blood pressure of 130–140 mmHg systolic), and she was tachycardic, with a temperature of 37.8°C. Physical examination was unremarkable, except for marked suprapubic tenderness. Routine blood tests were collected as well as blood and urine samples for microbiological culture. A urine dip stick test was positive for leucocytes and nitrites.

The clinical diagnosis was urosepsis in a diabetic. The patient was treated with intravenous (IV) fluids, intravenous co-amoxiclav and one dose of intravenous amikacin in line with the hospital policy for presumed urosepsis. She was started on an insulin sliding scale.

Her full blood count revealed a neutrophilia, raised CRP, and raised urea and creatinine. Previous results indicated that she was suffering from acute renal impairment (Table 26.1).

The patient responded well initially to the medical management: she became normotensive and her pulse settled. She was admitted to the acute medical unit on regular intravenous co-amoxiclav and as she was doing well no further doses of amikacin were given. An ultrasound of her renal tract was arranged to take place the next morning to exclude renal tract obstruction or collections.

> **⑥ Expert comment**
>
> The choice of a β-lactamase inhibitor in combination with an aminoglycoside as used in this case is a reasonable empiric treatment option for urosepsis. The specific choice of agents recommended in the hospital antibiotic guidelines will be informed by local resistance rates. In areas where there are high rates of resistance to gentamicin, amikacin is advocated in some hospital policies. Given the history of recurrent UTIs previously treated by her GP, it would have been useful to find out previous culture results and which antibiotics she had received to assess whether she had failed treatment with a particular antibiotic, as this information might have influenced initial antibiotic choice.

> **⑥ Expert comment**
>
> In a lady with diabetes plus acute renal impairment who has stabilized, it is possible to see why the team may have been cautious about writing up a further dose of amikacin. In areas where resistance to co-amoxiclav is low this would have been a reasonable decision. However, in areas where resistance is higher the combination of these two antibacterial agents is necessary to cover the possibility of resistant organisms. Multiple courses of antibiotics which had not worked should have raised a warning that the patient might have a resistant organism. Aminoglycosides can be dosed safely in renal impairment but if there were concerns about this factor the team should have discussed the case with the microbiology department to seek an alternative agent.

Table 26.1 Routine blood results from admission

Haematology		Biochemistry	
WBC	18.9×10^9/L	Urea	14.2 mmol/L
Hb	12.1 g/dL	Creatinine	210 µmol/L
Platelets	326×10^9/L	Na	142 mmol/L
Neutrophils	17.5×10^9/L	K	5.5 mmol/L
Prothrombin time	12.9 sec	ALT	45 iu/L
		ALP	140 iu/L
		Bilirubin	20 µmol/L
		Albumin	28 g/L
		CRP	345 mg/L

Early on the second day of admission she became profoundly septic. She suffered rigors and her blood pressure dropped to 60/30 mmHg. She was found to be acidotic with a blood pH of 6.9 and a blood lactate of 7 mmol/L. She was resuscitated with vigorous fluid management via central venous catheters and admitted to the intensive care unit (ICU). The ICU team discussed the patient with the consultant microbiologist on call. The microbiologist was able to access results that had not yet been released and reported that the urine culture had produced a heavy growth of *Escherichia coli*, and the blood culture had grown a GNB. No further information was available.

Considering the rapid deterioration and her risk factors for drug resistant *E. coli* including the risk of an extended spectrum β-lactamase (ESBL)-producing organism, the co-amoxiclav was stopped and meropenem was started. She was also given another dose of amikacin (less than 24 hours had passed since the first dose) and an urgent ultrasound of the renal tract was requested. The ultrasound did not reveal an obstructive cause or any collections.

⊕ **Clinical tip** Risk factors for ESBL carriage

The patient in this case had several risk factors for ESBL acquisition including age, sex, and, crucially, recurrent UTIs that had been treated with courses of different antibiotics. See Table 26.2.

The BSAC conducts annual bacteraemia surveillance (www.bsacsurv.org). The prevalence of ESBL was 9%, 8%, and 7% for *E. coli*, *Klebsiella*, and *Enterobacter* isolates, respectively, in 2011. These rates were similar to previous years [3].

Table 26.2 Risk factors for acquiring ESBL-producing organisms [1,2]

Community acquisition	Hospital acquisition
Age (>65 years old)	Intensive care admission
Sex (female)	Renal failure
Recurrent UTIs	Burns
Prior instrumentation to urinary tract	Urinary catheter
Diabetes mellitus	TPN
Previous antibiotic usage	Previous antibiotic usage

Source: Data from D. L. Paterson et al, International prospective study of *Klebsiella pneumoniae* bacteremia: implications of extended-spectrum β-lactamase production in nosocomial infections. *Annals of Internal Medicine*, Volume 140, Number 1, pp. 26–32, Copyright © 2004 The American College of Physicians; and Jesús Rodríguez-Baño et al, Community infections caused by extended-spectrum β-lactamase producing *Escherichia coli*. *Archives of Internal Medicine*, Volume 168, Number 17, pp. 1897–1902, Copyright © 2008 American Medical Association.

Table 26.3 Susceptibilities of *E. coli* identified in blood cultures taken on admission

Amoxicillin	Resistant	Tazocin	Sensitive
Co-amoxiclav	Sensitive	Cefpodoxime	Resistant
Cefuroxime	Sensitive	Cefoxitin	Sensitive
Cefotaxime	Resistant	Imipenem	Sensitive
Ceftazidime	Resistant	Meropenem	Sensitive
Gentamicin	Sensitive	Ciprofloxacin	Resistant
Amikacin	Sensitive	Trimethoprim	Resistant

Despite receiving optimum care on the ICU, later that day the patient suffered a cardiac arrest and died on the ICU. On the following day the GNB in the blood cultures was also identified as an *E. coli* and susceptibility testing to both isolates revealed the same antibiogram. The organism was resistant *in vitro* to amoxicillin, ciprofloxacin and the majority of the cephalosporins (Table 26.3). However, it was sensitive *in vitro* to co-amoxiclav and amikacin as well as meropenem.

❝ Expert comment

This susceptibility pattern suggests the presence of an ESBL enzyme. ESBLs confer resistance to penicillins, e.g. amoxicillin, ampicillin, and piperacillin, and second- and third-generation cephalosporins, e.g. cefuroxime, cefotaxime, and ceftazidime. Unfortunately CTX-M type ESBLs are now prevalent in the UK. The plasmids which carry the genes encoding these enzymes also include genes which confer resistance to other classes of antibiotics such as quinolones, trimethoprim, and aminoglycosides. This wide range of resistance mechanisms makes selecting appropriate empiric treatment difficult. Meropenem is an obvious choice but there are concerns regarding the overuse of carbapenems, particularly given the recent increasing rates of carbapenem resistance detected in the UK by PHE (previously the HPA). Since different strains are prevalent in different areas it is important to refer to your local antibiotic policy and liaise with your local microbiology department to ensure an appropriate empiric regime is chosen.

The microbiologist thought that the *E. coli* was likely to contain an ESBL due to the susceptibility pattern to the cephalosporins, and for surveillance purposes arranged confirmatory tests. The *E. coli* was confirmed as an ESBL producer.

✪ Learning point Definition and classification of ESBLs [4]

β-lactamases are enzymes that hydrolyse the β-lactam ring, leaving β-lactam antibiotics ineffective. β-lactamases can be carried chromosomally or on plasmids. The original plasmid-mediated β-lactamases identified in the 1960s in Gram-negative bacteria were active against amoxicillin and first-generation cephalosporins and were carried on plasmids (e.g. TEM1 and TEM2 in *E. coli*, SHV-1 in *K. pneumoniae*). The oxymino-cephalosporins (cefotaxime, ceftazidime, ceftriaxone) were introduced in the 1980s to counter these β-lactamases. Soon mutations in TEM1, SHV, and mutations in other plasmid-mediated β-lactamases (e.g. CTX-M) led to resistance to the oxyimino-cephalosporins and monobactams and these were labelled ESBLs. ESBLs remain sensitive to carbapenems and cephamycins [3] (cefoxitin) and *in vitro* they are inhibited by β-lactam β-lactamase inhibitors (BLBLI) such as clavulanate and tazobactam. ESBLs vary in their susceptibility *in vitro* to differing cephalosporins as in the case (sensitive to cefuroxime and resistant to the others). ESBLs have been identified in a broad range of Gram-negative bacteria including *E. coli*, *K. pneumoniae*, *Serratia* spp, *Enterobacter* spp, and PSA as well as many more. Treatment with carbapenems is effective and there is much ongoing debate about whether BLBLIs are also effective. (See Discussion.)

(continued)

Table 26.4 Classification of β-lactamase enzymes

Ambler group (molecular structure of active site)	A	B	C	D
Active site	Serine	Zinc binding thiol group	Serine	Serine
β-lactamase examples	TEM, SHV, CTX-M, carbapenemases (KPC)	Carbapenemases (VIM +IMP)	AmpC	OXA
In vitro response to β-lactamase inhibitors	Susceptible	Resistant	Resistant	Resistant
Bush-Jacoby-Medeiros (BJM) group	2 b, e, f	3	1	2d

Source: Data from *Mayo Clinic Proceedings*, Volume 86, Issue 3, Souha S. Kanj and Zeina A. Kanafani, Current Concepts in Antimicrobial Therapy Against Resistant Gram-Negative Organisms: Extended-Spectrum β-Lactamase-Producing Enterobacteriaceae, Carbapenem-Resistant Enterobacteriaceae, and Multidrug-Resistant *Pseudomonas aeruginosa*, pp. 250–259, Copyright © 2011 Mayo Foundation for Medical Education and Research. Published by Elsevier Inc. All rights reserved.

β-lactamases with extended spectrum activity can be chromosomally mediated, and inducible AmpC enzymes are an example. AmpC are found in certain Enterobacteriaceae such as *Enterobacter* spp, *Serratia* spp, *Citrobacter freundii*, *Acinetobacter* spp, *Proteus vulgaris*, *Providencia* spp, and *Morganella morganii* (ESCAPPM). In contrast to plasma-mediated ESBLs these are not inhibited by clavulanate *in vitro*, they hydrolyse the cephamycins (cefoxitin), and unlike ESBLs are sensitive to cefepime. Treatment with carbapenems is recommended.

β-lactamases have become increasingly recognized and expansive in number; much debate has taken place over how best to classify these enzymes. Essentially there are two schools of thought: one classification is by molecular structure of the active site (e.g. the Ambler classification) and the other by functional properties (e.g. BJM) [4]. The BJM grouping is based on the preferred substrate and inhibitor profiles of the ESBL. Group 1 are classically cephalosporinases which are not inhibited by β-lactamase inhibitors, group 2 are generally susceptible to β-lactamase inhibitors, and group 3 are metallo-β-lactamases (carbapenemases) which are not susceptible to β-lactamase inhibitors. See Table 26.4 [4].

⭐ **Learning point** Laboratory detection of ESBL [5]

Conventional laboratory detection of ESBLs may take up to 3–4 days. Automated systems (e.g. Vitek 2, Phoenix) speed detection considerably and molecular techniques are very likely to be of great importance in the future. In the UK the current recommendation from PHE is that, if an ESBL is identified, resistance to all cephalosporins should be reported.

Traditional disc diffusion methods for detection of ESBLs are based on identifying resistance to an indicator oxyimino-cephalosporin and then demonstrating inhibition of the resistance by its synergy (greater net effect of both agents) with a β-lactamase inhibitor, e.g. clavunate. It is recommended by PHE that cefpodoxime should be used as the indicator cephalosporin of choice, or ceftazidime (identifies TEM and SHV types) plus cefotaxime (identifies CTX-M).

Double disc tests: Two discs, one with the indicator cephalosporin and one with clavulanate, are placed a specified distance apart on an agar plate previously inoculated with the test organism. Synergy in the area between the two discs is observed if an ESBL is present. This method is not generally recommended due to its relative insensitivity.

Combination disc methods: Two discs, one with the indicator cephalosporin only and the other with the same cephalosporin plus clavulanate, are placed on the inoculated agar plate. The zone diameters around the two discs are measured and the zone around the combination disc should be larger than that around the other disc by a specified amount.

E-test ESBL strips: These strips are infused with two cephalosporin gradients, one at each end. One end is also infused with clavulanate. Two patterns indicate ESBL production and synergy. See Figure 26.1.

(continued)

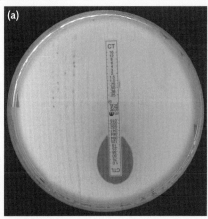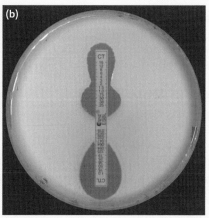

Figure 26.1 Both images demonstrate ESBL production. Mean inhibitory concentrations (MICs) that are more than eight-fold lower with clavulanate (a) or the presence of keyhole zones (b) imply ESBL production. CT, cefotaxime; CTL, cefotaxime + clavulanic acid.

✅ **Evidence base** Outcome of cephalosporin treatment for serious infections due to apparently susceptible organisms producing ESBL Implications for the clinical microbiology laboratory [6]

Study design: A prospective, multinational study on *Klebsiella pneumoniae* bacteraemia.

- 32 cases reviewed where ESBL-producing *Klebsiella pneumoniae* bacteraemia had been treated with cephalosporin.
- Isolates with an MIC ≤8 microgram/mL were considered sensitive, those with an MIC 16–32 microgram/mL were considered of intermediate sensitivity, and those with an MIC >64 microgram/mL were considered resistant in line with the pre-2011 recommendations of the CLSI.
- Clinical failure was defined as death within 14 days or persistence of fever/bacteraemia despite 48 hours of cephalosporin therapy.

Results
- The most commonly used cephalosporins were cefotaxime, ceftriaxone, ceftazadime, and cefepime. Cephamycins were not assessed.
- In the cases where the cephalosporin MIC was in the intermediate range (4 cases), there was 100% clinical failure rate.
- In the cases where the cephalosporin MIC was in the sensitive range *in vitro* (28 cases), there was 54% clinical failure rate.

Conclusions: This paper became the clinical basis on which the avoidance of cephalosporins (and reporting them all as resistant despite *in vitro* susceptibility) is founded.

Discussion

This case highlights some of the challenges surrounding the diagnosis and treatment of a patient with urosepsis due to an ESBL-carrying organism. One clear challenge is the retrospective nature of microbiological results and the need for faster diagnostics. Phenotypic microbiological results often take several days and therefore may not inform the acute treatment decisions. However, these results are very useful to inform local empirical prescribing policies and for de-escalation of antibiotic treatment. This case also demonstrates an example of the challenges of choosing empirical antimicrobials in the treatment of potentially highly resistant organisms.

Controlled trials to elicit the optimum treatment of ESBL-carrying organisms have not been performed and data is derived from clinical cohort and *in vitro* studies. The carbapenem group of antibiotics are stable to ESBL hydrolysis, demonstrate time-dependent killing, and are rapidly bactericidal *in vitro*. These antibiotics have produced the best outcomes *in vivo* and are currently the treatment drug of choice.

⊘ Evidence base Antibiotic therapy for *Klebsiella pneumoniae* bacteremia: implications of production of ESBL [7]

Study design: A subanalysis of 85 patient episodes of bacteraemia due to *Klebsiella pneumoniae* taken from a prospective study of 455 patient episodes performed in 7 countries during 1996 and 1997.

The primary endpoint was death from any cause in the first 14 days after the first blood culture was positive. Antibiotics were deemed active or inactive according to *in vitro* susceptibility findings.

Results
- The overall mortality was 23% (20 patients).
- Treatment with an antibiotic to which the isolate (or further isolates collected in the 1st 5 days) was resistant resulted in a mortality rate of 64% (7/11 patients). This value was significantly higher than the mortality rate of 14% (10/71 patients) found in those patients treated with an active antibiotic (OR 10.7; 95% CI 2.2–57.0; p = 0.001).
- Patients treated with monotherapy: treatment with a carbapenem was associated with a significantly lower mortality, 3.7% (1/27 patients), compared to 44% (4/9 patients) treated with an active cephalosporin or an active BLBLI and 36% (4/11 patients) treated with ciprofloxacin.

Conclusion: Carbapenems are associated with better outcomes in the treatment of ESBL *K. pneumoniae* bacteraemia than BLBLI, cephalosporins, or ciprofloxacin in this series. It must be noted that the numbers treated with antibiotics other than a carbapenem were small.

Possible physiological reasons why the non-carbapenem β-lactams were so poor could have been the inoculum effect for the β-lactams (at higher concentrations of organism *in vitro* the MIC increases) or inadequate dosing in the non-carbapenem groups.

---

❻ Expert comment

Carbapenems such as meropenem, imipenem, and ertapenem are stable to ESBL enzymes but decreased susceptibility is seen when the isolate loses porins, which decreases the permeability of the Gram-negative outer membrane. This mechanism appears to particularly affect ertapenem.

However, carbapenems are often the final option for many resistant Gram-negative organisms and overuse is already driving resistance through β-lactamases and other mechanisms. This challenge of antimicrobial-resistant organisms is not only true for Gram-negative organisms but also in Gram-positive organisms and mycobacteria.

★ Learning point Carbapenem resistance in Enterobacteriaceae [8]

Carbapenems are the final antibiotic defence for many Gram-negative bacteria and resistance to these agents can be categorized into two main groups:

- Porin loss plus ESBL plus AmpC: bacteria with porin loss show resistance only to ertapenem and are fully sensitive to meropenem and imipenem, classically seen with *Enterobacter* spp. These isolates do not usually require reference laboratory referral.
- Carbapenemases: β-lactamase enzymes that hydrolyse carbapenems and can be further divided into metallo-β-lactamases (MBLs) and non-MBLs.

Non-MBLs include class A and class D β-lactamases and of these the most clinically significant currently are the KPC (class A) and OXA (class D), although globally there are a plethora of other enzymes. These enzymes tend to be found in Enterobacteriaceae spp such as *Klebsiella* spp. Non-MBLs tend to be 'weak' enzymes, especially the OXA class, and rely on other resistance mechanisms such as porin loss and efflux pumps in addition to affect the resistance.

(continued)

MBLs have little in common with non-MBLs; they are molecularly diverse and have a unique hydrolytic action, which enables them to degrade all β-lactams, except monobactams. The most widely publicized MBL is NDM-1. Its spread within the Enterobacteriaceae from first isolation in New Delhi in 2008 to global occurrence within 2 years has caused great concern [9]. NDM-1 is carried on a plasmid, which confers resistance to a multitude of antimicrobials, leaving only colistin and tigicycline as active agents.

Levels of carbapenem resistance in the UK are low but rising with 339 Enterobacteriaceae (KPC 229, NDM1 44, OXA-48 29, VIM 26) containing carbapenemases reported to the HPA in 2010 [10].

Tight stewardship, de-escalation once susceptibility data is available, and appropriate dosing are all key factors in helping reduce the spread of carbapenem resistance. The use of an aminoglycoside plus a BLBLI combination (BLBLI) (as occurred in this case) as an empirical choice is also one method to reduce the use of carbapenems. In this case the isolate was sensitive to amikacin; however, in many ESBL-carrying organisms there is often associated aminoglycoside resistance and BLBLI is effectively left as monotherapy. There is debate over whether a BLBLI is appropriate therapy for ESBLs.

BLBLI show susceptibility *in vitro*, as in our case, and are probably used for the treatment of ESBLs more frequently than is recorded due to lack of a microbiological diagnosis and lack of specific testing for ESBLs in all laboratories. Despite *in vitro* sensitivity the MIC has been shown to be inoculum dose dependent [11] and treatment failures have been reported *in vivo* [7]. The advice is often that they are not suitable as treatment for severe infection caused by ESBL-carrying organisms. However, successful outcomes have been reported in certain situations, for example, in urinary tract infections [4]. Furthermore, two recent analyses suggest that the difference between carbapenems and BLBLI may be overestimated. The first study is a post hoc analysis of the data from 6 prospectively collected bacteraemia cohorts. Mortality at 30 days and hospital length of stay for patients with *E. coli* ESBL bacteraemia treated with either a BLBLI (amoxicillin-clavulanic acid and piperacillin-tazobactam) or carbapenem were compared. The analysis divided the patients into two groups according to whether the patients were treated empirically or definitively. There was a trend towards lower mortality rates in the BLBLI group compared to those in the carbapenem group for both empirical treatment and definitive treatment. Also on adjustment for confounders no association for increased mortality was found with BLBLI treatment compared to the carbapenem treatment [12]. The second study is a meta-analysis of 1,584 patients from 21 published reports of bacteraemia treated with carbapenems or BLBLI. Again no statistically significant difference was identified between the groups [13]. Although both these studies are analyses of data collected for other purposes and the usual caveats exist, they do provide increasing evidence that BLBLI may be a treatment option for ESBLs which are susceptible *in vitro*. Currently, although they may not be chosen for definitive (following antimicrobial susceptibility testing) treatment, they may be appropriate for empirical use in combination with an aminoglycoside.

Other available options include aminoglycosides and fluoroquinolones, but associated resistance is common. The newer drug tigicycline, a semi-synthetic derivative of minocycline, has excellent *in vitro* activity and was licensed for skin and soft tissue infections as well as complicated intra-abdominal sepsis caused by MDR organisms

🗨 Expert comment

β-lactamase inhibitors such as clavulanic acid and tazobactam inhibit ESBL enzymes; however, many CTX-M 15 ESBL producers (which is the commonest ESBL in the UK) also produce OXA-1, a β-lactamase inhibitor-resistant penicillinase which confers resistance to β-lactamase inhibitor combinations. They should not be used for severe infection caused by ESBL producers.

(including ESBLs). Reports of poor clinical outcomes with tigicycline compared to carbapenems in the treatment of severe infections led to the FDA issuing a warning against the use of tigecycline in severe infections [14]. The reasons for this reduced effectiveness *in vivo* are not established but options could include lack of urinary tract penetration and that it is only bacteriostatic. Other options for oral treatment of urinary tract infections from ESBLs include older agents such as fosfomycin and nitrofurantoin. Some suggest the use of cephalosporins to which the isolate retains *in vitro* sensitivity. However, this latter approach is controversial.

> **ⓕ Expert comment** Controversy on the clinical relevance of the laboratory detection of ESBL production
>
> There is currently a great deal of controversy and conflicting advice to diagnostic laboratories on whether they should carry out tests to detect ESBL production. Treatment failures have been described in cases where ESBL-containing isolates appeared sensitive to certain cephalosporins *in vitro*. In light of this finding, the BSAC, the EUCAST, and the CLSI recommended specific tests to detect ESBL production and the reporting of all producers as resistant to all cephalosporins and aztreonam regardless of the *in vitro* susceptibility test results.
>
> However, the most recent EUCAST and CLSI guidance no longer recommends specific ESBL detection tests. These organizations state that the introduction of the new, lower breakpoints used for *in vitro* testing of resistance to cephalosporins means that results can now be reported without further interpretation, and cephalosporins used in treatment if susceptible. The reason for this change is threefold and is summarized in Livermore et al. [15]. First, pharmacodynamic modelling with the new breakpoint shows serum concentrations over the MIC are achievable for over 40–50% of the time; second, animal models suggest that MIC is a better predictor of outcome than mechanism and there is nothing unique about the ESBL mechanism; and third, a reassessment of the reported cases of clinical failure show that failure occurred with isolates where the MIC was in the old CSLI intermediate range, which is above the new breakpoints.
>
> Current UK guidance published by the HPA (now PHE) [5] recommends to continue looking for ESBL production as treatment failures have been described even in low-MIC ESBLs and susceptibility tests (automated systems and disc zones) used in most laboratories often have poor reproducibility. An example of a low-MIC ESBL common in the UK and carried in *E. coli* ST131 (strain A) is CTX-M 15 which has the IS26 insertion between *bla*CTX-M-15 and its normal promoter in IS*Ecp1*. This insertion means that the cephalosporin MICs are lower than other CTX-M 15 strains.
>
> In the face of such contradictory advice and the absence of definitive clinical data, it would seem prudent to avoid cephalosporins in known ESBL-producing isolates when other treatment options are available.

The patient in the case had evidence of severe sepsis as noted by organ damage, high lactate level, and the need for ICU admission. All these features as well as her age and underlying diabetes put her at risk of a poor outcome. It is debatable whether the patient would have had a better outcome if she had received a carbapenem earlier rather than co-amoxiclav with amikacin. Choice of empirical agents must be determined by severity of clinical disease and local epidemiology of antimicrobial resistance. However, in view of the paucity of antibiotic choices for Enterobacteriaceae, there are concerns regarding the overuse of carbapenems.

A final word from the expert

This case highlights a number of issues surrounding the laboratory detection and treatment of ESBL-producing organisms. Indicator antibiotics are used for the detection of various resistance mechanisms, e.g. oxacillin for the detection of β-lactam resistance in *S. pneumoniae* and *S. aureus*, or Na for quinolone resistance in *Neisseria gonorrhoeae*. In these cases antimicrobials to which the organism may appear susceptible *in vitro* are reported as resistant if the indicator antibiotic suggests the presence of a certain resistance mechanism.

Currently there is a lack of consensus on whether this approach is required for ESBL and carbapenemase producers or whether *in vitro* susceptibility tests can be reported as read. This has led to uncertainty in the recommendations for definitive treatment in patients in whom these resistant organisms are detected.

Potentially of greater concern is the fact that the majority of antimicrobial prescribing is empirical and many patients do not have their pathogen isolated. The increasing prevalence of MDR organisms will lead to many patients receiving an ineffective empirical agent, and it has been shown that severely ill patients who receive inappropriate initial antimicrobial treatment have an increased mortality. New antimicrobial agents that are active against Gram-negative organisms resistant to current β-lactams are desperately needed [16].

References

1 Paterson DL, Ko WC, Von Gottberg A et al. International prospective study of *Klebsiella pneumoniae* bacteremia: implications of extended-spectrum β-lactamase production in nosocomial infections. *Ann Intern Med* 2004; 140: 26–32.

2 Rodríguez-Baño J, Alcalá JC, Cisneros JM et al. Community infections caused by extended-spectrum β-lactamase producing *Escherichia coli*. *Arch Intern Med* 2008; 168: 1897–1902.

3 Martin V, Mushtaq S et al. and the BSAC Extended Working Party on Resistance Surveillance. BSAC Bacteraemia Resistance Surveillance Update 2011. Available at http://www.bsacsurv. org/uploads/publications/publications/2012_FIS_bact_update.pdf

4 Kanj SS, Kanafani ZA. Current concepts in antimicrobial therapy against resistant gram-negative organisms: extended-spectrum β-lactamase-producing Enterobacteriaceae, carbapenem-resistant Enterobacteriaceae, and multidrug-resistant *Pseudomonas aeruginosa*. *Mayo Clin Proc* 2011; 86: 250–259.

5 Health Protection Agency. *UK Standards for Microbiology Investigations: Laboratory Detection and Reporting of Bacteria with Extended Spectrum β-Lactamases*. Available at http://www. hpa.org.uk/webc/HPAwebFile/HPAweb_C/1317135964970.

6 Paterson DL, Ko WC, Von Gottberg A et al. Outcome of cephalosporin treatment for serious infections due to apparently susceptible organisms producing extended-spectrum β-lactamases: Implications for the clinical microbiology laboratory. *J Clin Microbiol* 2001; 39: 2206–2212.

7 Paterson DL, Ko WC, Von Gottberg A et al. Antibiotic therapy for *Klebsiella pneumoniae* bacteremia: implications of production of extended-spectrum β-lactamases. *Clin Infect Dis* 2004; 39: 31.

8 Health Protection Agency. *UK Standards for Microbiology Investigations: Laboratory Detection and Reporting of Bacteria with Carbapenem-Hydrolysing β-lactamases (Carbapenemases)*. Available at http://www.hpa.org.uk/webc/HPAwebFile/HPAweb_C/1317138520481.

9 Yong D, Toleman MA, Giske CG et al. Characterization of a new metallo-β-lactamase gene, bla(NDM-1), and a novel erythromycin esterase gene carried on a unique genetic structure in *Klebsiella pneumoniae* sequence type 14 from India. *Antimicrob Agents Chemother* 2009; 53: 5046.

10 Health Protection Agency. Epidemiological data (carbapenem resistance and NDM-1). Available from http://www.hpa.org.uk/Topics/InfectiousDiseases/InfectionsAZ/ CarbapenemResistance/EpidemiologicalData/.

11 Thomson KS, Moland ES. Cefepime, piperacillin-tazobactam, and the inoculum effect in tests with extended-spectrum β-lactamase-producing Enterobacteriaceae. *Antimicrob Agents Chemother* 2001; 45: 3548.

12 Rodríguez-Baño J, Navarro MD, Retamar P et al. β-Lactam/β-lactam inhibitor combinations for the treatment of bacteremia due to extended-spectrum β-lactamase-producing *Escherichia coli*: a post hoc analysis of prospective cohorts. *Clin Infect Dis* 2012; 54: 167–174.

13 Vardakas KZ, Tansarli GS, Rafailidis PI, Falagas ME. Carbapenems versus alternative antibiotics for the treatment of bacteraemia due to Enterobacteriaceae producing extended-spectrum β-lactamases: a systematic review and meta-analysis. *J Antimicrob Chemother* 2012; 67: 2793–2803.

14 Food and Drug Administration. *Drug Safety Communication: Increased risk of death with Tygacil (tigecycline) compared to other antibiotics used to treat similar infections.* Available at http://www.fda.gov/Drugs/DrugSafety/ucm224370.htm.

15 Livermore DM, Andrews JM, Hawkey PM et al. Are susceptibility tests enough, or should laboratories still seek ESBLs and carbapenemases directly? *J Antimicrob Chemother* 2012; 67: 1569–1577.

16 Livermore DM. Has the era of untreatable infections arrived? *J Antimicrob Chemother* 2009; 64 (suppl 1): i29–i36.

27 Multidrug-resistant *Pseudomonas aeruginosa* infection in cystic fibrosis

James Hatcher

Expert commentary Michael Loebinger

Case history

A 22-year-old male was bought to his local emergency department by ambulance with a 3-day history of productive cough and shortness of breath. He described copious amounts of purulent green sputum with no blood, and shortness of breath associated with mild left-sided pleuritic chest pain. There was an associated fever and lethargy for 48 hours, but no night sweats, weight loss, or rigors.

The patient had a history of cystic fibrosis (CF). Throughout childhood he developed multiple respiratory tract infections with frequent courses of antibiotics, hospital admissions, and progressive deterioration in lung function.

> ⊕ **Clinical tip** Pathogens in cystic fibrosis lung disease
>
> The prevalence of each pathogen leading to lung disease in CF changes over time. *S. aureus* and *Haemophilus influenzae* are frequently isolated in infancy and childhood (Figure 27.1).
>
> Colonization with PSA occurs during childhood with 30% of children colonized by the end of the first year of life [1]. In adults PSA is the most common pathogen isolated with up to 80% of patients colonized [5]. PSA colonization is associated with faster deterioration in lung function and is an independent risk factor and in the vast majority of cases the cause of death. Patients are usually infected with a non-mucoid strain which over time develops into a mucoid phenotype which has a worse prognosis and cannot usually be cleared [1].
>
> *Burkholderia cepacia* complex is a group of environmental opportunistic pathogens that lead to particularly poor prognosis in CF patients. *B. multivorans* and *B. cenocepacia* are the most commonly isolated subtypes. Survival after infection with *B. cenocepacia* has been shown to be 67% at 5 years compared to 85% in patients colonized with PSA [2]. The number of exacerbations and clinic appointments have also been shown to increase with *Burkholderia cepacia* complex infection. *B. cenocepacia* ET12 stain has been shown to be highly transmissible between patients, with segregation of patients at clinic appointments recommended.
>
> Other pathogens associated with CF at much lower rates are *Stenotrophomonas maltophilia*, *Achromobacter xylosoxidans*, *Ralstonia pickettii*, *Pandorea apista*, *Aspergillus* spp, and atypical mycobacteria. The full impact of these pathogens is unknown.

The patient was currently on the waiting list for lung transplantation. At home he took regular nebulized saline with accompanying chest physiotherapy, bronchodilators, and had been increasing his use of home oxygen therapy.

① Expert comment

Standard respiratory care for a CF patient such as this would usually include in addition the mucolytic DNAse, oral azithromycin, and an inhaled antibiotic such as the polypeptide colistin (sometimes called colomycin) or the aminoglycoside tobramycin.

Inhaled antibiotics have the advantage of achieving high levels in the lung without the side effects or need for intravenous administration. There is evidence for the use of inhaled antibiotics in two situations in CF. First, in patients with chronic PSA infection (as in this case) inhaled antibiotics have been shown to improve lung function and to reduce the number of exacerbations, need for intravenous antibiotics, and hospital visits.

The second use of inhaled antibiotics in CF is for eradication after the first isolation of PSA in sputum to prevent chronic infection occurring. There is no evidence for the use of inhaled antibiotics in acute infections.

✔ Evidence base Intermittent administration of inhaled tobramycin in patients with cystic fibrosis [3]

This is one of the many studies showing that inhaled antibiotics in CF patients colonized with PSA improve lung function and reduce morbidity.

Study design: A multicentre double-blind placebo-controlled trial performed at 69 cystic fibrosis centres in the USA between 1995 and 1996.

Method: 520 patients (mean age 21) were enrolled and were randomly assigned to receive either 300 mg inhaled tobramycin or placebo twice daily for 4 weeks followed by no drug for 4 weeks. This on/off cycle was continued for 24 weeks.

Outcomes were assessed at week 20 and compared to those at week 0.

Results
- Treatment with tobramycin led to an increase in forced expiratory volume in one second (FEV_1) of 10%. Those in the placebo arm had a reduction of FEV_1 of 2% ($p < 0.001$).
- Patients in the treatment group were 26% (95% CI 2–43%) less likely to be hospitalized.
- The density of PSA in the sputum of the treatment group dropped by 0.8 $\log_{10}$ compared to an increase of 0.3 $\log_{10}$ CFU in the placebo group ($p < 0.001$). However, when PSA density was examined, at the end of each cycle of tobramycin the effect was less after the last cycle compared to the first cycle.
- No ototoxicity or renal impairment was detected; however, there were slightly higher rates of tinnitis.
- There was a trend towards an increase in MIC in the treatment group whereas there was a fall in MIC of isolates in the placebo group. The proportion of patients with PSA isolates with an MIC over 8 microgram/mL increased from 25% to 32% in the treatment group compared to 20% in PSA isolates in the tobramycin group.

A non-randomized follow-up study over 96 weeks showed that FEV_1 improvements continued and there was increased weight gain over this period. A decrease in tobramycin susceptibility was seen over time though the clinical consequences of this were not apparent.

Four months ago he had started a trial of long-term azithromycin although he did not feel that this antibiotic had helped his condition.

> **☢ Learning point** Macrolides in cystic fibrosis
>
> Macrolides have been shown to be beneficial in preventing exacerbations and preserving lung function in CF patients infected with PSA. The mechanism leading to improvement has not been fully established. One suggestion is that, although PSA is resistant *in vitro* to macrolides, *in vivo* macrolides may be able to inhibit PSA growth in the biofilm possibly by inhibiting quorum sensing. There is some experimental evidence to support this theory. Another theory is that the immune modulating effects of macrolides dampen the excessive inflammatory response to PSA and other respiratory pathogens.
>
> A Cochrane review published in 2012 looked at 10 RCTs that included 959 patients [4]. Five studies comparing azithromycin to placebo demonstrated consistent improvement in lung function (FEV_1) over 6 months; mean difference at 6 months 3.97% (95% CI 1.74–6.19%; n = 549, from four studies). Patients treated with azithromycin were twice as likely to have not had an exacerbation at 6 months, OR 1.96 (95% CI 1.15–3.33). Treatment with azithromycin was associated with a reduction in identification of *S. aureus* from respiratory culture, but also a significant increase in macrolide resistance. It was concluded that there was evidence of improved respiratory function after 6 months of azithromycin. However, data beyond 6 months is less clear, and there is a concern regarding emergence of macrolide resistance.

Three days earlier, at the beginning of his recent deterioration, he had started taking oral ciprofloxacin prescribed by his CF physician. The CF physician had looked after the patient since he had transferred to adult care 4 years earlier and he had been colonized with PSA for all this time. Eradication of PSA had been attempted by the paediatric team but had not been successful (Box 27.1).

> **Box 27.1** Infection control: PSA infection prevention and eradication [5]
>
> Once PSA is established in patients with CF it is almost impossible to eradicate and colonization has a deleterious effect on morbidity and mortality. Infection prevention and eradication are preferable.
>
> **Prevention:** The majority of PSA acquisition likely occurs from the environment. However, there have been examples of sibling-to-sibling transmission and hospital spread of certain strains. Good microbiological surveillance of current PSA types among CF patients, methods to reduce cross-infection including hand hygiene, cleaning of equipment, and consideration of segregation of patients with PSA from those not infected is recommended. Many of the studies in support of segregation introduced multiple infection control measures simultaneously and so the benefits are still debated. Certain strains seem more transmissible than others, and segregation in these instances is recommended. Segregation may prove to be impossible in many institutions as there is likely to be variation in PSA type, resistance profiles, and other co-infections. Other methods to reduce patients mixing, such as asking patients to obtain prescribed medication from a local pharmacy instead of the hospital pharmacy, are advised.
>
> All CF patients admitted to hospital should be treated in a side room.
>
> Prophylactic antibiotics to prevent the acquisition of PSA have been attempted without success. In one RCT children newly diagnosed with CF were given a 3-week course of oral ciprofloxacin and inhaled colistin, or placebo, every 3 months for 3 years. At the end of the period there was no significant difference in the annual rates of acquisition in either group [6].
>
> **Eradication:** Aggressive treatment of PSA on initial isolation may result in eradication in up to 80% of instances [5]. There are varied eradication regimens; however, a combination of oral ciprofloxacin and 3 months of inhaled colistin is commonly used. Multiple studies have shown that eradication can be effective, and this is supported by a Cochrane review. The UK recommendations are based on a
>
> (continued)

study from Copenhagen which compared 48 patients treated with 3 months of oral ciprofloxacin and inhaled colistin with 43 historical controls. After 3.5 years 16% of treated patients developed chronic *P. aeruginosa* infection compared to 72% of untreated historical controls (p <0.005) [7]. Furthermore, treatment maintained or increased pulmonary function during the year after inclusion compared to the control group.

On arrival at hospital, the patient was found to be in respiratory distress with tachycardia and tachypnoea. There were widespread coarse crepitations on auscultation. He was pyrexial (38.2°C), hypoxic (SpO$_2$ 84%) and had a CRP of 60 mg/L. The chest radiograph demonstrated widespread bronchiectasis and mucus plugging. Arterial blood gas analysis on room air was consistent with type I respiratory failure with a PaO$_2$ of 6.8. The patient was resuscitated with oxygen, and fluid and co-amoxiclav 1.2 g three times daily and clarithromycin 500 mg twice a day were started according to the hospital guidelines for severe community-acquired pneumonia. Cultures were sent to the microbiology department.

> ### ✚ Clinical tip
>
> The following antibiotics have anti-pseudomonal activity and can be considered for treatment in sensitive isolates:
> - β-lactams—ceftazidime, piperacillin-tazobactam, ticaricillin-clavulanic acid, meropenem, imipenem, doripenem, aztreonam
> - Aminoglycosides—tobramycin, amikacin, gentamicin
> - Fluoroquinolones—ciprofloxacin
> - Polymyxin—colistin sulphate
> - Miscellaneous—fosfomycin

❻ Expert comment

Following hospital guidelines for community-acquired pneumonia are not appropriate for infective exacerbations of CF. Co-amoxiclav and clarithromycin would not be suitable first-line antibiotics and would not give cover for the Gram-negative organisms such as PSA. It is likely that this patient was known to be a PSA carrier because the CF physicians had started him on ciprofloxacin as an outpatient. Always look up previous microbiological results or contact the hospital microbiology department where the patient is treated for CF. The patient is likely to be aware of his PSA status so it is always worth asking the patient, especially if you are not able to look up past microbiology results. First-line treatment in these patients would typically consist of ceftazidime or meropenem plus tobramycin for 14 days [8]. Tobramycin is preferred over gentamicin as it is thought to have fewer adverse effects, in particular, renal toxicity [9].

✪ Learning point Virulence factors of PSA

There is a complicated interaction of host- and organism-derived factors that contribute to the pathogenicity of *P. aeruginosa*. The organism needs to attach, colonize, and evade the host defences, leading to dissemination and systemic disease.

- **Surface components:** Pili on the surface of the organism attach to eukaryotic cells. The polar flagella are critical for motility initiating pulmonary infection. Flagella expression is switched off after lung colonization, followed by expression of genes involved in bioflim production.
- **Type III secretion system (TTSS):** *P. aeruginosa* encodes a TTSS that is a major determinant of virulence. These systems produce syringe-like structures, which penetrate the host cell and inject toxins, leading to cellular toxic effects such as irreversible damage to cellular membranes, and induction of cytokines such as TNF-α. The neutralization of the TTSS has been shown to prevent septic shock, leading to improved survival.
- **Extracellular products:** Exotoxin A is a potent enzyme that inhibits protein synthesis, causing direct tissue damage and necrosis. Pyocyanin is secreted, giving a blue-green pigment and causes a proinflammatory effect, disrupting bronchial epithelium and impairing ciliary function. Pyocyanin is found in high levels in patients with cystic fibrosis. *P. aeruginosa* produces two major siderophores that efficiently bind iron: pyochelin and pyoverdin. These are important virulence factors as they also help to control the expression of other factors such as exotoxin A and proteases.
- **Biofilms and quorum sensing:** *P. aeruginosa* grows as a biofilm in the CF lung and over time changes to a mucoid phenotype. Biofilm development is under quorum sensing control, which allows bacteria to coordinate behaviour by secretion of small diffusible molecules. Biofilms increase resistance to antimicrobials by decreasing the penetration of the drug into the extracellular matrix; they also inhibit the ability for destruction by the innate immune system.

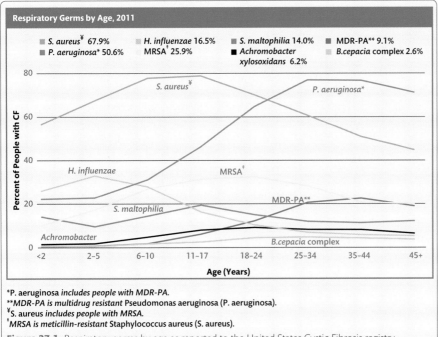

Figure 27.1 Respiratory germs by age as reported to the United States Cystic Fibrosis registry. Reproduced with permission from *Cystic Fibrosis Foundation Patient Registry 2011 Annual Data Report*, Bethesda, Maryland, USA, Copyright ©2012 Cystic Fibrosis Foundation. Available from http://www.cff.org/UploadedFiles/research/ClinicalResearch/2011-Patient-Registry.pdf

The next day the patient clinically deteriorated and began to develop type 2 respiratory failure necessitating non-invasive ventilation. After discussion with the on-call microbiologist his therapy was changed to intravenous ceftazidime 2 g three times daily, intravenous amikacin 15 mg/kg, and nebulized colistin 2 million units three times daily. At this stage a pseudomonas had been identified in the sputum but susceptibilities were not known.

Due to his profound hypoxia and decreasing respiratory effort he was semi-electively intubated and transferred to the intensive care unit.

The patient continued to deteriorate and the intravenous ceftazidime and amikacin was changed to intravenous meropenem 1 g three times a day and intravenous tobramycin 10 mg/kg based on the susceptibility pattern of the PSA isolated from the sputum on day 4 of admission, after discussion with the microbiology team (Table 27.1).

🄯 Expert comment

The decision to admit to ICU is not an easy one to make as classically CF patients on the waiting list for transplantation would not be deemed suitable. There are recent changes in thinking to this blanket policy, driven by the possible use of extracorporeal membrane oxygenation and the ability to perform transplantation in a ventilated patient.

Table 27.1 Sensitivity patterns of PSA that was isolated from sputum on days 1, 4, and 11. The PSA was reported as having two phenotypes: one was mucoid.

Antibiotic	Sputum day 1	Sputum day 4	Sputum day 11
Ciprofloxacin	Resistant	Resistant	Resistant
Piperacillin-tazobactam	Resistant	Resistant	Resistant
Gentamicin	Resistant	Resistant	Resistant
Amikacin	Resistant	Resistant	Resistant
Ceftazidime	Sensitive	Resistant	Resistant
Colistin sulphate	Sensitive	Sensitive	Sensitive
Tobramycin	Sensitive	Sensitive	Resistant
Meropenem	Sensitive	Sensitive	Resistant

⊕ **Clinical tip** PSA in the microbiology laboratory

P. aeruginosa is a non-sporing, non-capsulate, strictly aerobic GNB. A monotrichous flagellum provides mobility and kinetic activity. The organism grows in the routine microbiology laboratory easily, on a wide range of conventional media over a wide temperature range. It omits a sweet grape-like odour and most strains produce a diffusible pigment, typically a green-blue colour caused by pyocyanin or a yellow-green colour caused by fluorescein. The colonial appearance of *Pseudomonas* can vary considerably and can appear as discrete colonies of differing sizes or in a mucoid form. *P. aeruginosa* derives energy from carbohydrates by oxidative fermentation, unlike Enterobacteriaceae, which use fermentative metabolism. It gives a rapid positive reaction to the oxidase test which is a useful preliminary diagnostic test.

★ **Learning point** PSA drug resistance in the CF population

P. aeruginosa lives in complex communities within biofilms, with planktonic forms being released, and a sputum sample often contains mixed populations with a wide variety of antibiotic susceptibilities. In addition there are hypermutators, PSA bacteria that have reduced ability to repairs errors in DNA during replication, and so mutations accumulate at a higher rate than usual. Sensitivity testing can be difficult, with different results being obtained on different days. Furthermore, a subpopulation of bacteria resistant to a particular antibiotic may be present at the start but only multiply to high enough levels to be detected once selective pressure is exerted through the use of antibiotics. Drug resistance is common (see Table 27.2). Definitions of drug resistance are not standardized. The US Cystic Fibrosis Foundation defines multiple drug resistance as resistance to two of the three main classes of antibiotics, and panresistance as resistance to all three where the drug classes are aminoglycosides, pseudomonal penicillins, and fluoroquinolones. However, in some European studies multiple antibiotic resistance in PSA (MARPA) is defined as resistance to a pseudomonal penicillin plus resistance to tobramycin or amikacin as well as gentamicin.

Table 27.2 Percentage of isolates showing resistance to the stated antimicrobial agent using standardized breakpoints defined by the British Society of Antimicrobial Chemotherapy [10]

Antibiotic	Rates of resistance
Gentamicin	50%
Ceftazidime	39%
Piperacillin	32%
Ciprofloxacin	30%
Tobramycin	10%
Colistin	3%

Source: Data from Pitt TL et al, Survey of resistance of *Pseudomonas aeruginosa* from UK patients with cystic fibrosis to six commonly prescribed antimicrobial agents, *Thorax*, Volume 58, Issue 9, pp. 794–796, Copyright © 2003 BMJ Publishing Group Ltd & British Thoracic Society. All rights reserved.

Mechanisms of resistance [11]

PSA can acquire resistance through mutational changes or by gaining exogenous resistance genes (e.g. plasmids carrying the extended β-lactamases and metallo-β-lactamases). In CF mutational changes are more common. Derepression of inducible β-lactamases, reduction in permeability, and upregulation of efflux pumps are the main mechanisms of resistance. Upregulation of efflux pumps is particularly important and upregulation of certain pumps can affect all three of the main classes of antibiotics. For example, upregulation of MexAB-OprM leads to reduced fluoroquinolone, aminoglycoside and penicillins, cephalosporins and meropenem (not imipenem) activity.

Mutational mechanisms of resistance in PSA

β-lactam resistance
- Upregulation of efflux pumps (e.g. MexAB-OprM)
- Loss of porins (e.g. loss of OprD leads to resistance to the carbapenems)

(continued)

- De-repression of intrinsic β-lactamases (e.g. AMP C) leading to resistance to penicillins and cephalosporins

Fluoroquinolone resistance
- Mutations in topoisomerase II and IV lead to reduced affinity
- Upregulation of efflux pumps

Aminoglycoside resistance
- Reduced aminoglycoside transport possibly by loss of porins
- Upregulation of efflux pumps

If upregulation of the efflux pump MexAB-OprM occurs with the loss of porin OprD and the acquisition of aminoglycoside impermeability occurs, resistance to all classes can easily emerge, leaving only the polymyxin, colistin, to be used.

Despite the change in antibiotics, discussion with the transplant team, and ICU-level care, the patient died on day 14 after admission.

Discussion

This case highlights inadequate antibiotic prescribing for a patient known to be colonized with PSA when he acutely presented with a respiratory exacerbation to a hospital not experienced with treating CF patients. Unfortunately, this situation is not uncommon; due to patients with CF living longer, having better quality of life, and travelling more, this situation is likely to occur with increasing frequency.

The UK Cystic Fibrosis Trust guidelines suggest that on admission a patient with a respiratory exacerbation in whom microbiological results are unknown should be treated with a β-lactam active against PSA plus an aminoglycoside, preferably tobramycin [8].

Although the traditional interpretation is that susceptibility testing can closely guide antibiotic choice, there is some evidence in CF that the correlation between susceptibility and clinical effect is not so clear. In a retrospective study of 77 patients treated with intravenous ceftazidime and tobramycin, no correlation was found between improvement in lung function and the MIC of these antibiotics to PSA in sputa taken prior to the exacerbation [12]. In this study there were only four patients with isolates that had resistance over the breakpoint for both tobramycin and ceftazidime and so the results may not be reproducible in a larger trial. However, all four patients did improve. As there were no controls it is difficult to know if they would also have improved with no antibiotics or antibiotics that did not cover PSA (like those our patient received). One possibility is that it is not always the PSA that is responsible for the exacerbation. As such, antibiotics are often given irrespective of the susceptibility patterns, and in practice combinations that patients have found most efficacious in the past are frequently used.

Guidelines suggest that two anti-pseudomonas antibiotics from two classes should be used to get the benefits of synergy and reduce the risk of further resistance occurring. However, there is little evidence that two antibiotics act synergistically *in vivo* to produce improved outcomes. A systematic review in 2005 of single versus combination antibiotics found no difference in efficacy or safety, but there was a trend towards higher antimicrobial resistance with single agent use [13]. Aminoglycosides should be given as od dosing which is as efficacious but associated with fewer adverse effects compared to multiple doses [14].

A final word from the expert

This case highlights many of the complex issues surrounding management in cystic fibrosis and particularly focuses on PSA, which is the most prevalent problematic microbe in this population. It is worth summarizing treatment of this microbe on first isolation, in chronic colonization, and in acute exacerbations.

It has been well documented that the clinical state in CF patients deteriorates following PSA acquisition with increased morbidity and mortality (5). Neonatal screening has provided a unique opportunity to assess the impact of PSA and causality of this association. Studies from the Wisconsin CF Neonatal Screening Project have demonstrated an increased morbidity and more rapid decrease of lung function and CXR score after PSA isolation [1]. As such, significant efforts are made to eradicate this microbe on first isolation which can postpone colonization. In addition studies have demonstrated that this management can prevent clinical deterioration [7]; however, it is important to bear in mind that this study utilized historical controls. Various eradication protocols are utilized including combinations of oral ciprofloxacin and inhaled colomycin for up to 3 months [7], inhaled tobramycin for 1 month, and combinations of intravenous and inhaled therapy.

Patients with chronic PSA colonization are managed with long-term inhaled antibiotics (in addition to other agents which would commonly include azithromycin and DNase) which are documented to improve lung function and reduce exacerbations [3]. Practically, in the UK this normally consists of nebulized colomycin twice a day; however, other options include alternate month nebulized tobramycin or aztreonam lysine.

Acute exacerbations should be treated with two intravenous agents of differing class. Although there is no evidence of increased efficacy with two agents, there is evidence for a reduction in the development of resistance. There is presently no evidence for the use of inhaled antibiotics for the management of an acute infective exacerbation of CF.

There are significant recent developments in antibiotic therapy for PSA in CF patients, particularly surrounding the delivery of inhaled antibiotics. Inhaler (as opposed to nebulizer) versions of tobramycin and colomycin have been developed, with other agents such as inhaled ciprofloxacin in the pipeline.

Finally, it is important to remember that, aside from antimicrobials, airway clearance and chest physiotherapy are key in the management of both chronic and acute CF.

References

1 Li Z, Kosorok MR, Farrell PM et al. Longitudinal development of mucoid *Pseudomonas aeruginosa* infection and lung disease progression in children with cystic fibrosis. *JAMA* 2005; 293: 581.

2 Jones AM, Dodd ME, Govan JR et al. *Burkholderia cenocepacia* and *Burkholderia multivorans*: influence on survival in cystic fibrosis. *Thorax* 2004; 59: 948–951.

3 Ramsey BW, Pepe MS, Quan JM et al. Intermittent administration of inhaled tobramycin in patients with cystic fibrosis. Cystic Fibrosis Inhaled Tobramycin Study Group. *N Engl J Med* 1999; 340: 23–30.

4 Southern KW, Barker PM, Solis-Moya A, Patel L. Macrolide antibiotics for cystic fibrosis. *Cochrane Database Syst Rev* 2012; (11): CD002203.

5 Report of the UK Cystic Fibrosis Trust Antibiotic Working Group. Pseudomonas aeruginosa *infection in people with cystic fibrosis: Suggestions for prevention and infection control*, 2nd edition. November 2004. Available at http://www.cftrust.org.uk (accessed 2 March 2013).

6 Tramper-Stranders GA. Controlled trial of cycled antibiotic prophylaxis to prevent initial *Pseudomonas aeruginosa* infection in children with cystic fibrosis. *Thorax* 2010; 65: 915.

7 Frederiksen B, Koch C, Hoiby N. Antibiotic treatment of initial colonization with *Pseudomonas aeruginosa* postpones chronic infection and prevents deterioration of pulmonary function in cystic fibrosis. *Pediatr Pulmonol* 1997; 23: 330–335.

8 Report of the UK Cystic Fibrosis Trust Antibiotic Working Group. *Antibiotic treatment for cystic fibrosis*, third edition. May 2009. Available at http://www.cftrust.org.uk (accessed 16 December 2012).

9 Smyth A, Lewis S, Bertenshaw C et al. Case-control study of acute renal failure in patients with cystic fibrosis in the UK. *Thorax* 2008; 63: 532–535.

10 Pitt TL, Sparrow M, Warner M, Stefanidou M. Survey of resistance of *Pseudomonas aeruginosa* from UK patients with cystic fibrosis to six commonly prescribed antimicrobial agents. *Thorax* 2003; 58: 794–796.

11 Livermore D. Multiple mechanisms of antimicrobial resistance in *Pseudomonas aeruginosa*: our worst nightmare? *Clin Infect Dis* 2002; 34: 634–640.

12 Smith AL. Susceptibility testing of *Pseudomonas aeruginosa* isolates and clinical response to parenteral antibiotic administration: lack of association in cystic fibrosis. *Chest* 2003; 123: 1495–502.

13 Elphick H, Tan A. Single versus combination intravenous antibiotic therapy for people with cystic fibrosis. *Cochrane Database Syst Rev* 2005; CD002007.

14 Smyth A, Tan KH, Hyman-Taylor P et al. Once versus three-times daily regimens of tobramycin treatment for pulmonary exacerbations of cystic fibrosis—the TOPIC study: a randomised controlled trial. *Lancet* 2005; 365: 573–578.

28 The treatment of *Mycobacterium abscessus* lung disease

Mariyam Mirfenderesky

Expert commentary David E. Griffith

Case history

A 64-year-old white woman with *Mycobacterium abscessus* repeatedly isolated from sputum samples was referred to a specialist unit for consideration of treatment. The patient had been diagnosed with cryptogenic bronchiectasis 10 years previously. Treatment included an ipratropium bromide inhaler and a mucolytic, with daily postural drainage. There was also a history of hypertension for which she took bendroflumethiazide 2.5 mg and atenolol 50 mg.

When reviewed in clinic the patient reported that her bronchiectasis had been relatively stable until 2 years previously when she began to notice an increase in sputum production and frequency of exacerbations. Most recently she had suffered with small volume haemoptysis which settled spontaneously. On average antibiotics were prescribed every 4–6 months for exacerbations but hospitalization was never required. The patient described herself as 'lethargic' and 'failing to thrive' but denied a history of fevers or sweats. Her weight remained constant at 36 kg. On examination she was thin with lung signs compatible with bronchiectasis.

Investigations revealed that six expectorated sputum samples submitted for analysis over the past 18 months had isolated *M. abscessus*. Recent imaging including a CXR and CT scan of the chest had shown progressive lung disease with bilateral patchy infiltrates and pulmonary nodules, compatible with non-tuberculous mycobacterial infection (NTM) (see Figure 28.1). Baseline blood tests were unremarkable apart from a mildly elevated CRP of 42 mg/L. A full cystic fibrosis mutation analysis did not reveal any mutations.

✪ Learning point *Mycobacterium abscessus*

M. abscessus is the third most commonly recovered NTM respiratory pathogen after MAC and *Mycobacterium kansasii*, and accounts for 80% of rapidly growing mycobacterial (RGM) respiratory disease isolates [1].

There is growing recognition that *M. abscessus* is an important human pathogen responsible for a wide spectrum of diseases including pulmonary, skin and soft tissue, and disseminated infection [1]. By its nature *M. abscessus* causes a slowly progressive lung disease, with estimated mortality rates of 15% [2]. The largest group of patients with *M. abscessus* lung disease are white, female non-smokers, older than 60 years of age, with no predisposing lung disease.

M. abscessus is also of concern in the cystic fibrosis (CF) population. While *M. abscessus* (18%) is second only to MAC (76%) in prevalence in this cohort, a decline in lung function is most likely seen with *M. abscessus* [3]. *M. abscessus* has been associated with life-threatening disseminated infection in CF patients after lung transplant, and it is for this reason that many transplant centres consider active *M. abscessus* lung disease a contraindication to listing for lung transplantation [3].

> **✦ Learning point** NTM
>
> The NTM are a diverse group of organisms with differing disease potentials and virulence. It is assumed that the source of NTM is environmental, particularly from water sources (e.g. household plumbing systems) where significant biofilms can form.
>
> Traditionally mycobacterial isolates were classified into RGM or 'slow growing mycobacteria' according to whether they form colonies on subculture within 7 days. Although this distinction is no longer routinely used in the laboratory it still proves a useful broad classification for NTMs, particularly for the RGM [1]. See Table 28.1.
>
> **Table 28.1 Growing characteristics of non-tuberculous mycobacteria**
>
> | RGM | Slow growing mycobacteria |
> | --- | --- |
> | M. chelonae | MAC |
> | M. abscessus | M. kansasii |
> | M. fortuitum | Mtb |
>
> Over the years significant achievements have been made in the isolation and identification of NTMs, leading to increased awareness. Advances in molecular typing techniques, particularly 16S rRNA gene sequencing, have resulted in a dramatic rise in the number of speciated mycobacteria, currently in excess of 160, of which 40 have been associated with lung disease [4].
>
> Determining the incidence and prevalence of NTM infection remains difficult. Unlike *Mtb*, there is no mandatory reporting and not all isolated NTMs are significant or associated with true disease. Recent data supports the widely held view that NTM disease prevalence is increasing, with rates between 5.5–8.6 cases/100,000 and >20 cases/100,000 population in those above 50 years of age [5]. Due to the rising prevalence and difficulty in treating and curing patients, many authorities now regard NTM as a significant and growing public health concern [4].

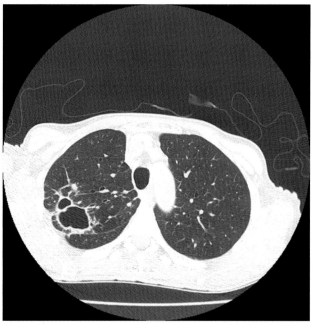

Figure 28.1 Moderate bronchiectasis with thick-walled cavity in right upper lobe. Multiple nodules in both lung fields.

> **Learning point** Clinical and radiological findings in NTM disease
>
> Symptoms of NTM lung disease are variable and non-specific. They range from cough, fatigue, malaise, dyspnoea, to fever, haemoptysis, chest pain, and weight loss. Constitutional symptoms are common with advancing NTM lung disease. It is often difficult to separate symptoms due to coexisting lung disease from NTM disease. Physical findings are non-specific and are related to the underlying lung pathology.
>
> Radiological findings can be difficult to differentiate from tuberculous signs and a variety of findings can be found. HRCT of the chest is now routinely recommended to demonstrate the characteristic abnormalities of nodular/bronchiectatic NTM lung disease. Radiology of *M. abscessus* is similar to other forms of NTM lung disease including multilobar, patchy, reticulonodular or mixed interstitial-alveolar opacities with an upper lobe predominance. Cavitation occurs in 15% of cases [6].

> **Learning point** Risk factors for NTM infection
>
> Lung disease due to NTM infection occurs commonly in those with structural lung disease such as bronchiectasis and previous mycobacterial infection. Bronchiectasis and NTM infection often coexist, making causality difficult to determine. NTM lung disease also occurs in women without clearly defined risk factors [1].
>
> Abnormal cystic fibrosis (CF) genotypes, alpha 1-antitripsin, and certain body habitus may predispose to NTM infection [1]. The prevalence of NTM infection in patients with CF has risen over the past two decades, ranging from 4% to 20% depending on the centre. Prevalence correlates with age, rising to 40% in patients above 40 years of age [3]. NTMs tend to infect those with milder lung disease, with one study finding that 20% of adults with bronchiectasis and /or pulmonary NTM infection had undiagnosed CF. It is thus recommended that all individuals presenting with bronchiectasis who are culture positive for NTM should be screened for CF regardless of age [7].
>
> Recently TNF-α blockers have been implicated in predisposing to serious and occasionally fatal NTM disease. TNF-α blocking agents should be used with extreme caution in patients with active NTM disease and only if they are also receiving adequate therapy for their NTM disease or prophylaxis if they have had NTM in the past [1].

> **Clinical tip** Current work-up advised for suspected NTM lung disease [1]
>
> - A CT scan of the chest should be performed prior to initiation of therapy and used to assess radiological response to treatment.
> - Send three or more sputum samples for AFBs. Isolation of NTM in culture is essential for the diagnosis of NTM lung disease. There is no role for empirical therapy. A single positive culture is generally regarded as indeterminate.
> - When collecting sputum samples do not allow patients to drink or rinse their mouth with tap water prior to collecting an expectorated sample, due to the risk of environmental contamination with NTM.
> - Consider bronchoscopy or induced sputum sampling when the patient is not spontaneously productive. Bronchoscopy may be more sensitive and less prone to environmental contamination with NTM than sputum samples obtained conventionally.
> - Exclude other lung pathologies such as TB or lung cancer.
> - Consider lung biopsy in patients with non-diagnostic microbiological and radiological criteria or where there is a concern regarding another disease process.
> - Screen all patients who present with bronchiectasis and are culture-positive for NTM, regardless of age, for CF with both a sweat chloride test and genotyping.
> - Monitor closely those patients that do not meet all of the American Thoracic Society (ATS) criteria with serial CT scans and sputum cultures, as NTM lung disease is characteristically slowly progressive.
> - If the diagnosis remains in doubt refer the patient for expert opinion.

> ⊕ **Clinical tip** Summary of ATS guidelines for the diagnosis of NTM pulmonary disease [1]
>
> See Table 28.2.
>
> **Table 28.2 Summary of ATS Guidelines for the Diagnosis of NTM Pulmonary Disease**
>
> | | |
> |---|---|
> | Clinical | Pulmonary symptoms: cough, haemoptysis, fever, breathlessness, night sweat, reduction in lung function
Exclusion of other diagnoses |
> | Radiological | CXR: nodular or cavitatory lesions
CT: multiple small non-calcified nodules, multifocal bronchiectasis with or without cavitation |
> | Microbiological | Two positive sputum cultures or one positive bronchial lavage or biopsy specimen showing typical histopathological features with positive culture on transbronchial or lung biopsy |
>
> Source: Data from Griffith DE et al, An official ATS/IDSA statement: diagnosis, treatment, and prevention of nontuberculous mycobacterial diseases, *American Journal of Respiratory and Critical Care Medicine*, Volume 175, Number 4, pp. 367–416, Copyright © 2007.

The case was discussed at a multidisciplinary meeting where it was agreed that she met the criteria for invasive non-tuberculous mycobacterium (NTM) infection according to the ATS guidelines, 2007. The patient had clear evidence of microbiological infection with, and progressive radiological changes secondary to, *M. abscessus*. Due to the widespread nature of the disease, thoracic surgery was not an option. The patient was offered a trial of treatment but was warned of poor cure and high relapse rates. Treatment was planned for a minimum of one year, starting with multiple parenteral agents, and would require an initial period of hospitalization.

> ⊕ **Clinical tip** Which NTM are significant?
>
> Deciding which NTM species is clinically significant remains a challenging problem. Knowing the potential virulence of the NTM isolated along with information about the site of isolation and characteristics of the individual are required to make this decision. *M. kansasii* and *M. szulgai* are almost always associated with significant disease when isolated from respiratory samples, whereas *M. gordonae* and *M. terrae* usually represent contamination of respiratory samples. *M. simiae* and *M. fortuitum* are not typical respiratory pathogens even if the NTM diagnostic criteria are met [4]. Recent evidence suggests that *M. abscessus*, when isolated from respiratory samples, has significant pathogenic potential, leading some authorities to view its isolation, even in a single sputum sample, as evidence of indolent disease.

> ⊕ **Expert comment**
>
> *M. abscessus* likely ranks in the mid-range of NTM respiratory pathogens in terms of virulence and as a potential cause of lung disease in non-cystic fibrosis patients. I think it is generally regarded as having virulence for humans similar to that of *M. avium* complex (MAC). This designation is important because it allows a more measured approach to the diagnosis of the patient and the determination of the need for therapy. This organism may, however, be more virulent than MAC in cystic fibrosis patients and requires very careful evaluation in that population. Molecular speciation of *Mycobacterium abscessus* in patients with cystic fibrosis has demonstrated the close link of this organism in the environment, particularly in therapeutic areas where the crucial respiratory therapy of such patients is undertaken. The potential for environmental transmission is of great importance in this chronic condition.

Table 28.3 Drug sensitivities of patient's *M. abscessus* isolate according to agar disc diffusion

Antibiotic		Antibiotic	
Amikacin	I	Clarithromycin	S
Gentamicin	R	Erythromycin	R
Tobramycin	R	Linezolid	R
Cefoxitin	I	Ciprofloxacin	R
Cefuroxime	R	Moxifloxacin	R
Imipenem	I	Ofloxacin	R
Co-trimoxazole	R	Doxycycline	R
Trimethoprim	R	Minocycline	R
Vancomycin	R	Tigecycline	S
Azithromycin	I	Roxithromycin	S

I, intermediate; R, resistant; S, sensitive.

Further species identification of the *M. abscessus* isolate could not be performed by the regional Mycobacterium reference laboratory and *in vitro* susceptibilities were determined by agar disc diffusion (Table 28.3).

> ⭐ **Learning point** *Mycobacterium abscessus* molecular epidemiology
>
> *M. abscessus* has been identified as a species in its own right since its separation from the *M. chelonae* group in 1992. More recently, using molecular techniques, it has been subdivided into three closely related species: *M. abscessus* subspecies (ssp) *abscessus* (formerly *M. abscessus*), *M. abscessus* ssp *bolletii* (formerly *M. massiliense*), and the organism previously identified as *M. bolletii* which is awaiting further taxonomic clarification [5]. Proportions of these species accounting for *M. abscessus* complex are variable and region specific. Rates for *M. abscessus* ssp *bolletii* range from 18% to 55% [8]. Clinically this is an important differentiation to make. *M. abscessus* ssp *abscessus* has a functioning *erm* gene whereas *M. abscessus* ssp *bolletii* does not. This inducible resistance to macrolides seen with *M. abscessus* ssp *abscessus* isolates means that they are much more difficult to treat, with lower response rates (88% vs. 25%; p <0.001, in terms of culture conversion maintained at one year) [8]. Unfortunately this differentiation is not yet routinely made by the majority of reference units.

> 💬 **Expert comment**
>
> This case highlights current shortcomings in current laboratory support for clinicians caring for patients with NTM diseases in general, and specifically for patients with *M. abscessus* lung disease. First, the species identification of *M. abscessus* isolates is of more than academic interest. Admittedly, even using molecular techniques for species identification, there is still controversy surrounding the nomenclature of *M. abscessus* isolates. Even given that limitation, clinicians require accurate identification of *M. abscessus* isolates to make reasonable treatment decisions. For instance, an isolate identified as *M. abscessus* ssp *bolletii* (*M. massiliense*) would very likely be susceptible *in vitro* to macrolide based on the assumption that, even though an *erm* gene is present, it is very likely inactive. Alternatively, if the isolate is identified as *M. abscessus* ssp *abscessus* the isolate probably has an active *erm* gene so that macrolide therapy would very likely *not* be of benefit. That finding would not necessarily preclude the use of macrolide for other indications (such as an immune-modulating drug for bronchiectasis) but would be a strong indication that macrolide could not be counted on as an effective component of a multidrug treatment regimen. Even if the isolate is identified as *M. abscessus* ssp *abscessus* it is conceivable that a mutation in the *erm* gene has rendered it inactive, which raises the second important area where laboratory support must be improved. The presence of an active *erm* gene can be detected by simply incubating the *M. abscessus* isolate in the presence of macrolide and then measuring the MIC of the macrolide for that isolate. In this case, for instance, it appears that only one MIC for macrolide was
> (continued)

> 💬 **Expert comment**
>
> This is not only a confusing area, it continues to evolve. The major source of confusion is that the organism that most investigators identify as *M. massiliense* is officially designated taxonomically as *M. abscessus* ssp *bolletii*. That designation is likely to change at some point to *M. abscessus* ssp *massiliense*. In the meantime, what is most important is not the taxonomic designation for an isolate but its *erm* gene status and activity.

determined prior to exposure of the isolate to macrolide. An alternative strategy would be to re-measure the MIC of the isolate after the patient has received several weeks of macrolide as part of a multidrug regimen for treatment of the *M. abscessus* infection. The clinician needs to know the functionality of the *erm* gene in all clinical *M. abscessus* isolates. Recent evidence suggests that information strongly influences treatment outcomes for these patients with macrolide-containing regimens. This patient's response to macrolide-based therapy strongly suggests that her *M. abscessus* isolate was most likely *M. abscessus* ssp *bolletii* (*M. massiliense*) rather than *M. abscessus* ssp *abscessus*.

Overall, it is not acceptable any longer to identify *M. abscessus* isolates without subspecies identification. Sadly, many laboratories still identify these isolates as only '*M. chelonae/M. abscessus* complex' which is 20 years out of date. It is also unacceptable to measure one pretreatment macrolide MIC for *M. abscessus*. The activity of the *erm* gene must be ascertained for each isolate. Microbiology laboratories, which are frequently ahead of clinicians in the management of mycobacterial diseases, must in this case catch up with the needs of clinicians.

⭐ **Learning point** Antimicrobial susceptibility testing (AST) of RGM

The gold standard method for RGM AST is broth microdilution; however, many laboratories may still use agar disc elution, diffusion or, more recently, E-tests [1,9]. These techniques are not recommended due to problems with standardization.

Further complicating this is the current mismatch between *in vitro* and *in vivo* drug susceptibility testing (DST) [1]. *In vitro* testing does not guide therapy in the same way as in the therapy of TB [1]. Recent work with the RGM has identified several inducible resistance genes. Erythromycin methylase (*erm*) genes impair binding of macrolides to their target ribosomes. The presence of this inducible *erm* gene is the primary mechanism of clinically significant macrolide resistance for some NTMS, particularly the RGMs such as *M. abscessus* and *M. fortuitum* [10]. However, not all *M. abscessus* or *M. fortuitum* isolates develop *in vivo* macrolide resistance. While the isolate may appear susceptible *in vitro*, it may or may not respond to the macrolide *in vivo*; so-called 'cryptic resistance' [4].

Based on susceptibility data it was decided to commence an initial regime of intravenous amikacin 15 mg/kg (3 times per week), imipenem 500 mg twice a day (low body weight), tigecycline 50 mg twice daily, with oral clarithromycin 500 mg twice daily (Table 28.4). She was admitted as an inpatient to a side room.

Table 28.4 Typical agents used in the treatment of *M. abscessus* and their side effects

Antibiotic	Dose	Tip
Amikacin	10–15 mg/kg daily to achieve peak serum levels in low 20-mg/mL range or 25 mg/kg 3 times/week. Although unproven, od dosing appears reasonable	Needs baseline audiogram. Repeat at 1 month intervals while on drug to monitor for ototoxicity. Reduce frequency to 3 times per week to prevent this
Cefoxitin	12 g daily IV in divided doses	Not routinely available in the UK. Associated with high rates of termination due to hypersensitivity (rash, fever, eosinophilia)
Imipenem	1–2 g daily in 2–4 times divided doses	Nausea and vomiting, can lower seizure threshold; hypersensitivity
Tigecycline	50 mg twice daily	Nausea and vomiting. Reducing dose may improve tolerability
Linezolid	600 mg twice daily; anaemia, peripheral neuropathy, nausea and vomiting Not licensed for more than 28 days	Consider 300–600 mg od when using long-term (use with pyridoxine to reduce effects of peripheral neuropathy). Other side effects: blood disorders requiring frequent monitoring of FBC, optic neuropathy, nausea and vomiting

> **✪ Learning point** Infection control
>
> NTM do not seem transmissible from person to person, nor do they reactivate following latent infection. This is also the case in the cystic fibrosis population where strains causing infection are predominately non-clonal, suggesting acquisition from the environment rather than patient-to-patient spread [3].
>
> When collecting respiratory samples (spontaneous, induced, bronchoscopy) due to the similarities between NTM lung disease and TB, appropriate precautions to prevent the nosocomial transmission of TB should be followed. This patient was admitted to a side room until sputum samples on this admission were negative for TB, in case she had both TB and *M. abscessus*. It's always worth discussing with infection control colleagues to ask their preference.
>
> Healthcare-associated pseudo-outbreaks have most commonly been associated with bronchoscopy and the use of tap water, which may contain environmental NTM. The use of tap water should be avoided in automated endoscopic washing machines as well as in manual cleaning.
>
> Outbreaks of hospital-acquired infection have occurred causing soft tissue, bone, and indwelling line infections following the use of contaminated surgical equipment, particularly in health tourists. Avoid contact or contamination of equipment or indwelling lines with tap water, avoid multidose vials, and always follow recommended sterilization procedures [1].

> **❝ Expert comment**
>
> Tigecycline is very poorly tolerated because of severe nausea and vomiting in the typical older patient with low body mass who has *M. abscessus* lung disease. One option is to start with tigecycline 25 mg per day and increase the dose to 50 mg per day if possible. However, it is unusual for patients to tolerate a dose greater than 25 mg per day over long periods of time.

The goal was to continue the parenteral agents for as long as possible up to a maximum of 6 months with the intent to cure. A PICC line was inserted and an audiogram was performed at baseline and again on a monthly basis to monitor for possible amikacin-induced ototoxicity. The patient suffered initially with persistent nausea and vomiting and thus the dose of tigecycline, thought to be the most likely culprit, was decreased to 50 mg od with good effect. After a period of 2 weeks the patient was transferred back to her referring hospital where arrangements were made to receive OPAT.

While on the parenteral agents the patient was seen in clinic at monthly intervals when sputum samples were obtained and submitted for mycobacterial culture. When she could not expectorate, induced sputa were obtained. Microbial culture conversion was achieved after 2 weeks of therapy and the patient remained sputum culture-negative at the 6-month point. A repeat CT of the chest performed at this stage showed improvement in the extent of the lung disease (Figure 28.2). In herself she reported a marked decrease in her cough with no recent exacerbations, and a rise in her energy levels.

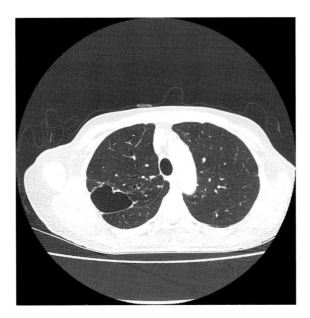

Figure 28.2 Partial resolution of nodules throughout both lung fields with improvement in areas of previous consolidation.

All parental agents were stopped after 6 months. Oral clarithromycin 500 mg twice daily was continued, with doxycycline 100 mg twice per day and moxifloxacin 400 mg od (ECGs required to monitor for long QT) added, despite *in vitro* resistance, to complete a further 6 months. At 12 months sputum samples remained culture negative for *M. abscessus* and the patient reported feeling the best she had in years. All treatment was stopped at this stage. The patient remains under life-long follow-up.

Discussion

This case highlights the difficulties physicians encounter when dealing with pulmonary cases of *M. abscessus*. When compared with the treatment of drug-sensitive TB, the treatment of *M. abscessus* is longer, more expensive, more toxic, and significantly more likely to fail [5].

Controversies exist in all aspects of this field, from the microbiological diagnostics, to when to treat, and what to treat with. There are no RCTs to guide treatment and, for the most part, the investigation, management, and treatment of cases is based on expert opinion.

M. abscessus is one of the most antibiotic-resistant organisms to treat. It is uniformly resistant to all standard anti-tuberculous agents and most other antimicrobials. Traditionally macrolides form the backbone of all NTM treatment regimes. In *M. abscessus* they are the only oral option reliably active *in vitro*. Challenging this dogma was the recent discovery of the *erm* gene or macrolide resistance gene. Isolates, while initially appearing to have susceptible or intermediate MICs to macrolides, soon develop resistance after prolonged incubation. At present, detecting for inducible macrolide resistance or full species identification which can be used to guess inducible macrolide resistance is not routinely performed by reference laboratories.

Detecting for the actual gene via molecular methods is also not helpful as the gene may not be 'switched on' or functioning. This leaves the physician in the unfortunate position of having to second guess the likely resistance pattern. It is because of the *erm* gene that treatment for *M. abscessus* now necessitates a prolonged parenteral drug regime, and not relying on a single agent macrolide as was done in the past.

The current ATS/IDSA guidelines for the treatment of NTM disease states that 'At present, there is no reliable or dependable antibiotic regime, to produce cure for *M. abscessus* lung disease' [1]. The chance of cure is quoted as 8%, as defined by the return of respiratory symptoms to baseline and culture conversion for at least one year [11].

The guidelines suggest a combination of amikacin, cefoxitin or imipenem for 2–4 months, with prolonged oral therapy using drugs to which the organism is susceptible. Surgical options should also be explored as cure rates are improved in this cohort. However, for most patients the consensus is that *M. abscessus* lung disease is a chronic incurable infection.

Over the past few years several new studies have been published which are beginning to shed new light on treatment options with improved response and cure rates than those suggested in the guidelines. For example, we now know that microbiological response rates can be as high as 88% in patients with *M. abscessus* ssp *bolletii* but remain low at 25% in those with *M. abscessus* ssp *abscessus* lung disease. Again, these differences are thought to be due to inducible macrolide resistance genes found in all *M. abscessus* ssp *abscessus* isolates but not in *M. abscessus* ssp *bolletii* [8].

⚖ Expert comment

These data are from a study in the early 1990s and are probably a worst-case scenario. Better outcomes are quoted below and are almost certainly more realisitic for current management. The statement is also made that *M. abscessus* infection is an incurable chronic disease. This patient shows that is not necessarily the case. Bronchiectasis is without question a chronic, incurable disease, but *M. abscessus*, especially without an active *erm* gene, is far from universally incurable.

Regimes now consist of prolonged parenteral courses with use of aggressive adjunctive surgery where possible.

> ✅ **Evidence base** Outcomes in patients with *Mycobacterium abscessus* pulmonary disease treated with long-term injectable drugs [12]
>
> Lyu et al. reported the response of 41 patients with *M. abscessus* lung disease assigned to a treatment regime consisting of a macrolide and either one (amikacin) or two (amikacin and cefoxitin or imipenem) parenteral agents. The median duration of parenteral antibiotic treatment was 230, 83, and 511 days for amikacin, cefoxitin or imipenem, and total antibiotic treatment, respectively. Thirteen patients underwent adjunctive surgical resection. Drug termination was necessary in 43% due to adverse side effects. Culture conversion was achieved in 80.5% (33/41), which did not differ significantly between the one and two parenteral agent groups, nor between patients treated medically or surgically. Median follow-up was 445 days during which 4 patients subsequently relapsed. The authors attribute the high response rates to the prolonged administration of parenteral agents.

> ✅ **Evidence base** Clinical and microbiologic outcomes in patients receiving treatment for *Mycobacterium abscessus* pulmonary disease [2]
>
> Jarand et al. treated 107 patients with *M. abscessus* lung disease with antibiotic regimes individualized according to known drug susceptibilities and patient tolerance. Just over a quarter received surgery (24) in addition to medical treatment. Sixteen different antibiotics were used in 42 different combinations with an average of 4.6 drugs per person and an average parenteral treatment course of 6 months. The commonest parenteral agents were amikacin (71%), imipenem (55%), and cefoxitin (30%). Drug intolerance and side effects were common with at least one drug stopped in 65% of patients. Cefoxitin and amikacin were the most common culprits. A total of 69 patients completed follow-up. In total 49 patients (71%) culture-converted of which 16 (23%) subsequently relapsed. Significantly more surgical patients who had culture-converted remained negative for at least 1 year compared with medical patients (57% vs. 28%; p = 0.022). In both these studies speciation into subspecies *M. abscessus* ssp *abscessus* or *M. abscessus* ssp *bolletii* was not performed.

What parenteral agents to use and how long to use them remains at the discretion of the acting physician with the information gained from results of susceptibility testing. Most experts would recommend a combination of at least two parenteral drugs based on *in vitro* MIC with a macrolide and would continue therapy for one year after culture conversion. Once the parenteral stage is over, some would advocate a consolidative oral phase. In known macrolide-resistant cases, options are more limited because there is often no oral drug available which is reliably sensitive *in vivo*. Choices include:

* continuing parenteral agents for as long as possible (over 1 year);
* adding in other oral agents (with or without known resistance *in vitro*) to the macrolide, as happened in this case;
* viewing treatment complete at the time parenteral agents are stopped.

Before embarking on such intense treatment regimes both the physician and patient need to be clear about the achievable goal. Six to twelve months of negative sputum cultures post-treatment for *M. abscessus* ssp *bolletii* maybe a reasonable goal. In the case of *M. abscessus* ssp *abscessus*, no antimicrobial regimes are sufficient to achieve this, thus 6 months of negative sputum cultures while on treatment may be all that is achievable. Other endpoints may include symptomatic improvement, radiological improvement, transient sputum conversion, or suppressive therapy with episodic antibiotics.

Returning to our patient, the goal was to treat with intention to cure. Three parenteral agents were chosen for a prolonged course of 6 months. Whether three agents were better than two is not known. Increases in drug toxicity, drug interactions, and side-effect profiles may have occurred, but was this a gamble worth taking? The patient tolerated the regime without major complication and sputum conversion was achieved rapidly and maintained, which was promising. Unfortunately subspeciation of the *M. abscessus* isolate could not be performed. As there was no way to predict whether macrolides would prove useful or not, a decision was made to add doxycycline and moxifloxacin to clarithromycin in the event that a functioning *erm* gene was present despite resistance *in vitro* to these antibiotics. Since termination of treatment the patient remains under 6-monthly follow-up with regular sputum cultures and imaging if necessary.

⑯ Expert comment

The therapy of NTM diseases presents some interesting paradoxes for clinicians. By far the most vexing is the frequently encountered disparity between *in vitro* susceptibilities and *in vivo* response to individual antimicrobial agents. In this case, the initial therapeutic regimen was chosen based on the *in vitro* susceptibility results for the patient's *M. abscessus* isolate. The initial parenteral therapy was followed by oral therapy with two agents (doxycycline and moxifloxacin) to which the organism did not appear to be susceptible *in vitro*. Again, this apparent paradox suggests that the patient's isolate was *M. abscessus* ssp *bolletii*. It also reinforces our limited understanding of the role of *in vitro* susceptibility testing for guiding therapy of this difficult organism. It is rather perplexing that the initial therapeutic choices for the patient were based on *in vitro* susceptibility results for the patient's isolate while at least two and possibly all three of the chronically administered oral medications (if the isolate had an active *erm* gene that was not detected initially) were not active *in vitro*. And yet, the patient did well. To further complicate this already confusing picture, recent data suggests that azithromycin is a less potent inducer of the *erm* gene than clarithromycin and should probably be the macrolide of choice for all *M. abscessus* infections.

A final word from the expert

The case is typical of *M. abscessus* lung disease in almost all aspects save the patient's very favourable response to therapy, which is unfortunately not the norm. While there is little doubt that the patient discussed in this report had progressive *M. abscessus* lung disease and required therapy for *M. abscessus*, not all respiratory *M. abscessus* isolates are a harbinger of progressive disease. Fortunately, *M. abscessus* lung disease is generally an indolent process so that there is usually time (months) to carefully assess the significance of an *M. abscessus* respiratory isolate for each patient. The indolent nature of the disease process combined with the very difficult and poorly tolerated treatment regimens essentially mandates that both physician and patient should be convinced of the need for therapy, which will inevitably require significant sacrifices on the patient's part.

The choice of therapeutic regimens remains problematic. Mounting evidence suggests that lung disease due to *M. abscessus* ssp *bolletii* (*M. massiliense*) is considerably more responsive to current therapeutic regimens than disease due to *M. abscessus* ssp *abscessus*, likely due in no small part to the absence of a functional *erm* gene in *M. abscessus* ssp *bolletii*. This recent observation has important implications. First, microbiology laboratories must identify *M. abscessus* isolates to the species level, and must identify the activity status of the *erm* gene for each isolate. Second, physicians can probably treat the isolates with an inactive *erm* gene less aggressively (i.e. with less aggressive parenteral therapy) than isolates with an active *erm* gene, usually *M. abscessus* ssp *abscessus*.

References

1 Griffith DE, Aksamit T, Brown-Elliott BA et al. An official ATS/IDSA statement: diagnosis, treatment, and prevention of nontuberculous mycobacterial diseases. *Am J Respir Crit Care Med* 2007; 175: 367–416.

2 Jarand J, Levin A, Zhang L, Huitt G, Mitchell JD, Daley CL. Clinical and microbiologic outcomes in patients receiving treatment for *Mycobacterium abscessus* pulmonary disease. *Clin Infect Dis* 2011; 52: 565–571.

3 Hauser AR, Jain M, Bar-Meir M, McColley SA. Clinical significance of microbial infection and adaptation in cystic fibrosis. *Clin Microbiol Rev* 2011; 24: 29–70.

4 Griffith DE. Nontuberculous mycobacterial lung disease. *Curr Opin Infect Dis* 2010; 23: 185–190.

5 Griffith DE, Aksamit TR. Therapy of refractory nontuberculous mycobacterial lung disease. *Curr Opin Infect Dis* 2012; 25: 218–227.

6 Griffith DE, Girard WM, Wallace RJ. Clinical features of pulmonary disease caused by rapidly growing mycobacteria. An analysis of 154 patients. *Am Rev Respir Dis* 1993; 147: 1271–1278.

7 Rodman DM, Polis JM, Heltshe SL et al. Late diagnosis defines a unique population of long-term survivors of cystic fibrosis. *Am J Respir Crit Care Med* 2005; 171: 621–626.

8 Koh W-J, Jeon K, Lee NY et al. Clinical significance of differentiation of *Mycobacterium massiliense* from *Mycobacterium abscessus*. *Am J Respir Crit Care Med* 2011; 183: 405–410.

9 Brown-Elliott BA, Nash KA, Wallace RJ. Antimicrobial susceptibility testing, drug resistance mechanisms, and therapy of infections with nontuberculous mycobacteria. *Clin Microbiol Rev* 2012; 25: 545–582.

10 Nash KA, Brown-Elliott BA, Wallace RJ. A novel gene, erm(41), confers inducible macrolide resistance to clinical isolates of *Mycobacterium abscessus* but is absent from *Mycobacterium chelonae*. *Antimicrob Agents Chemother* 2009 Apr; 53(4):1367–76.

11 Griffith DE. The talking *Mycobacterium abscessus* blues. *Clin Infect Dis* 2011; 52: 572–574.

12 Lyu J, Jang HJ, Song JW et al. Outcomes in patients with *Mycobacterium abscessus* pulmonary disease treated with long-term injectable drugs. *Respir Med* 2011; 105: 781–787.

29 Multidrug-resistant tuberculosis

Caoimhe Nic Fhogartaigh

🕐 **Expert commentary** Mike Brown

Case history

A 24-year-old student from Mumbai presented to hospital in London with a 3-week history of dry cough, fever, and night sweats. There was associated lethargy, anorexia, weight loss, and increasing shortness of breath. A few days previously, she developed right-sided pleuritic pain, visited her general practitioner, and was commenced on amoxicillin, but subsequently developed haemoptysis. She had no history of TB or TB contact. Neither had she been vaccinated with BCG. She had no past medical history, and was not on any medication.

On examination, temperature was 38.7°C, respirations 18/minute, oxygen saturations 98% on air, heart rate 130 beats/minute, blood pressure 127/67 mmHg, no lymphadenopathy; respiratory and cardiovascular examinations unremarkable. Weight 38 kg.

Blood tests revealed a low haemoglobin at 10.7 g/dL, but the remaining full blood picture, renal function, and electrolytes were all normal. The ALT was slightly raised at 50 iu/L, the albumin low at 34 g/L, and CRP raised at 33 mg/L. An HIV antibody test was negative. The chest radiograph showed an infiltrate in the right upper lobe with cavitation (Figure 29.1).

Sputum microscopy revealed numerous acid and alcohol-fast bacilli (AFB). She was admitted to a negative pressure room, and after counselling was started on quadruple anti-tuberculous therapy. As she was living in university accommodation she was kept in hospital until established on treatment for 2 weeks, and contact tracing was commenced. Four weeks later the culture and drug susceptibility results became available:

- *Mtb tuberculosis* complex
- RIF, INH, and streptomycin—highly resistant
- Pyrazinamide—resistant; ethambutol and second-line sensitivities pending

> ✪ **Learning point** MDR TB
>
> MDR TB is defined as any strain of *Mtb* displaying *in vitro* resistance to at least the two most effective first-line anti-tuberculous drugs, RIF and INH. Extensively drug-resistant (XDR) TB is additionally resistant to a fluoroquinolone and one of the injectable aminoglycosides. Development of drug resistance depends on the initial burden of actively multiplying organisms, the rate of spontaneous mutations for each drug, drug concentration and exposure time, and pharmacodynamic factors such as absorption, diffusion into lesions, and maintenance level of drug. The problem of drug resistance is a consequence of many factors including poor compliance, poor prescribing practice, insufficient supplies of drugs, and inadequate public health measures in low-resource settings, as well as onward community transmission of undiagnosed or partially treated cases. MDR TB accounts for approximately 3.6% of all TB globally, with 650,000 cases reported in 2010, and many more are estimated to be unreported [1]. Prevalence varies geographically, with regions of the Russian Federation reporting up to 28.3% MDR TB [1]. In the UK, MDR TB accounted for 1.6% of laboratory-confirmed TB cases in 2011 [2].

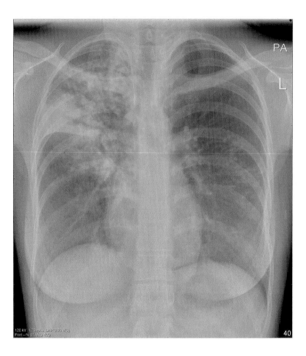

Figure 29.1 CXR: infiltrate in right upper lobe with cavitation.

⊕ Clinical tip Culture confirmation

Early diagnosis of drug resistance is important in all new TB diagnoses; hence the recommendation for sampling for mycobacterial culture and phenotypic DST **before treatment is initiated**. However, these investigations may take 1–3 months, and earlier diagnosis of MDR TB is important.

❝ Expert comment

Most patients with MDR TB will have one or more risk factors:

- History of previous TB treatment, or treatment failure
- Contact with a known case of drug-resistant TB
- Birth in a foreign country, especially those of high TB prevalence
- HIV
- Residence in London

However, significant rates of primary MDR TB have also been seen in cases with no apparent risk factors [3]. Modelling has shown that early rapid testing for RIF and INH resistance on smear-positive material is cost effective in reducing mortality and acquisition of MDR TB when background prevalence of MDR TB is greater than 1% and INH monoresistance greater than 2% [4]. Consequently, many hospitals have a policy that all smear-positive samples undergo rapid molecular resistance testing, either on site or by request to the reference laboratory.

★ Learning point Rapid molecular diagnosis of MDR TB

The RNA polymerase b-subunit (*rpo*B) gene encodes RIF resistance in 95% of cases. RIF resistance predicts MDR TB as approximately 90% of all RIF-resistant isolates are also INH resistant [5]. Real-time PCR assays, such as GeneXpert MTB/RIF (Cepheid), may be used at the point of care, by operators with minimal expertise, on unprocessed samples to amplify MTB-specific sequences and the *rpo*B gene, providing TB identification and RIF resistance results within 2 hours, with 98% sensitivity when performed on smear-positive samples and 72.5% in smear-negative cases. The Genotype MTBDR line probe assay (Hain Lifescience) can detect INH and RIF resistance in 84.2% and 96.2% of smear-positive samples, respectively [7].

> **ⓘ Expert comment**
>
> Once MDR TB is suspected on the basis of rapid molecular tests for RIF resistance (and INH if available), additional molecular tests for resistance to second-line drugs (see Table 29.1) may be performed by the reference laboratory on special request, in order to select optimal second-line drug therapy for the individual.
>
> **Table 29.1 Molecular resistance mechanisms to first and second-line anti-tuberculous drugs [8]**
>
> | Drug | Target | Mechanism | Resistance gene |
> |---|---|---|---|
> | RIF | β-subunit of RNA polymerase | Inhibition of RNA synthesis | rpoB |
> | INH | Catalase peroxidase | Inhibition of mycolic acid biosynthesis | katG |
> | INH (protionamide can exhibit cross-resistance with this mutation) | Enoyl ACP reductase | Inhibition of mycolic acid biosynthesis | inhA |
> | Pyrazinamide | Nicotinamidase, pyrazinamidase | Depletion of membrane energy | pncA |
> | Ethambutol | Arabinosyltransferase | Inhibition of arabinogalactan synthesis | embB |
> | Streptomycin | Ribosomal protein, 16S rRNA, rRNA methyl transferase | Inhibition of protein synthesis | rpsL, rrs, gidB |
>
> From Zhang Y and Yew WW, Mechanisms of drug resistance in *Mycobacterium tuberculosis*, *International Journal of Tuberculosis and Lung Disease*, Volume 13, Issue 11, pp. 1320–30, 2009. Reprinted with permission of the International Union Against Tuberculosis and Lung Disease. Copyright © The Union.

Conventional TB DST is notoriously difficult to perform, interpret and standardize, and therefore is only performed in a few reference laboratories. *Direct* DST refers to the inoculation of smear-positive clinical samples into culture media with various concentrations of anti-tuberculous drugs, and incubating so that the susceptibility information is available at the time of culture positivity. *Indirect* methods are applied once positive cultures are available, of which the proportion method is the most established. Ten-fold dilutions of culture suspension are inoculated into control and drug-containing media, and the comparison between the number of colonies on the drug and control media used to estimate the proportion of colonies resistant to each drug, expressed as a percentage of the population tested. For example, at INH 0.2 mg/L and RIF 40 mg/L concentrations, 1% or more colony growth constitutes resistance. The critical concentrations for each drug are those that have been shown to most reliably discriminate between probably susceptible strains of MTB, derived from untreated new diagnoses, and probably resistant strains from patients experiencing treatment failure with a regimen containing the drug in question. DST for RIF and INH are more reliable than for other anti-tuberculous drugs in accurately predicting resistance in terms of clinical failure. The absolute concentration method is another method, not routinely used in the UK, which determines the MIC of each drug, and may become a useful tool in the future for more pharmacologically based management of individual MDR and XDR TB cases.

At the time of receiving the susceptibility results, the patient had ongoing fevers, failed to gain weight, and was poorly tolerating her medication due to GI upset. Physical examination remained normal, but consolidation on CXR had progressed.

> **✪ Learning point**
> **Mycobacterial culture and DST**
>
> To shorten the long turnaround time associated with conventional Lowenstein Jensen culture, methods using liquid media, and indicators such as carbon dioxide or oxygen consumption for automated positive results, for example BACTEC and Mycobacterial Growth Indicator Tube (MGIT), have been developed.

The implications of the MDR diagnosis for prolonged treatment and monitoring were explained. Based on the first-line drug susceptibilities, molecular tests for resistance were requested upon discussion with the Mycobacterial Reference Laboratory, the results of which were available before phenotypic susceptibilities to second-line drugs. The *rpo*B, *inh*A, *kat*G, *pnc*A, and *gyr*A resistance genes were detected. Quadruple therapy was discontinued and she was commenced on moxifloxacin, intravenous amikacin, cycloserine, prothionamide, para-aminosalicylic acid (PAS), and linezolid.

> **⦿ Expert comment**
>
> In MDR TB cases, pyrazinamide and ethambutol are often continued (in addition to at least four second-line drugs), as DST results for these drugs are poor predictors of clinical response. In this case, there was both phenotypic and genotypic evidence of pyrazinamide resistance, which meant that she had effectively been receiving ethambutol monotherapy for one month, and so may have developed ethambutol resistance. The *gyr*A mutation suggested fluoroquinolone resistance and, therefore, possible pre-XDR TB. In a South African XDR TB cohort, use of moxifloxacin, in spite of apparent resistance, was associated with better culture conversion and mortality outcomes [9]; therefore, the patient was commenced on a high dose of 600 mg daily. The addition of linezolid was to ensure she was receiving adequate drug therapy in case of more extensive resistance.

> **✚ Clinical tip**
> **Monitoring MDR TB treatment**
>
> As well as daily clinical review, the patient underwent regular monitoring investigations: full blood picture and biochemistry three times weekly, amikacin (trough) and cycloserine (peak) level twice weekly until stable then weekly, sputum for AFB twice weekly, weight weekly, ECG weekly, and thyroid function tests monthly. Audiometry was performed at baseline, and then every 2 weeks.

Four weeks later, second-line susceptibility results became available:

- Moxifloxacin, ofloxacin—resistant
- Amikacin, kanamycin, capreomycin—sensitive
- Protionamide, ethionamide, PAS—sensitive
- Linezolid—sensitive

Six weeks into the MDR treatment regimen her cough became less productive, weight stabilized, CXR appearances improved, but she still had intermittent fevers and remained sputum smear and culture positive. She developed sensory disturbance in her feet, which progressed to a burning discomfort up to her thighs, despite pyridoxine and addition of amitryptiline. This was attributed to linezolid which was discontinued, leaving her on four effective second-line drugs, as well as high-dose moxifloxacin. Three months into treatment, she developed hypothyroidism, presumably secondary to protionamide and PAS, and started thyroxine replacement. At 4 months she developed pain in her left hip and Achilles tendon. Ultrasound was normal, and she was suspected to have tendinopathy secondary to moxifloxacin. Shortly afterwards she developed tinnitus and dizziness with reduced hearing bilaterally at > 2000 Hz on audiometry. It was also noted that the time to culture positivity, which had been gradually increasing, had plateaued, leading to concern that she was failing on the current regimen.

After discussion with the TB MDT, the decision was made to stop amikacin, and replace with clofazimine and the diarylquinoline TMC 207, if application for compassionate use was successful. Starting TMC 207 would require cessation of moxifloxacin due to the additive effect on QT-prolongation.

⊕ Clinical tip Preventing and managing adverse drug reactions

Current second-line anti-tuberculous therapy has been compared to chemotherapy with regard to the degree of side effects (see Table 29.2) and the importance of continuing medication. Many of the GI effects can be managed with timing modifications, anti-emetics, and anti-diarrhoeals. Peripheral neuropathy may be ameliorated with high doses of pyridoxine (up to 300 mg), and neuropathic pain medications such as amitryptiline. Oncology/palliative care services may be able to provide advice on pharmacotherapy to help counteract side effects. High frequency hearing loss on audiometry appears before symptomatic hearing loss at lower frequencies, emphasizing the importance of regular audiometry for early detection of toxicity and termination of therapy.

Table 29.2 Second-line drug toxicities, prevention, and management

Drug/class	Adverse effects	Monitoring/prevention
Amikacin, kanamycin (injectable aminoglycosides)	Reversible nephrotoxicity in 10–20% Irreversible ototoxicity (cochlear damage: tinnitus, high frequency hearing loss; vestibular damage: vertigo, dizziness, ataxia, nausea) Neuromuscular blockade	Trough drug levels, renal function and electrolytes Avoid nephrotoxic drugs Maintain hydration and electrolytes Audiometry at baseline and then every 2 weeks Reduce dose frequency to 3–5/week if possible Contraindicated in myasthenia gravis
Capreomycin	Reversible nephrotoxicity and electrolyte loss: hypomagnesaemia, hypocalcaemia, hypokalaemia Rarely ototoxicity	No need for levels Regular electrolyte monitoring Baseline audiometry repeated at three and 6 months of treatment
Levofloxacin, moxifloxacin (3rd & 4th generation fluoroquinolones)	GI upset, rarely hepatitis (moxifloxacin) CNS: headache, dizziness, tremor, rarely seizures Rash and photosensitivity Prolongation of QT interval (rarely arrhythmias) Musculoskeletal: arthralgia, tendonopathy, rarely tendon rupture	Anti-emetic Liver function monitoring Avoid in elderly, cardiac arrhythmias, epilepsy Serial ECGs
Protionamide	GI Reversible hepatotoxicity in 5% Peripheral neuropathy Psychiatric Hypothyroidism (increased risk with concomitant PAS) Rash Hyperglycaemia	Anti-emetics Pyridoxine Thyroid function tests
Para-amino salicylic acid (PAS)	Severe GI intolerance Hypersensitivity Drug-induced lupus and mononucleosis-like syndromes	Anti-emetics Divided doses
Cycloserine	Peripheral neuropathy CNS effects incl. irritability, confusion, and psychiatric disturbance (psychosis in up to 10%)	Contraindicated in patients with epilepsy or severe depression Monitor drug levels
Linezolid	Bone marrow suppression; peripheral neuropathy; blindness	Reduce dose to 600 mg od Monitor full blood count
Clofazimine	Reversible skin pigmentation (up to 100% of cases) Enteropathy	Avoid sun exposure

⟨⟨ Expert comment

It is important that a single drug is never added to a failing regimen due to the risk of further resistance and treatment failure. If TMC 207 had not been available, an option would have been to replace amikacin with capreomycin which has much lower rates of ototoxicity. Also, although moxifloxacin is not recommended with TMC 207, levofloxacin (even at high doses) is permitted and using this drug could have enabled the physicians to continue a fluoroquinolone with TMC 207.

Once established on the regimen of protionamide, cycloserine, PAS, clofazimine, and TMC 207 she converted to culture negativity at 6 months into treatment. She was discharged back to her student accommodation with follow-up in TB clinic weekly. Ultimately, she wanted to return to her family and complete treatment in India (Box 29.1).

Box 29.1 Infection control and public health issues

Patients with suspected or confirmed MDR TB should be admitted to an airborne infection isolation room (AII). These rooms receive 6–12 air changes per hour and are under negative pressure, that is, air flows from the outside area into the room. The air may be exhausted to the outside, or recirculated if filtered through a high efficiency particulate respirator (HEPA filter). Until a room is available, the patient should wear a surgical mask. When entering AII rooms, healthcare workers should wear FFP3 (filtering face piece) masks. The continued use of AII rooms and masks is advised in cases of confirmed MDR TB, even if the patient is smear negative. According to WHO guidelines, MDR TB cases are considered non-infectious once two consecutive sputum samples, at least 1 week apart, are confirmed to be culture negative after 6 weeks of incubation.

Once an MDR TB case is confirmed or suspected, it should be notified to the public health department, and a case conference convened involving the consultant in communicable disease control, the TB physician, TB nurse, and any other relevant staff, such as the local microbiologist, representatives of hospital infection control, or the patient's GP. The objectives of this meeting should be:

- To confirm the diagnosis of MDR TB
- To nominate the clinician responsible for treatment, TB nurse, and location of treatment
- To agree definitions for contact-tracing (including staff contacts)
- To ensure immediate adequate isolation
- To agree criteria for discharge to the community

✔ Evidence base MDR TB and international travel

The best evidence for onward transmission of MDR TB on flights comes from a retrospective screening exercise of 925 passengers after a patient with smear-positive MDR TB died 13 days after air travel [10]. On three flights, all under 8 hours' duration, only 14 passengers had positive tuberculin skin tests (TST), and no conversion was recorded (skin tests were offered immediately and then at 12 weeks). All but one had other risk factors for a positive TST. On the fourth flight, which was over 8 hours long, 15 passengers were identified with positive TST, and in six of these conversion was observed. Of the six, four were seated within two rows of the case, and the other two were in the same section but reported visiting friends near the case for prolonged periods. Although this shows that transmission can occur during a flight, rates are very low, and there has not been a case of active TB attributed to exposure in an aircraft. In our case, it was agreed with the HPA (now PHE) that the patient could travel once she had two consecutive negative cultures.

At TB clinic follow-up, the patient reported palpitations. ECGs showed persistently prolonged QTc interval at 486 ms. Electrolytes remained within normal range. Over 8 weeks the QTc interval reached a peak of 588 ms, at which stage the TMC 207 was discontinued due to risk of cardiac arrythmias. When QTc normalized, moxifloxacin 800 mg daily was reintroduced, and was better tolerated.

❝ Expert comment

The concern with using moxifloxacin in the case of proven resistance is that exposing mycobacteria to subinhibitory concentrations of fluoroquinolone has been shown to significantly increase mutation rates *in vitro* [11]. However, given the evidence of the importance of fluoroquinolones for drug-resistant TB treatment [9,12], moxifloxacin levels were measured over 24 hours after an 800 mg dose, and demonstrated levels above the MIC of the isolate (1 mg/L) for at least 16 hours (see Figure 29.2), supporting the use of the drug.

(continued)

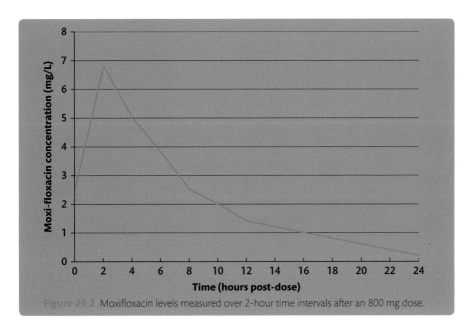

Figure 29.2 Moxifloxacin levels measured over 2-hour time intervals after an 800 mg dose.

She was referred to a physician in India with a stable supply of second-line TB medications, and facility for close monitoring, to continue on the consolidation phase for 18 months from culture conversion. At 18 months, she is asymptomatic, has normal CXR appearances, and remains sputum smear and culture negative.

Three close contacts were found to have evidence of latent TB infection and are under regular follow-up to ensure early diagnosis of active disease, as there is no latent TB treatment regimen for contacts of MDR TB.

Discussion

This case illustrates the difficulties of constructing a suitable regimen in drug-resistant TB due to limited choice of efficacious drug, significant drug toxicity, costs, and duration of therapy. As a result, MDR TB is associated with such adverse outcomes as treatment failure, default from treatment, increased mortality, and more extensive drug-resistance patterns. Efforts have been made by the WHO to formulate guidelines for the management of MDR TB [13,14]; however, as yet there have been no RCTs to compare the efficacy of one regimen to another, and guidance is based on expert opinion and systematic reviews of data from observational studies. These are limited by the ability to analyse only pooled outcome data from heterogeneous cohorts associated with *proportions* of patients with specific clinical features, or on a specific treatment. A recent *individual patient* meta-analysis has attempted to provide a more accurate illustration of the impact of treatment factors on MDR TB outcomes (Evidence base: MDR pulmonary TB treatment regimens and patient outcomes).

> **✓ Evidence base** MDR pulmonary TB treatment regimens and patient outcomes: an individual patient data meta-analysis of 9,153 patients [15]
>
> **Study design:** From three systematic reviews, 67 MDR TB cohorts with satisfactory clinical and treatment outcome data were identified. Individual patient information was requested from each cohort; 35 studies were subsequently excluded due to non-response, no information on drug susceptibility, or cohort size <25. However, the excluded studies did not differ in clinical characteristics or treatment outcomes. Patients with XDR TB, extrapulmonary TB only, or missing data were excluded, leaving a total of 9,153 patients from 23 countries.
>
> **Method:** Data such as age, sex, HIV infection, AFB smear, culture, DST (first- and second-line), drugs used and duration for intensive and continuous phases, and outcomes were collected. Definitions for treatment success and failure were well-defined for each cohort and considered comparable to WHO definitions; however, relapse was only ascertained in 14 studies. Random effects multivariable logistic meta-regression was used to estimate adjusted odds of treatment success associated with different clinical and treatment covariates. Attempts were also made to account for inter-centre variability.
>
> **Results:** Overall, 54% were treated successfully, 8% failed/relapsed, 23% defaulted, and 15% died. Patients who died were older, more likely to have HIV, and had previous treatment, particularly with second-line drugs. Treatment success (compared with failure/relapse) was associated with use of later-generation fluoroquinolones (adjusted OR 2.5; 95% CI 1.1–6.0), ethionamide/protionamide (aOR 1.7; CI 1.3–2.3). Patients requiring group 5 drugs had worse outcomes, probably biased by the fact that these were more complicated cases in terms of drug resistance, disease severity, and co-morbidity.
>
> The use of ≥4 likely effective drugs in the intensive phase was associated with treatment success (OR 2.3; CI 1.3–3.9) and odds did not increase significantly with the use of more drugs. Similarly, ≥3 likely effective drugs in the continuation phase was associated with success (OR 2.7; CI 1.7–4.1) and odds did not increase significantly with more drugs. However, in patients previously treated with second-line drugs, the maximal odds of success was seen with 5 effective drugs in both the intensive and continuation phases. This result was based on only 18 studies for intensive phase, and 15 for continuation phase, with adequate data on number of effective drugs, and therefore analysed a smaller number of patients.
>
> Odds of success were greatest with 7–8.4 months of intensive phase therapy (OR 4.8; CI 1.9–11.8) and total duration of 24.6–27.5 months (OR 11.7; 4.5–30.2). In patients receiving later-generation quinolones, maximal odds for success occurred at shorter treatment durations, but was not statistically significant. It must be noted that the effect of duration after microbiological sputum conversion could not be analysed due to limited microbiological data.
>
> The authors conclude that at least 4 likely effective drugs (including a later-generation quinolone and protionamide) should be used in the intensive phase, and at least 3 in the continuation phase, where DST is available, for the durations described above. The benefits of long duration of therapy must be weighed against risks to patients and burdens on health systems. RCTs are required to address optimal drug therapy and duration, particularly in relation to culture conversion.

Therapy may be individualized or standardized, depending on the approach of the relevant national health system. In developed countries where second-line DST is available, individualized regimens are preferable, as this prevents development of further resistance on a suboptimal regimen, and prevents exposure to toxic second-line drugs to which the isolate may be resistant. Meta-analysis of 33 retrospective reviews of MDR TB treatment cohorts reported success rates of 64% with individualized treatment, and 54% with standardized treatment, although this difference was not statistically significant [16].

DST for the second-line drugs is particularly challenging due to lack of standardization, low reproducibility, and poor clinical predictive values. Attempts have been made to define critical concentrations predictive of resistance to second-line drugs considering both clinical and laboratory defined resistance of study samples [17].

Rapid tests for molecular markers of second-line drug resistance (Table 29.1) have increasing utility.

When formulating an individualized regimen, at least 4 drugs to which the isolate is likely to be susceptible must be selected. The choice of drugs is based on DST results, treatment history, susceptibility pattern of TB contacts, national drug resistance patterns, and existing evidence for drug efficacy, safety, and cost. Table 29.3 summarizes an approach to formulating an MDR regimen.

The regimen must include a fluoroquinolone and an injectable agent. Later generation fluoroquinolones, such as moxifloxacin and levofloxacin, have been associated with significantly increased cure rates in MDR TB [16]. Ciprofloxacin is not effective. The newer fluoroquinolones have lower mean inhibitory concentrations, improved activity against TB *in vitro* and in animal models, and early bactericidal activity comparable to INH, as well as a suggestion of early sterilization. Fluoroquinolones exhibit dose and concentration-dependent killing of TB and further pharmacokinetic and pharmacodynamic studies are required to establish optimum dosing regimens and safety profiles.

The injectable aminoglycosides (kanamycin, amikacin) and polypeptides (capreomycin) display excellent extracellular bactericidal activity and are essential components of MDR TB therapy. Streptomycin should never be used as resistance is very common, but does not correlate with resistance to other injectables. Amikacin has shown slightly better *in vitro* activity against MDR TB compared with capreomycin, and is often the first-line injectable in developed regions; however, capreomycin may be preferred in view of the more favourable side-effect profile. Kanamycin is reserved for resource-poor settings where cost is an issue.

Group 4 second-line anti-tuberculous drugs include thioamides (ethionamide and protionamide), cycloserine, and para-aminosalicylic acid (PAS). These drugs are bacteriostatic, and are less effective than injectables and fluoroquinolones, but each has a different mechanism of action, so in theory use of two or more drugs from this group may improve efficacy. There may be some cross-resistance between thioamides and INH in the presence of an *inh*A gene mutation (see Table 29.1). Cycloserine is a structural analogue of D-alanine which competitively inhibits mycobacterial cell wall synthesis. Mechanisms of cycloserine resistance have not been clearly elucidated but may be due to genetic mutations in D-alanyl-D-alanine synthetase. There is no cross-resistance with other drugs. Neuro-psychiatric side effects are the main drawback.

Expert comment

Where there is doubt about the efficacy of any of the drugs, it is reasonable to increase the number of second-line agents empirically until DST results are available, bearing in mind the increased risk of intolerance and toxicity. Pyrazinamide and ethambutol, if continued, should be in addition to at least four second-line drugs, in an attempt to prevent development of further resistance. Some experts advise that drugs from group 5 should only count as half a drug in the MDR regimen, due to the lack of efficacy data.

Table 29.3 Classes of anti-tuberculous drugs and construction of an MDR TB regimen

Group/drug class	Examples	How to construct an MDR regimen
1. First-line therapy	INH, RIF, pyrazinamide, ethambutol	Stop RIF and INH. Continuation of pyrazinamide is recommended, ignoring the DST result
2. Fluoroquinolones	Levofloxacin, moxifloxacin	Choose one of these
3. Injectables	Amikacin, capreomycin, kanamycin	Choose one of these
4. Second-line therapy	Protionamide, cycloserine, PAS	Choose up to three (should include protionamide) to make a ≥4 drug regimen
5. Reinforcement drugs (less effective/less evidence)	Clofazimine, amoxicillin-clavulanate, linezolid, meropenem, clarithromycin, thioacetazone	Choose as many as required to make ≥4 drug regimen (2 of these is equivalent to one group 4 drug)

PAS is a very old anti-tuberculous drug which acts preferentially on extracellular organisms, though the exact mechanism of action is unclear. The main drawback is nausea, which can be severe.

Data for the heterogeneous group 5 drugs is limited and some suggest using two of these drugs to make up one of the group 1–4 drugs. Linezolid may be more effective than many of the other drugs in this group.

New drugs are in development such as TMC 207, a diarylquinoline which acts by inhibiting mycobacterial ATP synthase. In a small, phase 2 RCT it significantly reduced the time to culture conversion compared to placebo when added to a standard five-drug second-line regimen in newly diagnosed MDR TB, with 48% of cases converting to negative culture at 2 weeks in the TMC 207 group compared with only 9% in the placebo group [18].

Microbiology plays a key role in monitoring response to therapy. Sputum AFB smear *and* culture, at least monthly (and preferably weekly) during therapy, should be performed to detect treatment failures in a timely manner. Clinical features such as sputum production, fever, and weight should also be carefully monitored, with serial imaging at appropriate intervals used to aid clinical monitoring.

Meta-analyses of MDR TB cohorts have provided some information on optimum duration of MDR TB therapy (see Evidence base: MDR pulmonary TB treatment regimens and patient outcomes). WHO recommend an intensive phase (including an injectable agent) lasting 8 months, and a total treatment duration of 20 months (with the intensive phase continuing until at least 4 months post culture conversion, and the consolidation phase for at least 18 months post culture conversion) [14]. However, the quality of evidence for this recommendation is low, and with increasing use of newer generation fluoroquinolones, and the improved culture conversion rates seen with TMC 207 and other second-line anti-tuberculous drugs in development, there is a need to perform RCTs to assess the safety and effectiveness of shorter treatment regimens.

The role of surgery has been assessed in several case series and cohort studies, the majority of which were performed in specialist thoracic surgery centres. The indications are outlined below.

✚ Clinical tip Surgical management in MDR TB [19]

Indications

Localized disease and any of the following:

- Persistent positive smear or sputum culture despite appropriate chemotherapy
- High risk of relapse based on drug-resistance profile and radiological findings
- Complications including bronchiectasis, empyema, haemoptysis
- Sufficient perioperative drug treatment should be available (to reduce bacterial burden and allow healing of bronchial stump)

Perioperative work-up:

- CT scan to assess extent and guide resection
- Pulmonary function tests to ensure adequate pulmonary reserve
- Bronchoscopy to rule out endobronchial TB, contralateral disease, or malignancy
- Echocardiogram to exclude heart failure or pulmonary hypertension
- Optimization of nutrition

The tuberculous cavity is an ideal environment for mycobacterial growth, as the thick wall acts as a barrier to host defences and drug penetration, which may lead to the development of resistance. Removal of lesions reduces bacillary burden and facilitates host immune responses against remaining disease. Lobectomy, followed by pneumonectomy, are the most common procedures. Timing of surgery is usually between 2 and 6 months from the start of treatment, and therapy is usually continued for 12–24 months postoperatively. Success rates range from 47% to 100%, with more unfavourable outcomes seen in those with severe, bilateral disease, more extensive resistance (especially XDR), poor lung function, and poor nutritional status. Median perioperative morbidity and mortality rates are 23% and 1.3%, respectively. Complications include prolonged air leak, empyema, bronchopleural fistula, infection, and bleeding [19]. The availability of experienced surgeons and specialist thoracic surgery facilities are extremely important in order to optimize outcomes.

Compliance with MDR TB treatment regimens may be a problem once patients are discharged from hospital, and so assessment and management of drug side effects during the hospital stay is crucial, as well as close follow-up in the community. Directly observed therapy is standard practice, either by a TB nurse, district nurse, or responsible family member or friend, and weekly TB clinic follow-up in the initial stages is advisable. Psychological support and incentives may be required. Contact tracing is as for non-MDR TB, but no prophylactic regimen is advised due to lack of efficacy data and risks of toxicity. Rather, long-term clinical follow-up for symptoms, supplemented by radiological investigations, is the preferred approach.

Only physicians experienced with drug-resistant TB should be responsible for the clinical management of such cases. A multidisciplinary approach involving TB physician, TB nurse, microbiology, infection control, and public health specialists is necessary to ensure optimum diagnosis and management, as well as prevention of transmission and surveillance. In the UK, the British Thoracic Society [20] provides an online forum for confidential case management discussion with a team of experts.

A final word from the expert

This case highlights the significant challenges associated with management of MDR TB, even in a well-resourced setting. This patient's successful outcome was supported by access to rapid diagnostics, detailed phenotypic sensitivity testing, therapeutic drug level monitoring, and the availability of a new anti-tuberculous drug. Ongoing clinical trials of these new drugs, and further dose-ranging studies on existing drugs to define optimal regimens, are likely to transform the management of both sensitive and resistant TB over the next decade.

References

1 World Health Organization. *Multidrug-Resistant Tuberculosis Report, 2010*. Available at http://www.who.int/tb/publications/2010/mdrtb2010report_executive_summary.pdf.
2 Health Protection Agency. *Tuberculosis in the UK 2012 Report*. Available at http://www.hpa.org.uk/webc/HPAwebFile/HPAweb_C/13171349134044.
3 Otero L, Krapp F, Tomatis C et al. High prevalence of primary multidrug resistant tuberculosis in persons with no known risk factors. *PLoS ONE* 2011; 6: e26276.

4 Oxlade O, Falzon D, Menzies D. The impact and cost-effectiveness of strategies to detect drug-resistant tuberculosis. *Eur Respir J* 2012; 39: 626–634.

5 Wright A, Zignol M, Van Deun A et al. Epidemiology of antituberculosis drug resistance 2002–07: an updated analysis of the Global Project on Anti-Tuberculosis Drug Resistance Surveillance. *Lancet* 2009; 373: 1861–1873.

6 Boehme CC, Nabeta P, Hillemann D et al. Rapid molecular detection of tuberculosis and rifampin resistance. *N Engl J Med* 2010; 363: 1005–1015.

7 Somoskovi A, Dormandy J, Mitsani D, Rivenberg J, Salfinger M. Use of smear-positive samples to assess the PCR based genotype MTBDR assay for rapid, direct detection of the *Mycobacterium tuberculosis* complex as well as its resistance to isoniazid and rifampin. *J Clin Microbiol* 2006; 44: 4459–4463.

8 Zhang Y, Yew WW. Mechanisms of drug resistance in *Mycobacterium tuberculosis*. *Int J Tuberc Lung Dis* 2009; 13: 1320–1330.

9 Dheda K, Shean K, Zumla K et al. Early treatment outcomes and HIV status of patients with extensively drug-resistant tuberculosis in South Africa: a retrospective cohort study. *Lancet* 2010; 375: 1798–1807.

10 Kenyon TA, Valway SE, Ihle WW, Onorato IM, Castro KG. Transmission of multidrug-resistant *Mycobacterium tuberculosis* during a long airplane flight. *N Engl J Med* 1996; 334: 933–938.

11 Gillespie SH, Basu S, Dickens AL, O'Sullivan DM, McHugh TD. Effect of subinhibitory concentrations of ciprofloxacin on *Mycobacterium fortuitum* mutation rates. *J Antimicrob Chemother* 2005; 56: 344–348.

12 Johnson JC, Shahidi NC, Sadatsafavi M, Fitzgerald JM. Treatment outcomes of multidrug-resistant tuberculosis: a systematic review and meta-analysis. *PLoS One* 2009; 4: e6914.

13 World Health Organization. *Guidelines for the programmatic management of drug-resistant tuberculosis. Emergency update 2008.* Available at http://whqlibdoc.who.int/ publications/2008/9789241547581_eng.pdf.

14 World Health Organization. *Guidelines for the programmatic management of drug-resistant tuberculosis, 2011 update.* Available at http://whqlibdoc.who.int/ publications/2011/9789241501583_eng.pdf.

15 Ahuja SD, Ashkin D, Avendano M et al. on behalf of the Collaborative Group for Meta-Analysis of Individual Patient Data in MDR-TB. Multidrug resistant pulmonary tuberculosis treatment regimens and patient outcomes: an individual patient data meta-analysis of 9,153 patients. *Plos Med* 2012; 9: e1001300.

16 Orenstein EW, Basu S, Shah NS et al. Treatment outcomes among patients with multidrug-resistant tuberculosis: systematic review and meta-analysis. *Lancet Infect Dis* 2009; 9: 153–161.

17 Kam KM, Sloutsky A, Yip CW et al. Determination of critical concentrations of second-line anti-tuberculosis drugs with clinical and microbiological relevance. *Int J Tuberc Lung Dis* 2010; 14: 282–288.

18 Diacon AH, Pym A, Grobusch M et al. The diarylquinoline TMC207 for multidrug-resistant tuberculosis. *N Engl J Med* 2009; 360: 2397–2405.

19 Kempker RR, Vashakidze S, Solomonia N, Dzidzikashvili N, Blumberg HM. Surgical treatment of drug-resistant tuberculosis. *Lancet Infect Dis* 2012; 12: 157–166.

20 British Thoracic Society. Multidrug-Resistant Tuberculosis Clinical Advice Service. Available at http://www.brit-thoracic.org.uk/delivery-of-respiratory-care/tuberculosis/ mdrtb-clinical-advice-service.aspx.

30

Diagnostic and management issues in tuberculous meningitis

Naghum Dawood

🔢 **Expert commentary** Catherine Cosgrove

Case history

A 23-year-old man of Zimbabwean origin presented with confusion to his local emergency department. His mother reported that he had complained of a headache for 6 days and had malaise and vomiting for the last 2 days. He had not complained of fever.

He had emigrated to the United Kingdom from Zimbabwe 8 years previously and had not travelled outside the UK since. He worked from home for an insurance company, where he lived with his mother, her partner, and his younger sister. He was otherwise fit and well.

In the emergency department, examination revealed him to be confused with a GCS of 14/15. He had a temperature of 36.6°C and he was not haemodynamically compromised. Neurological examination was abnormal with neck stiffness. Examination of other systems was normal. A chest radiograph was normal and the urine dipstick test was unremarkable.

Acute meningitis was suspected despite the lack of fever and he was commenced on intravenous ceftriaxone. His blood results revealed a CRP and WCC in normal range.

He underwent a CT scan and LP (Table 30.1) which showed a proteinaceous lymphocytic picture.

> 🔢 **Expert comment**
>
> A Normal WCC and CRP are unlikely in classical bacterial meningitis so there is a need to think of alternative infective causes or non-infective causes of reduced GCS. Infective causes with a normal WCC include TB meningitis [1], viral meningitis or encephalitis, *Legionella, Mycoplasma, Listeria,* or cryptococcosis. A low WCC in classical bacterial meningitis is associated with a poor prognosis. A low or normal CRP is common in TBM and viral meningitis [2].

> ➕ **Clinical tip** Differential diagnosis for a lymphocytic proteinaceous CSF
>
> - **Mycobacterium:** TB
> - **Bacterial:** *Listeria* meningitis/encephalitis, brucellosis, Lyme disease, partially treated acute bacterial meningitis, paraspinal abscess, brain abscess
> - **Viral meningoencephalitis:** herpex simplex virus, varicella zoster virus, mumps, other viruses (typically less proteinaceous and normal glucose ratio)
> - **Fungal meningitis:** cryptococcosis, histoplasmosis, coccidioidomycosis
> - **Spirochaete:** syphilis
> - **Parasite:** toxoplasmosis
> - **Malignant:** lymphoma, leukaemia, leptomeningeal carcinomatosis (breast, lung, and melanoma)
> - **Autoimmune/inflammatory:** sarcoidosis, Behcet's disease, systemic lupus erythematosus

After LP, he was commenced on intravenous high-dose acyclovir (10 mg/kg three times a day) because the team considered a viral encephalitis as part of the differential diagnosis. The following morning he underwent an MRI scan of the brain. The MRI showed multiple ring-enhancing lesions within the cerebellar and cerebral hemispheres and, on enhancement, subtle diffuse meningeal enhancement was noted throughout (Figure 30.1 and 30.2).

The radiologist suggested TBM was in the differential diagnosis of the findings.

At this point, one day after admission, the diagnosis of possible TBM was made on the basis of the MRI findings, the CSF, the history, and the patient's negative HIV test result.

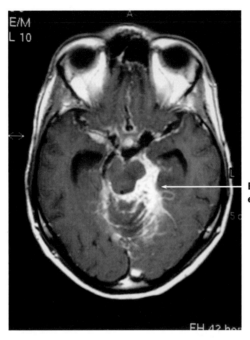

Basal meningeal enhancement

Figure 30.1 Example of an MRI of brain, showing basal meningeal enhancement.
Image courtesy of Royal Free Hospital.

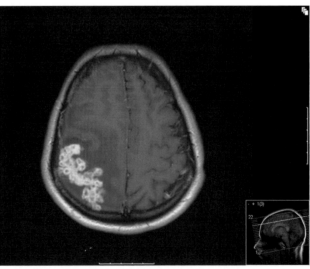

Figure 30.2 Example of an MRI of brain, showing meningeal enhancement and ring-enhancing lesions (tuberculomas), sometimes compared to a 'bunch of grapes'.
Image courtesy of Royal Free Hospital.

Table 30.1 Typical CSF findings in TBM

Typical CSF findings in TBM	Frequency/range of findings
Appearance: clear	80–90%
Opening pressure >25 cmH$_2$O	50%
Cells (usually lymphocytes)	5–1000 × 10^3/mL
Any lymphocytes	30–90%
Any neutrophils	10–70%
CSF to plasma glucose ratio <50%	95%
CSF glucose <2.2 mmol/L	Not quoted
Elevated protein (usually over 0.4 g/L)	0.45–3 g/L; can be as high as 10 g/L in spinal block
Xanthochromia occasionally	

The patient was commenced on first-line anti-TB treatment of Rifater® (RIF, INH and pyrazinamide) and ethambutol. He was also commenced on high-dose intravenous dexamethasone. The patient was immediately transferred to a tertiary ID centre for further care.

Learning point Steroids and TBM

Adjunctive corticosteroids have been shown to improve mortality at 9 months in a RCT from Vietnam. Although there was no improvement in severe disability in the study, a Cochrane review of

Table 30.2 Steroid regimes in management of TBM

Organization/trial	Steroid regimen
NICE [6]	Prednisolone 20–40 mg if on RIF, otherwise 10–20 mg. Children equivalent to prednisolone 1–2 mg/kg, maximum 40 mg, with gradual withdrawal of the glucocorticoid considered, starting within 2–3 weeks of initiation
Thwaites et al. [7] (BIA option 3 [3])	Grade 1 week 1: 0.3 mg/kg/day IV dexamethasone week 2: 0.2 mg/kg/day IV week 3: 0.1 mg/kg/day oral week 4: 3 mg total/day oral week 5– reducing by 1 mg each week over 2 weeks
	Grade 2–3 week 1: 0.4 mg/kg/day IV dexamethasone week 2: 0.3 mg/kg/day IV week 3: 0.2 mg/kg/day IV week 4: 0.1 mg/kg/day IV week 5: 4 mg total/day oral week 6: reducing by 1 mg each week over 3 weeks
IDSA 2003 [8]	Dexamethasone 12–16 mg/day IM for 3 weeks Then tapered down over a further 3 weeks to stop

(continued)

three trials (including this one) suggests that when data is combined an improvement in rates of death or disabling residual neurological deficit is observed [4].

Whether the mortality benefit observed in the original Vietnam study continues after the first 2 years from diagnosis has been called into question by the follow-up study of the same patient group. This study shows that mortality benefits are only seen up to 2 years when the cohort is looked at as a whole. However, subgroup analysis suggests that the mortality benefit continues to 5 years for patients with TBM grade 1. The reason for the benefit in TBM 1 rather than more severe disease could be because these patients have not suffered irreversible damage by the time treatment is initiated [5].

There are no trials comparing corticosteroid type, doses, or formulation and so the steroid dose can be chosen from different guidelines based on the trials (see Table 30.2). All patients with TBM should be given steroids [3]. The largest trial is the Thwaites trial and many would follow their protocol.

✔ Evidence base Dexamethasone for the treatment of TBM in adolescents and adults [7]

This landmark study provides evidence that the use of adjunctive glucocorticoids in TB meningitis reduces risk of death at 9 months.

Study design: A multicentre randomized, double-blind, placebo-controlled trial which took place in Vietnam and was published in 2004.

Method: The study compared 274 patients who received dexamethasone (for 6–8 weeks at tapering doses) to 271 who received placebo. Both groups also received standard quadruple TB therapy. Patients were over the age of 14 years and were suffering with TBM classified according to diagnostic criteria as 'definite', 'probable', or 'possible'. Mortality and disability were assessed at 9 months. Outcomes were assessed according to intention-to-treat analysis.

Results: At 9 months 10 patients (1.8%) were lost to follow-up. Adjunctive dexamethasone was associated with a reduced risk of death at 9 months (relative risk 0.69; 95% CI 0.52–0.92; p = 0.01) and reduced rate of side effects from TB medications. There was no reduction in the numbers of patients with severe disability, nor in the numbers with severe disability or death.

Conclusions: Adjunctive dexamethasone reduces the risk of death at 9 months for adult patients with TBM but probably does not alter the rate of severe disability. Possible reasons why disability was not reduced are insensitivity of the disability assessment measure and only 34% of patients had CSF culture confirmation of the diagnosis, which may have diluted the effect [9].

At the ID unit he was noted to no longer be confused and further history revealed that he had lived with an aunt who had pulmonary TB when he was 7 years old. Clinical examination again revealed him to be apyrexial, with a normal cardiovascular, respiratory, and abdominal examination with no organomegaly, but with widespread tender cervical lymphadenopathy and a BCG scar on his right arm. Neurological examination revealed disdiadochokinesis bilaterally, dysmetria in finger–nose pointing, and diplopia on left gaze consistent with a left sixth (abducens) nerve palsy.

★ Learning point Pathophysiology, signs, and prognosis of TBM

The clinical manifestations and neurological complications of TBM can be explained by the pathogenesis. Primary infection (in children) and reactivation of infection (in immunocompromised older hosts) results in bacteraemia leading to the formation of tubercles on the meninges and in the brain. The rupture or caseation of a subependymal tubercle (known as the Rich focus) into the

(continued)

subarachnoid space leads to a hypersensitivity reaction resulting in inflammation. Foci that caseate away from the subarachnoid space form tuberculomas.

1. Inflammation in the subarachnoid space leads to meningitis and a gelatinous fibrous mass at the base of the brain which encases the cranial nerves leading to cranial nerve palsies. Cranial nerve abnormalities are usually reversible.
2. Inflammation of the blood vessels results in vasculitis, thrombosis, aneurysms, and infarction leading to symptoms of stroke.
3. Inflammation extending to the basal cisterns results in a communicating hydrocephalus.

See Table 30.3.

Table 30.3 Frequency of neurological symptoms and signs in TBM [3]

Symptoms and signs	Frequency
Headache	50–80%
Fever	60–95%
Vomiting	30–60%
Anorexia/weight loss	60–80%
Neck stiffness	40–80%
Confusion	10–30%
Coma	30–60%
Cranial nerve palsy	30–50%
CVI	30–40%
CIII	5–15%
CVII	10–20%
Hemiparesis	10–20%
Paraparesis	5–10%
Seizures: Children	50%
Seizures: Adults	5%

Adapted from *Journal of Infection*, Volume 59, Issue 3, Guy Thwaites et al, British Infection Society guidelines for the diagnosis and treatment of tuberculosis of the central nervous system in adults and children, pp. 167–197, Copyright © 2009 The British Infection Society with permission from Elsevier. http://www.sciencedirect.com/science/journal/01634453

Prognosis is related to the clinical stage at presentation. The British Medical Research Council classifies the clinical presentation of TBM accordingly [10]:

- Stage I—alert, no focal neurology, no hydrocephalus on imaging
- Stage II—mild confusion, lethargy, isolated focal neurological signs, cranial neuropathies/hemiparesis
- Stage III—severe confusion and stupor, coma, seizures, multiple focal neurological signs. This is advanced disease.

Attempts were made to confirm or at least add weight to the diagnosis of TBM. A Mantoux test was performed and revealed a 22 mm scar at 48 hours.

A full body CT scan confirmed lymphadenopathy throughout the chest but no other changes consistent with TB. An induced sputum, repeat LP, and FNA from an axillary lymph node were performed.

AFB using auramine stains and cytology were negative on all these samples. CSF CrAg test was negative and a sample sent to the reference laboratory for GeneXpert® PCR analysis for *Mtb* were negative. Other diagnoses were considered and a full panel of serological tests (including Brucella and Lyme) were negative. An autoimmune screen was negative.

❝ Expert comment

It is well-known that there is a substantial false-positive and false-negative rate when using tuberculin skin tests (e.g. Mantoux). The rate of skin test positivity in TBM in studies has varied from 10% to 50% [3]. The commercially available IGRAs have only been licensed for detecting latent disease, rather than active TB disease. Some clinicians do use them to investigate active disease but at best they can only suggest prior contact with TB. No currently available test takes away the need to culture all possible specimens.

❝ Expert comment

In patients in whom an LP is undertaken with TBM as part of the differential, at least 6 mL of fluid should be removed [3]. The larger the quantity of CSF taken, the more likely a positive diagnosis will occur. It is generally considered safe to remove 15–17 mL at one time.

✪ Learning point Laboratory diagnosis on CSF

Microscopy and culture traditionally have a low sensitivity with rates reported as low as 37% and 53%, respectively. Sensitivity of microscopy can be increased to 80% by taking at least 6 mL of CSF for centrifugation prior to staining, looking at a slide for over 30 mins, using fluorescence, sending for analysis the last fluid removed at LP, and repeating samples. Rates of culture positivity can be increased by using liquid broth media [9].

Nucleic acid tests

Currently NAATs have not been shown to be more sensitive than microscopy or culture. One comparison using the Gen-Probe amplified *Mtb* direct test (MTD) on CSF showed that there was a trend towards a lower sensitivity; with the molecular test detecting 25/66 (38%) compared to microscopy 34/66 (52%) (p = 0.15) before anti-tuberculous chemotherapy had started [9,11]. However, 5–15 days into treatment, sensitivity was better in the NAAT (28%) than with microscopy (2%) suggesting NAATs may be useful once treatment has started [9]. Combining microscopy with NAAT gave a combined sensitivity of 45/66 (68%). The GeneXpert MTB/RIF (Xpert), an automated cartridge-based NAAT, has been shown in pulmonary specimens to have a higher sensitivity than conventional NAATs; it is awaited to see whether this test will have a higher sensitivity than microscopy for CSF samples.

Over the next few days the patient developed several symptoms that were thought to be side effects of the anti-tuberculous medication.

✚ Clinical tip Side effects of first-line TB drugs

It is reported that 10% of people starting quadruple TB therapy develop side effects [12]. See Table 30.4 [13].

Table 30.4 Side effects of first-line TB drugs

INH	Peripheral neuropathy, hepatitis
	Rare: agranulocytosis, optic neuritis
RIF	Hepatitis, thrombocytopenia, rash, GI upset
	Rare: renal impairment, haemolytic anaemia
Pyrazinamide	Hepatitis, vomiting, high urate levels, rash
	Rare: photosensitivity, gout
Ethambutol	Retrobulbar neuritis, arthritis
	Rare: hepatitis, photosensitivity

Source: Data from Chan SL, in *Clinical Tuberculosis*, Davies PDO (ed), Chapman Hall, London, UK, Copyright © 1994.

He complained of paraesthesia in his fingers and toes, presumed to be due to INH-induced neuropathy, and the medical team increased the vitamin B6 (pyridoxine) from 10 mg to 50 mg.

✚ Clinical tip

Peripheral neuropathy due to INH is dose-related and uncommon (<0.2%) at doses currently prescribed [8]. INH competes with vitamin B6 (pyridoxine) in its role as a co-factor in the synthesis of neurotransmitters, resulting in peripheral neuropathy (painful), paraesthesia, and rarely ataxia. Rates of peripheral neuropathy are increased in rapid acetylators, those with low pyridoxine levels or those with other conditions which predispose to peripheral neuropathy. These conditions include alcohol consumption, chronic liver or renal disease, malnutrition, pregnancy, and breast feeding. Children also have increased risk. Only those with risk factors should be given prophylactic pyridoxine at 10 mg per day (UK) or 25 mg (USA). In reality it is often routinely given to all patients [8,12].

He developed joint aches with no associated swelling. Pyrazinamide therapy was stopped; however, the uric acid level was normal. Joint pains improved and he was commenced on non-steroidal anti-inflammatory drugs (NSAIDs).

> **❝ Expert comment**
>
> Pyrazinamide is a synthetic analogue of nicotinamide that is only weakly bactericidal against extracellular *Mtb* organisms, but it has potent intracellular bactericidal activity, particularly in the relatively acidic intracellular environment of macrophages and areas of acute inflammation. In the treatment of TB its role is thought to be as a sterilizing agent acting on the slowly replicating populations. The addition of pyrazinamide to RIF and INH regimens in the 1980s led to a reduction in treatment duration from 9 months to 6 months for pulmonary TB. Pyrazinamide frequently causes joint symptoms. Often these can be mitigated by simple analgesia. Pyrazinamide inhibits renal tubular excretion of uric acid by blocking its renal tubular secretion, resulting in some degree of hyperuricaemia that is often asymptomatic. Uric acid plasma concentration tends to increase as the length of time on therapy increases. Whether joint symptoms warrant discontinuation of therapy, especially without elevated uric acid levels, is a matter for debate and clinical judgement. The BTS suggests increasing the duration of medication for TBM from 12 months to 18 months in patients who cannot tolerate pyrazinamide [12].

On day 10 into treatment for TBM, he developed nausea and vomiting with abdominal tenderness. The patient's transaminase level had steadily risen and was now 5 times the baseline value. An abdominal ultrasound was normal and a full liver screen including viral hepatitis and autoimmune screens were all negative. Drug-induced hepatitis secondary to the anti-tuberculous medication was diagnosed and all drugs were stopped except ethambutol.

> **✪ Learning point** Drug-induced hepatitis
>
> Patients on anti-tuberculous therapy commonly experience a self-limiting, asymptomatic increase in transaminases. Drug-induced hepatitis, however, usually symptomatic with an increase in transaminases over three times the upper limit of normal (3× ULN), is associated with 9.25-fold increased risk of unsuccessful TB outcomes, and mortality risk of 2% [14]. It occurs in approximately 2% of European TB treatment cohorts, and in up to 28% of Asian cohorts with higher rates of malnutrition, viral hepatitis, and HIV [15]. It usually occurs within 2 months of starting TB therapy, but may occur at any stage. Pyrazinamide appears to be the most hepatotoxic, then RIF and INH. There is no hepatotoxicity associated with ethambutol.
>
> The British Thoracic Society 1998 guideline recommends withholding all drugs if transaminases increase to >5× ULN, or 3× ULN in the presence of symptoms, until transaminases return to <2× ULN [8,12]. Reintroduction of drugs in a stepwise manner beginning with INH, the least toxic, is advised.
>
> Risk factors for drug-induced hepatitis include:
>
> - Age over 60 years
> - Female sex
> - Asian ethnicity
> - Low body mass index or malnourishment
> - Excessive alcohol use
> - HIV
> - Viral hepatitis
> - Abnormal baseline liver function
> - Slow acetylator status
> - Concurrent use of other hepatotoxic drugs
>
> (continued)

As some cases may be asymptomatic, monitoring of those at risk is essential to detect drug-induced hepatitis at an early stage. Pre-treatment LFT should be performed, and if normal there is no need to repeat unless the patient has risk factors, or symptoms/signs of hepatotoxicity. If baseline function is abnormal, there is underlying liver disease, or risk factors exist, it is advisable to repeat every 2 weeks to monitor for the development of hepatotoxicity [8,12].

He was commenced on second-line TB drugs: moxifloxacin and capreomycin. On day 17, ALT peaked at 884 iu/L. There was a discussion as to whether to stop the moxifloxacin, but it was continued. ALT improved over the next few days.

ⓕ Expert comment

The doses and best treatment regime in TBM has been controversial, with concerns surrounding the choices likely to best penetrate the CSF and the need for combination therapy to prevent drug resistance. Most clinical guidelines suggest the standard three drugs (RIF, INH, pyrazinamide) plus an extra such as ethambutol [3]. Of the standard drugs, INH and pyrazinamide penetrate the CSF well. In the past there have been advocates of higher dose INH (10 mg/kg compared with conventional dose of 5 mg/kg), although levels above the MIC are found in the CSF with standard doses. RIF penetrates the CSF less well and there have been advocates for higher doses of this antibiotic in CNS disease; intravenous RIF should be strongly considered at the initiation of treatment if there are concerns about absorption of medications.

Ethambutol does not penetrate into the CSF well and is a relatively weak antimycobacterial agent and so there has been considerable interest in moxifloxacin as an alternative agent. Moxifloxacin has been shown to have good antimycobacterial activity and good CSF penetration [16].

Capreomycin is a cyclic polypeptide and one of the injectable agents used in drug-resistant TB. CSF penetration by streptomycin and capreomycin is poor; however, the hope is that in the presence of inflammation enough will get through to prevent mono-treatment with moxifloxacin. Capreomycin and streptomycin are anti-TB medications that can be used in patients with liver impairment; capreomycin was chosen over streptomycin as it causes less hearing damage.

On day 17 the original CSF revealed *Mtb*. The isolate culture sample was analysed by PCR and found to be negative for RIF resistance genes, but TB-PCR positive.

On day 28, the patient's renal function deteriorated. Plasma creatinine rose to 240 μmol/L. The cause of the renal impairment was thought to be non-steroidal anti-inflammatories (NSAIDs) and capreomycin. The NSAIDs and capreomycin were stopped and the INH and RIF were gradually reintroduced as the ALT had reduced to 36 iu/L.

He developed a cushingoid appearance and the dexamethasone was weaned according to protocol. He was discharged on a 12-month course of daily oral RIF 600 mg, INH 300 mg, ethambutol 1 g, moxifloxacin 400 mg, and pyridoxine 50 mg. Pyrazinamide was not restarted (Table 30.5).

ⓕ Expert comment

A review and meta-analysis has suggested that 6 months of therapy may be sufficient; however, most guidelines suggest a full year of therapy for TBM [17]. Reasons given for the prolonged course in TBM include disease severity, CNS drug penetration, undetected drug resistance, and patient adherence.

Discussion

The major challenges in this case were confirming the diagnosis of TB meningitis and managing the side effects of TB medications started empirically. Unlike the

Table 30.5 Results of LP, day 1 and day 3

Parameter (units)	Reference range	Day 1	Day 3
Opening pressure (cmwater)	10–15 cmH$_2$O	32	30
WCC/mm^3	0–4/mm^3	177	230
Lymphocytes (%)/mm^3	0/mm^3	100	90
Polymorphs (%)/mm^3	0/mm^3	0	10
Microscopy		NOS	NOS
Routine culture		No growth	No growth
Auramine stain for AFB		Negative	Negative
Mycobacterial culture		Awaited	Awaited
Protein (g/L)	0.15–0.45 g/L	>2	1.96
Glucose CSF (mmol/L)	½ to 1/3 blood glucose	1.4	1.5
Glucose serum (mmol/L)	<5.6	*	8
CSF CrAg and viral PCR (VZV, HSV, ENT)		*	Negative
Cytology		*	No malignant cells

NOS, no organism seen; * not performed.

management of pulmonary TB where there is often time to collect samples over a few days and gain evidence for the diagnosis of TB, TBM is a medical emergency and samples should be collected as quickly as possible and TB medications started on presentation. Early detection is critical, as outcome depends on initiation of early therapy. Diagnosis of TBM is based on three factors: clinical presentation and suspicion, radiological findings, and CSF parameters and microbiology [3]. However, lack of specificity in the clinical history and examination signs and lack of sensitivity in the laboratory tests make a firm diagnosis difficult, especially in the early stages.

So, are there ways to make a firm diagnosis more likely? Clinically a high index of suspicion for TBM in a patient from an area of high TB prevalence is important, especially when the clinical and laboratory features do not fit other infectious or non-infectious causes. A good history can often help with the identification of risk factors for TB. For example, in the case, the household TB contact was not identified until he was transferred for tertiary care. Laboratory features like a low WCC or CRP in the presence of fever may also be useful. CSF analysis is always important and a high opening pressure, high protein, normal or slightly raised WCC with or without lymphocytes, and a low glucose is very suspicious of TB. Algorithms designed to help the clinician identify cases that may have TBM rather than acute bacterial meningitis have been devised. Although these lack sensitivity and specificity and have not been validated in the low-prevalence high-resource setting, they may help physicians in the early stages of an admission [1].

> **✓ Evidence base   Diagnosis of adult TBM by use of clinical and laboratory features [1]**
>
> **Background:** Until more sensitive diagnostic methods are available, a large proportion of patients with suspected TBM are treated empirically. This study aimed to look for clinical and laboratory features which could be used as an aid to help diagnose TBM, particularly in resource-poor settings.
>
> **Methods:** Data collected prospectively in a teaching hospital in Vietnam on 143 patients who satisfied diagnostic criteria for TBM (37 with culture confirmed TBM and 106 with clinical ± radiological diagnosis) and 108 patients with bacterial meningitis was used to compare clinical and laboratory
>
> (continued)

features between groups. Features compared included duration of headache, fever, presence of neck stiffness, GCS on presentation, blood pressure, cranial neuropathies, serum WCC (percentage neutrophils), CSF opening pressure, CSF WCC/neutrophils/lymphocytes, CSF to blood glucose ratio, and CSF lactate. Features independently associated with TBM were used to create two diagnostic aids/algorithms.

Results: Younger age, longer length of history, lower WBC count, lower total CSF WCC, and lower CSF neutrophil proportion were all independently associated with TBM. A diagnostic rule based on a scoring system was developed. Scores were as follows, points allocated are in brackets: age ≥36 (2), blood WCC ≥15,000 10^3/mL (4), duration of illness ≥6 days (−5), CSF total WCC ≥ 900 × 10^3/mL (3), CSF % neutrophils ≥75% (4). Using a score of 4 or less for TBM produced a sensitivity of 86% and a specificity of 79% with prospective test data.

Conclusion: Certain clinical and laboratory features are useful in differentiating between TBM and bacterial meningitis. The diagnostic rule may be useful in areas of high TB prevalence and poor laboratory resources.

Imaging is important to add to diagnostic clues and to identify areas which could be sampled for further microbiological and histological specimens. Chest radiography may be positive in around 50% of cases of active or past TB [9]. Signs of parenchymal, pleural, or lymph node disease should be looked for and a sputum sample obtained for AFB analysis. Further chest and abdominal imaging may be necessary to identify other clues such as lymphadenopathy. Patients with suspected TBM should have brain imaging performed before LP. Enhanced CT scan and diffusion-weighted MRI may show leptomeningeal enhancement, tuberculomas, or stroke [9,18] which are suggestive of the diagnosis.

Microbiological diagnostic yield from CSF can be improved by maximizing the number of specimens sent to the laboratories through repeating the CSF sampling, and sending sufficient samples (6 mL) of CSF. Samples from other sites should also be cultured.

A final word from the expert

TBM is easily missed, with catastrophic consequences. It is often a diagnosis of exclusion, having ruled out all other more likely diagnoses. Often the CT scan of the head will be normal, and even changes on the MRI may be subtle. AFB on direct CSF smear may not be seen, and in cases of suspected TBM the bacilli may not even be cultured. In the case discussed, the positive Mantoux test was helpful, but this may often be negative, and a negative test would certainly not rule out TB. The lymphadenopathy is a helpful pointer but, again, may not be present. If there were concerns about lymphoma as an alternative diagnosis then formal node biopsy should be performed, with a sample also for TB culture.

When considering a diagnosis of TBM a careful hunt should be made for clues and possible specimens to culture. Thus sputum specimens should be taken, examined, and cultured, any nodes should be sampled, and repeated LP may need to be performed. Consideration should be made of CT scan investigation of chest and abdomen to detect pathology not detected by other means, and in children bone marrow aspiration and gastric washings may be helpful. While it is not usually possible to wait for the results of mycobacterial culture prior to initiating treatment, subsequent culture results help guide therapy.

The side effects of anti-tuberculous chemotherapy are well-known and documented. In non-life-threatening TB we have the luxury of withholding TB medication while side effects dissipate and then gentle re-introduction in a stepwise fashion. In TBM we do not have the luxury of time, and difficult decisions need to be made regarding the most likely drug to cause the side effect. In this case pyrazinamide caused joint symptoms and usually these can be managed with analgesia without stopping the drug. Moxifloxacin is a useful drug in cases with hepatitis as it can almost always be safely given, as can the injectable drugs.

In summary, TB is an important cause of lymphocytic meningitis which throws up difficult diagnostic and management dilemmas. Due to its significant mortality and morbidity, treatment is often commenced empirically, but all efforts should be made to acquire a culture diagnosis.

Acknowledgements

We thank Dr Caoimhe Nic Fhogartaigh for the Learning point: Drug-induced hepatitis. We thank the Royal Free Hospital, London, for MR images of the brain showing TBM.

References

1 Thwaites GE, Chau TT, Stepniewska K et al. Diagnosis of adult tuberculous meningitis by use of clinical and laboratory features. *Lancet* 2002; 360: 1287-1292

2 De Beer FC, Kirsten GF, Gie RP, Beyers N. Strachan AF. Value of C reactive protein measurement in tuberculous, bacterial, and viral meningitis. *Arch Dis Child* 1984; 59: 653–656.

3 Thwaites G, Fisher M, Hemingway C, Scott G, Solomon T, Innes J; British Infection Society. British Infection Society guidelines for the diagnosis and treatment of tuberculosis of the central nervous system in adults and children. *J Infect* 2009; 59: 167–187.

4 Prasad K, Singh MB. Corticosteroids for managing tuberculous meningitis. *Cochrane Database Syst Rev* 2008; (1): CD002244.

5 Török ME, Nguyen DB, Tran TH et al. Dexamethasone and long-term outcome of tuberculous meningitis in Vietnamese adults and adolescents. PLoS One. 2011;6(12):e27821. Epub 2011 Dec 8.

6 National Institute for Health and Clinical Excellence. Clinical diagnosis and management of tuberculosis, and measures for its prevention and control. Clinical guidelines, CG117 - Issued: March 2011. Available at Guidance.nice.org.uk/CG117/

7 Thwaites GE, Nguyen DB, Nguyen HD et al. Dexamethasone for the Treatment of Tuberculous Meningitis in Adolescents and Adults. *N Engl J Med* 2004; 351: 1741–1751.

8 Treatment of tuberculosis. American Thoracic Society, CDC, and Infectious Diseases Society of America, *MMWR Recommendations and Reports* June 20, 2003 / 52(RR11);1–77. Available at http://www.cdc.gov/mmwr/preview/mmwrhtml/rr5211a1.htm.

9 Thwaites GE, Tran TH. Tuberculous meningitis: many questions, too few answers. *Lancet Neurol* 2005; 4: 160–170.

10 Medical Research Council Report. Streptomycin treatment of tuberculosis meningitis. *Lancet* 1948; 1: 582–596.

11 Thwaites GE, Caws M, Chau TT et al. Comparison of conventional bacteriology with nucleic acid amplification (amplified mycobacterium direct test) for diagnosis of tuberculous meningitis before and after inception of antituberculosis chemotherapy. *J Clin Microbiol* 2004; 42: 996–1002.

12 Chemotherapy and management of tuberculosis in the United Kingdom: recommendations 1998. Joint Tuberculosis Committee of the British Thoracic Society. *Thorax* 1998; 53: 536–548.

13 Chan SL, in Clinical tuberculosis, Davies PDO (ed), Chapman Hall, London, 1994.

14 Shang P, Xia Y, Liu F et al. Incidence, Clinical features and impact on anti-tuberculosis treatment of anti-tuberculosis drug induced liver injury (ATLI) in China. *PLoS One* 2011; 6: e21836.

15 Tostmann A, Boeree MJ, Aarnoutse RE, De Lange WCM, Van Der Ven, Dekhuijzen R. Antituberculosis drug-induced hepatotoxicity: Concise up-to-date review. *J Gastroenterol Hepatol* 2008; 23(2): 192–202.

16 Donald PR. Cerebrospinal fluid concentrations of antituberculosis agents in adults and children. *Tuberculosis (Edinb)* 2010; 90: 279–292.

17 van Loenhout-Rooyackers JH, Keyser A, Laheij RJ, Verbeek AL, van der Meer JW. Tuberculous meningitis: is a 6-month treatment regimen sufficient? *Int J Tuberc Lung Dis* 2001; 5: 1028–35.

18 Misra UK, Kalita J, Maurya PK. Stroke in tuberculous meningitis. *J Neurol Sci* 2011; 303: 22–30.

31 Treated pulmonary tuberculosis complicated by sarcoidosis

Georgina Russell and Sally O'Connor

Expert commentary Felix Chua

Case history

A 29-year-old white South African man presented to the ID clinic with a persistent cough, night sweats, and 18-kg weight loss. He had resided in the United Kingdom for 6 years but returned frequently to his homeland. His wife had completed treatment for culture-proven pulmonary TB 3 years earlier although he himself did not have a significant medical history. Initial investigations showed a 10-mm TST reaction in the absence of a BCG scar, negative HIV serology, and radiographic evidence of right upper lobe consolidation (Figure 31.1). A well-defined rounded opacity and non-specific nodularity were present in the contralateral lung, which appeared diminished in volume. Fluorescence microscopy of sputum demonstrated the presence of AFB.

Standard daily anti-tuberculous therapy was commenced and fully sensitive *Mtb* was subsequently cultured in sputum. Clinical response was prompt and at completion of 6 months of therapy, resolution of the radiological abnormalities was noted. Onset of new exertional breathlessness several months later led to a repeat chest radiograph which demonstrated new nodular consolidation in the left upper lobe. Induced sputa subsequently cultured fully sensitive *Mtb* although microscopically clear of visible AFB. He reported that his wife was receiving treatment for reactivated pulmonary TB (also to fully sensitive *Mtb*) in Kwazulu-Natal. The couple had previously tested negative for HIV.

The patient was recommended on quadruple anti-TB agents but soon afterwards returned to South Africa to join his wife. While there, serial plain radiographs disclosed progressive radiological deterioration with development of confluent bilateral airspace consolidation, numerous lung nodules, and moderate bihilar lymphadenopathy (BHL). A differential diagnosis of MDR TB, atypical non-TB infection, lymphoma, and sarcoidosis was considered. Fibreoptic bronchoscopy performed 5 months into the course of anti-tuberculous treatment showed widespread mucosal nodularity, extrinsic airway compression of both main bronchi, and a non-obstructing soft tissue mass within the right bronchus. Luminal washings subjected to PCR were negative for *Mtb* and failed to culture AFB. Biopsy of the endobronchial lesion demonstrated granulomatous inflammation with focal caseous necrosis and a possible solitary AFB on Ziehl-Neelsen (ZN) staining. Culture of biopsied material was sterile.

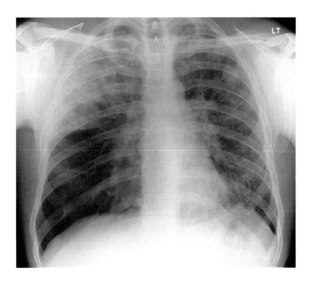

Figure 31.1 Chest radiograph from first presentation showing right upper lobe consolidation.

> ⭐ **Learning point** Differential diagnosis for intrathoracic lymphadenopathy
>
> The main differential diagnosis of intrathoracic lymphadenopathy includes sarcoidosis, mycobacterial disease (particularly TB), lymphoma, other malignancies (particularly bronchogenic carcinoma), fungal disease, and chronic suppurative lung conditions such as bronchiectasis.
>
> In sarcoidosis, such lymphadenopathy is commonly bilateral and relatively symmetrical, with a predilection for the hilar, lower right paratracheal, aorto-pulmonary window and subcarinal stations. Unihilar, lone mediastinal and posterior mediastinal lymphadenopathy are highly unusual and more suggestive of another pathology. Nodal calcification in longstanding disease usually appears punctate or eggshell-like; a differential diagnosis for the latter would include silicosis although the parenchymal changes would be dissimilar.
>
> In TB, asymmetrical hilar adenopathy may be quite striking on plain radiography; on CT, such nodes often appear necrotic or peripherally enhancing. Prior active disease may be indicated by nodal calcification. Infections other than mycobacterial disease that can cause mediastinal lymphadenopathy include histoplasmosis, coccidioidomycosis, mycoplasma, and viral infections (e.g. EBV).
>
> Mediastinal rather than hilar adenopathy per se is a more frequent finding in lymphoma; where present, hilar lymphadenopathy tends to occur asymmetrically. Such nodes often expand along or around bronchovascular structures rather than invade them. Metastatic intrathoracic nodal disease occurs most commonly in primary lung cancer. Large volume lymphadenopathy is a well-recognized feature of small cell lung cancer. Other cancers that may spread to these nodes include breast, head and neck, GI, and melanoma. KS in patients with AIDS can also present with similar findings. Other rarer causes of mediastinal lymphadenopathy include broncholithiasis (usually calcified) and fibrosing mediastinitis.

Despite continuation of anti-TB treatment, radiological and clinical deterioration persisted. Following initial failure to isolate a pathogenic agent in numerous sputum samples, the patient underwent video-assisted thoracoscopic surgery (VATS) to obtain intrathoracic nodal and lung tissue. Histological examination showed prominent granulomatous inflammation with Langhans giant cells and scanty caseous necrosis. AFB were not isolated despite prolonged culture.

The patient completed 12 months of anti-TB drugs and returned to the UK for a further opinion. He reported residual breathlessness but was constitutionally

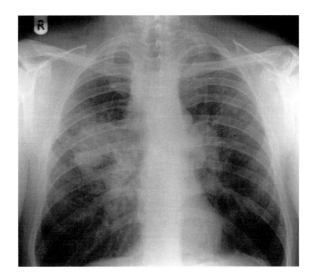

Figure 31.2 Chest radiograph at the end of 12 months of treatment for TB showing new bilateral hilar lymphadenopathy.

asymptomatic. New large-volume bilateral hilar lymphadenopathy was evident on his plain radiograph (Figure 31.2).

Cross-sectional imaging by CT showed patchy consolidation in the right lung and elsewhere, clusters of 'tree-in-bud' opacities suggestive of active mycobacterial disease in addition to the gross adenopathy. In the absence of bacteriological growth, he was maintained on standard anti-TB treatment and ultimately completed a total of 20 months of therapy. Throughout that period, numerous sputum specimens obtained by induction remained culture negative.

Over the ensuing year or so, the patient continued to experience episodic breathlessness but was able to resume his job as an administrator. A repeat CT 14 months after the first showed extensive mediastinal, hilar, and paratracheal adenopathy, prompting reconsideration of a lymphomatous malignancy as a potential aetiology (Figure 31.3).

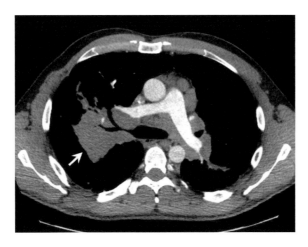

Figure 31.3 CT scan of the thorax showing mediastinal, hilar, and paratracheal adenopathy.

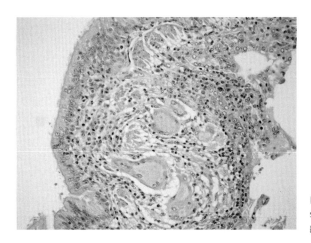

Figure 31.4 Histology specimen showing non-caseating granulomatous inflammation.

By this time, cervical and inguinal lymphadenopathy was also evident; ultrasound-guided FNA of these peripheral nodes demonstrated non-caseating lymphadenitis without any evidence of mycobacterial infection.

Following consultation with a respiratory physician, the patient underwent repeat VATS biopsy of the right lower lobe and mediastinal lymph nodes. Histological analysis of biopsied material demonstrated florid non-caseating granulomatous inflammation with numerous Langhans giant cells and lymphocytes as well as marked perilesional sclerosis of adjacent lung suggestive of established pulmonary sarcoidosis (Figure 31.4). Immunohistochemistry did not identify any malignant markers and special stains as well as subsequent cultures were negative for fungi and AFB.

⚙ **Learning point** Pursuing tissue/lymph node biopsy or aspiration

The wide range of disease patterns in sarcoidosis suggests that it may not be a single disease or, at the very least, may be triggered by more than one aetiological agent or set of pathological circumstances. A secure diagnosis of sarcoidosis therefore necessitates tissue evidence of epithelioid cell granulomatous inflammation in sites acknowledged to be susceptible to sarcoidal disease. Granulomatous inflammation is a pathological hallmark of disorders as varied as TB, berylliosis, schistosomiasis, Crohn's disease, and idiopathic granulomatous diseases (e.g. panuveitis), among others. It may also occur in the context of lymphoma or carcinoma, either occurring adjacent to the lesion itself or within the loco-regional lymph nodes. However, the granulomas in such situations are typically B-cell positive, as opposed to B-cell-poor reactions found in sarcoidosis.

Sarcoidal reactions may also arise in combined variable immunodeficiency (CVID). Approximately 5–10% of patients with CVID will develop granulomatous complications in one or more organs including the lungs, where the radiological appearances may look entirely similar to classical sarcoidosis. Thus, the finding of histological evidence of granulomatous inflammation in an individual with hypogammaglobulinaemia, a history of frequent infections, and atypical clinical features of sarcoidosis should prompt exclusion of CVID.

Obtaining biopsy material from an organ suspected as having sarcoidosis allows microbiological analysis to be undertaken to exclude ID that may be mimicked by the condition. Special stains for mycobacteria and fungi as well as substrate for microbial culture and molecular testing are among the investigations that can be performed.

● **Learning point** Sarcoidosis

Sarcoidosis is a multifaceted disorder of unclear aetiology that bears the pathological hallmark of non-caseating epithelioid cell granulomatous inflammation. It is believed to develop in genetically susceptible individuals following exposure to a persisting environmental, occupational, or infectious agent [1]. Its prevalence varies according to ethnicity—it is three times more common in black Americans than white Americans. Among Europeans and Asians, it is commonest in northern Sweden and Japan, respectively. Seasonal clustering (early > latter part of the year) and occupational clustering (automobile manufacturing and bird keeping, among others) have also been reported [2].

✓ **Evidence base** Infection as a cause of sarcoidosis

The role of a transmissible agent as a trigger for sarcoidosis has been postulated since the early 1900s [3]. Particular attention has been paid to mycobacteria (*Mtb*, *M. leprae*, and NTM) including acid-fast cell-wall-deficient forms ('L forms'), bacteria (*Propionibacteria*, *Yersinia* spp), fungi (*Histoplasma* spp, *Aspergillus* spp), metazoa (*Schistosoma*), protozoa (*Leishmania*), and several viruses (EBV, CMV). A permissive interplay of ethnic, genetic, geographic, and other environmental factors appears to still be necessary for any infectious agent to pathologically induce a sarcoidal phenomenon [1,2].

A mycobacterial-related role in the pathogenesis of sarcoidosis has long been postulated but remains unproven. Applying advanced molecular techniques to PBMCs isolated from patients with sarcoidosis, it has been shown that a certain percentage of such individuals mount strong Th1-type responses (e.g. interferon-gamma, IFNγ production) against mycobacterial antigens [2]. In a large meta-analysis of studies that used PCR to identify mycobacterial nucleic acid sequences in different tissues from sarcoid-affected patients, a positive signal was seen in just over a quarter of nearly 900 samples evaluated. Antibodies against *Mtb* catalase-peroxidase (mKatG) have also been found in a higher proportion of patients with sarcoidosis than the general population and mKatG itself has been identified in biopsied tissue from such individuals [4]. Moreover, about half of patients in some studies are 'mKatG responders' whose PBMCs induce classical Th1-type immune reactions in response to mKatG peptides. Although the 'Kveim antigen' has never been identified, mKatG peptides share some of the physico-chemical properties of Kveim homogenates [5].

Actual evidence that a viable infectious agent is necessary for inducing sarcoidosis is scant. The Kveim reagent does not contain live organisms yet consistently produces a granulomatous sarcoidal reaction. Thus, while mycobacterial peptides could represent persistent antigenic stimuli in sarcoidosis, there is as yet no evidence that live mycobacteria can or are a prerequisite for causing the disease.

The ACCESS (A Case Control Etiologic Study of Sarcoidosis) study failed to identify an infectious agent after a detailed analysis of blood by molecular techniques [6]. Further studies of affected tissues or organs are necessary if the infectious agent theory of the pathogenesis of sarcoidosis is to be tested further. Apart from mycobacteria, propionibacteria have also been closely scrutinized but, despite a growing number of studies, its DNA has only been found in the lymph nodes of Japanese and certain European patients.

❝ **Expert comment** Development of sarcoidosis post-TB

The development of sarcoidosis as a post-TB phenomenon is a widely held but challenging clinical concept. Its pathophysiological basis is certainly plausible as substantial similarities exist between sarcoidosis and mycobacterial infections with regard to immunopathological responses, epidemiology, and clinical presentation. A recent meta-analysis of 31 studies showed a 25.6% prevalence of mycobacterial DNA in patients with sarcoidosis; the OR of finding mycobacterial genes in samples from such patients was 10-fold that in control individuals [7]. Others have found a higher frequency of mycobacterial 16s rRNA in sarcoidosis patients. However, the potential for sample contamination limits the utility of nucleic acid amplification of stored tissue. It is also not a substitute

(continued)

for mycobacterial culture. Apart from the technical limitations of such studies, it remains possible that TB may be irrelevant to the pathogenesis of sarcoidosis. Studies probing for low-copy number mycobacterial nucleic acids have failed to convincingly demonstrate their presence in nodal tissue from sarcoidosis patients. Such studies, however, do not discount the possibility that sarcoidosis can develop after a variable period following active TB disease.

Case reports of concomitant sarcoidosis and TB also exist—that patients have developed sarcoidosis while being treated for TB might suggest that *Mtb* is unlikely to be the aetiological agent for sarcoidosis in these individuals [8]. However, it has been suggested that the situation of sarcoidosis may be similar to leprosy, a condition denoted by tuberculoid and lepromatous forms. In this analogy, sarcoidosis would represent the tuberculoid (pauci-bacillary) corollary of the pathological responses that arise following exposure to certain mycobacteria. It is also possible that the occurrence of certain HLAs associated with higher risk of developing TB in patients with sarcoidosis contributes to the subsequent development of TB in patients who first present with sarcoidosis.

Recommencement of systemic (oral) corticosteroids produced prompt clinical improvement. Early radiological improvement was also evident after 3 months; by 6 months, adjunct treatment with hydroxychloroquine and azathioprine was introduced to allow gradual tapering of the corticosteroid dose.

➕ **Clinical tip** Role and limitations of systemic corticosteroids in sarcoidosis

In pulmonary sarcoidosis, corticosteroids should be considered when lung function or radiological changes are clearly deteriorating over a 3–6-month interval. Although the decision to commence treatment for symptom control is often subjective, in general persistent cough, breathlessness, and chest pain are among the commoner reasons for starting systemic steroids [2]. A trial of inhaled steroids may be indicated for sarcoid-related cough in the absence of other symptoms. The role of inhaled therapy as maintenance treatment following an initial course of oral steroids is not established. Inhaled steroids have not been shown to improve lung function or radiographic abnormalities. Specific clinical situations in which systemic steroids should be commenced include airway obstruction, disease affecting the nervous system (including Bell's palsy), cardiac sarcoidosis, hypercalcaemia, renal disease, and severe protracted fatigue.

➕ **Clinical tip** Management of long-term steroids and how to wean

For most patients, an initial prednisolone dose of 30–40 mg/day is adequate but may need to be maintained for 2–4 weeks before it is gradually reduced. In most cases, it should be possible to reach a maintenance steroid dose of approximately 10 mg by the end of the third month of treatment. For others, it may be necessary to prescribe a 'holding' daily dose of 15–20 mg for a month or so before further dose reduction is undertaken. Decrements below 10 mg are typically achieved by reducing the daily dose by 1–2 mg every few weeks; even using this gentle protocol, some patients will report recrudescence of symptoms including arthralgia, fatigue, and non-specific pains when the daily prednisolone dose drops below a certain level. The use of non-steroidal agents or a steroid-sparing drug may facilitate the weaning process.

Discussion

Clinical presentation of sarcoidosis

One of the major challenges in diagnosing sarcoidosis relates to its variable presentation and clinical course. Although 90% of patients with the disease have thoracic involvement affecting the lungs and/or lymph nodes, such manifestations can themselves be heterogeneous.

The initial presentation of pulmonary sarcoidosis is often related to the patient's sex, race, and age. BHL is frequently diagnosed on plain chest radiography, either as an asymptomatic finding or in association with mild cough and exertional dyspnoea. Constitutional symptoms such as fatigue, fever, and weight loss are more common in African-Caribbean and Asian-Indian patients. Other symptoms include non-specific chest pain, dysphagia, and arthralgia (often of the ankles). Erythema nodosum is less common in African-Caribbean, Japanese, and Indian patients than in white individuals of northern European descent. An average of 6–9 months may separate symptom onset from a firm diagnosis of pulmonary sarcoidosis.

✔ **Evidence base** Genetic associations in sarcoidosis

Numerous reports have shown that familial clustering of cases occurs in sarcoidosis. The presence of the disease in a first-degree relative increases the risk several-fold. Among siblings, monozygotic twins have a much higher risk of developing the disease than dizygotic twins.

Research on gene variants that confer particular risk for sarcoidosis has strongly focused on human leucocyte antigen (HLA) genes. While a large number of polymorphisms are reported to be important in sarcoidosis, it is likely that there is broad heterogeneity in HLA-mediated susceptibility to both the disease and its progression. Carriage of HLA-DRB1*1101 is a strong risk factor for sarcoidosis in both white and black individuals. In Swedish subjects, carriage of HLA-DQB1*0201 and HLA-DRB1*0301 has been associated with a strong likelihood of developing acute sarcoidosis (Lofgren's syndrome) whereas carriage of HLA-DQB1*0602 has been linked to chronic and severe disease.

Polymorphisms of non-HLA genes implicated in sarcoidosis include genes encoding TNF-α, the T-cell receptor (TCR), co-stimulatory molecules involved in TCR activation and other chemokines. Of these, the TNF-308A allele has been associated with a greater predisposition to Lofgren's syndrome across several ethnic groups. Many such gene variants do not influence disease susceptibility as such but play a role in modulating the clinical phenotype of sarcoidosis.

Ethnic differences in disease rates, susceptibility, and possibly even treatment response may be influenced by genetics. Studies on a mutation in a putative immune-regulatory co-factor gene, butyrophilin-like 2 (BTNL2), have shown that such abnormalities obey strict ethnicity boundaries. An association of the role of BTNL2 in sarcoidosis has been described in white Americans but not those of black ethnicity.

Genome-wide screening may provide the means to identify a regulatory 'switch' or critical molecule responsible for the development of sarcoidosis but this disease is not likely to be a single-gene disorder. In other words, both the functional implication as well as the 'percentage attributable risk' of each genetic lesion must be established and validated before it can be considered aetiologically relevant to sarcoidosis.

Acute sarcoid presentations termed Löfgren's syndrome (erythema nodosum, BHL, and arthralgia) and Heerfordt's syndrome (uveitis, parotitis, fever and, in a minority of cases, facial nerve palsy) tend to occur in younger patients. Over 75% of those developing Löfgren's syndrome may spontaneously improve or remit within 2 years of presentation; of these, a small number will subsequently relapse. While the true rate of spontaneous disease remission is unknown, relapse does not necessarily signify a worse prognosis. Chronic pulmonary sarcoidosis progressing to lung fibrosis occurs in 10–20% of cases. Pulmonary hypertension may complicate fibrotic lung disease or develop separately as a result of infiltrative granulomatous vasculopathy affecting the pulmonary circulation.

Physical examination may reveal palpable lymphadenopathy in up to a third of patients at presentation, typically in the cervical, axillary, epitrochlear, and inguinal regions. Painful joint swelling, cutaneous manifestations, and splenomegaly may be evident although the last is rarely clinically significant. Digital clubbing is rare and auscultatory crackles are uncommon except in established lung fibrosis.

Investigations for pulmonary sarcoidosis

A firm diagnosis of pulmonary sarcoidosis is made when the usual histological characteristics are combined with compatible clinical and radiological features [1,2]. A confident diagnosis may also be reached clinico-radiologically without information from biopsy; for example, Löfgren's syndrome or pulmonary sarcoidosis with prior biopsy findings from an extrapulmonary site. However, negative microbiological cultures and histological confirmation is crucial when TB, other granulomatous diseases, (including mycobacterial, fungal, and parasitic infections) or lymphoma form part of the differential diagnoses.

Serum angiotensin converting enzyme (sACE) level has relatively low sensitivity and specificity for sarcoidosis, being elevated in only 40–60% of patients. Raised sACE may also be encountered in other granulomatous disorders such as TB and berylliosis. Moreover, phenotypic variations in sACE levels in both normal and sarcoid-affected individuals are affected by insertion (I) and deletion (D) polymorphisms of the ACE gene. However, normalization of a previously high sACE level may be a useful indicator of treatment response, particularly when accompanied by symptomatic improvement. Corrected serum calcium and urinary calcium should also be measured since untreated hypercalcaemia can cause renal failure. Increased serum calcium maybe seasonal in patients as increased vitamin D during the sunny months is hydroxylated to its active form by the sarcoidal granulomas.

The Mantoux (TST) test can be diagnostically helpful, not only in helping identify active TB disease but also because an anergic response is compatible with active sarcoidosis. Although no longer used, the Kveim test involving the injection of homogenized splenic tissue from a patient with sarcoidosis into a recipient suspected of having the disease remains the most specific test for sarcoidosis, with a false-positive rate of 0.5–1.5%. A positive test occurs more frequently in Löfgren's syndrome (70–90%) than in those with a stage III CXR (30–40%).

> ⊕ **Clinical tip** Interpretation of Mantoux test in sarcoidosis and TB
>
> Suppressed delayed-type hypersensitivity to tuberculin has long been recognized in those with active sarcoidosis. The mechanism underlying tuberculin anergy/hyposensitivity in this condition is poorly understood. Although some patients have been reported to 'restore' their sensitivity to tuberculin following successful steroid treatment for sarcoidosis, such observations remain inconclusive and, consequently, opinions differ as to how likely and for how long tuberculin anergy may persist in sarcoidosis and whether immunological recovery associated with restoration of tuberculin sensitivity might correlate with the activity of their sarcoid disease. Curiously, failure to mount a tuberculin response in sarcoidosis may persist even after repeated administration of the BCG vaccine.

Plain chest radiography is often the first diagnostic imaging performed in sarcoidosis but is inferior to CT in terms of diagnostic sensitivity and specificity. A contiguous ('volumetric') CT study is recommended to adequately demonstrate the entire lung and associated lymph node stations. HRCT is non-contiguous and is sufficient as a follow-up modality for those with predominantly parenchymal disease. Bilateral hilar or combined hilar-mediastinal lymphadenopathy, perilymphatic lung nodules, and symmetrical inflammatory or fibrotic opacities that emanate from both hila in a bronchocentric pattern are the most frequent findings in pulmonary sarcoidosis. Perilymphatic nodularity is easiest to discern along bronchovascular structures, where it is found adjacent to lobar fissures; the latter may appear 'beaded'. Larger mass-like densities, small cystic spaces, miliary nodules, and pleural thickening or effusion are unusual manifestations of the condition [9].

✪ Learning point plain CXR staging

Although the radiological manifestations of pulmonary sarcoidosis are heterogeneous, bilateral hilar lymphadenopathy (BHL) is the commonest radiographic finding, occurring in 50–75% of patients. BHL in sarcoidosis is usually symmetrical; fewer than 5% of cases present with unilateral hilar lymphadenopathy. The use of plain imaging remains a crucial part of the clinical workup of this condition, particularly with its advantages of low cost, low radiation, speed, and wide availability.

In the 1950s, a three-stage classification system was proposed to describe the most frequent hilar and parenchymal appearances of sarcoidosis. An extended (five-stage) system subsequently proposed by Scadding in 1961 remains in use today (stage 0, normal; stage I, BHL; stage II, BHL with parenchymal infiltrates or nodules; stage III, parenchymal changes alone; and stage IV, lung fibrosis) [10]. Both this and a subsequent staging system proposed by Siltzbach sought to highlight associations between radiographic abnormalities and clinical outcome. Not surprisingly, Scadding observed after monitoring patients for more than 5 years that patients with stage III or IV disease were more likely to be symptomatic and to do less well. Since that time, others have confirmed the view that radiographic stage III/IV pulmonary sarcoidosis is associated with a much worse long-term prognosis and excess mortality. In one meta-analysis, a mortality rate of 4.8% in referral centres versus 0.5% in community/population-based centres was attributed to a higher percentage of patients with stage III/IV disease.

Gallium-67 (^{67}Ga) radionuclide scans are now rarely used to diagnose sarcoidosis but may reveal particular scintigraphic patterns that are highly suggestive of the disease (e.g. 'panda' sign due to uptake in the lacrimal and parotid glands) [2]. ^{18}F-FDG PET has been shown to be useful in identifying occult sites of granulomatous disease and to reveal specific patterns of myocardial sarcoidosis. In most centres, however, cardiac MRI has superseded both echocardiography and gallium-67 scanning as the modality of choice for investigating cardiac sarcoidosis.

Endobronchial granulomatous inflammation may be apparent at fibreoptic bronchoscopy in up to a third of patients with pulmonary sarcoidosis. Chronic airway abnormalities may lead to airway hyper-reactivity, distortion, narrowing, or bronchiectasis. Bronchoscopic biopsy of the airway lining, even when the mucosa appears normal, may yield a positive result in 30–40% of cases. Transbronchial biopsy to obtain parenchymal granuloma has a positive yield of 40–90% in reported case series. Broncho-alveolar lavage (BAL) fluid demonstrating lymphocytosis supports (but does not prove) a diagnosis of sarcoidosis, particularly when a CD4:CD8 T-lymphocyte ratio of > 3.5 is present. The use of FNA of lymph nodes has gained popularity, particularly when combined with endobronchial ultrasound (EBUS-FNA) to enhance the accuracy of nodal sampling. Surgical biopsy is afforded by mediastinoscopy or anterior mediastinotomy to sample intrathoracic lymph nodes and VATS to obtain parenchymal lung tissue.

Treatment of pulmonary sarcoidosis

Not all patients with pulmonary sarcoidosis require treatment; for those who do, optimal treatment has not been defined [2,11]. The likelihood that the disease may spontaneously improve or remit must be considered before embarking on treatment. Immunomodulatory drugs including corticosteroids are not a cure for the disease—they provide symptomatic relief and may promote inflammatory resolution, occasionally in dramatic fashion. The most compelling reasons to commence treatment include severe or functionally significant symptoms, severely impaired or progressively worsening lung function, and progressive radiological abnormalities. Findings from a small number of randomized placebo-controlled trials of oral steroids suggest that symptoms and radiological changes are most likely to improve in those with radiographic stage II/III disease, but benefits for lung function are inconsistent.

Inhaled, oral, and parenteral corticosteroids are used for treating pulmonary sarcoidosis. The optimal dose and duration of systemic steroids have not been studied in randomized prospective trials. A starting dose of 20–40 mg prednisolone per day suffices for most patients; higher doses are required for concomitant cardiac, ocular, or cerebral disease. A short initial course of intravenous methylprednisolone is useful for gaining more rapid control of the disease and as a quicker means to evaluate 'steroid response'.

Once started, steroids may be difficult to wean off; it has been said that a strong determinant for steroid dependence is steroid commencement itself. Patients who respond initially to therapy may subsequently relapse even if they were successfully weaned off treatment previously. There is no evidence that treatment can prevent the progression of inflammatory to fibrotic sarcoidosis or reduce overall mortality.

Likewise, the decision to treat extra-pulmonary sarcoidosis is also considered from the perspective of 'threatened organ' function balanced against clinical expectations as well as possible deterioration in quality of life with treatment. Typical indications for treatment include disease affecting the nervous system (including ocular), cardiac disease, nephritis, recalcitrant hypercalcaemia, lupus pernio and other cutaneous complications, as well as severe constitutional symptoms including chronic unremitting fatigue.

A number of other agents have been employed in sarcoidosis both for their anti-inflammatory properties and because they are crucial for a successful 'steroid wean'. Such a role for methotrexate is based on findings from small studies including a single RCT; no such trials exist for azathioprine, mycophenolate mofetil (MMF), or cyclophosphamide. Results with chloroquine-based agents in treating sarcoid lung disease have been inconsistent; however, hydroxychloroquine is a useful adjunct for the management of constitutional symptoms such as tiredness and arthralgia. Methylphenidate has been used to successfully treat some patients with excessive fatigue. For a small number of patients, steroids are ultimately weaned off, allowing a non-steroid agent to remain as sole therapy for their pulmonary sarcoidosis. The risk of disease relapse in such cases is thought to be at least moderately high.

Trials of anti-TNF-α agents in sarcoidosis are currently in progress [12]. So far, infliximab appears to be more beneficial than etanercept but the cost of such drugs in general may prove too prohibitive for widespread use. Systemic TNF blockade is associated with a risk of reactivating latent TB, a consideration of vital clinical importance as TB may represent a potential pathogenetic factor in the development of this disease in some individuals.

Lung transplantation is performed for a small number of patients each year. The presence of right heart dysfunction and pulmonary hypertension may necessitate combined heart–lung transplantation. Sarcoidosis has been shown to redevelop in transplanted lungs.

A final word from the expert

Sarcoidosis can be an enigmatic disorder whose diagnosis can be difficult to ascertain. Delays in diagnosis are not uncommon as it may be mistaken for a number of other conditions due to its varied presentation. Pulmonary lymph node sarcoidosis in particular can be confused for intrathoracic nodal TB, lymphoma, histoplasmosis, or even silicosis. Rather than representing a single disease entity, sarcoidosis is believed to arise as a granulomatous manifestation in organs or lymph nodes exposed to poorly understood stimuli. The factors that determine whether such sarcoidal reactions ultimately resolve without tissue scarring or progress to fibro-inflammatory organ damage remain poorly understood.

As the present case illustrates, sarcoidosis can develop after prior active TB. This phenomenon renders diagnostic attempts to distinguish between the two pathologies even more challenging. During the diagnostic process, thorough consideration of a number of factors must be undertaken, including:

- a detailed history of symptom evolution, physical examination, and baseline investigations such as the tuberculin skin (Mantoux) test, sputum studies, blood tests including serum ACE level and inflammatory markers;

- recourse to tissue sampling/biopsy for histological and microbiological analysis when clinical and radiological considerations have been taken to their limits;

- the role of a careful trial of empiric treatment in cases where it is not possible to clearly differentiate between sarcoidosis and TB despite the above. In such instances, standard TB treatment is usually instituted before systemic corticosteroids are trialled.

It is crucial to fully explain to patients that, should it not be possible to confidently exclude active TB disease as the cause of their symptoms, a trial of empiric TB therapy is advisable to minimize the risk of activating subclinical TB by the use of potent systemic immune-modulatory agents more conventionally employed to treat sarcoidosis.

References

1 Baughman RP, Culver DA, Judson MA. A concise review of pulmonary sarcoidosis. *Am J Respir Crit Care Med* 2011; 183: 573–581.

2 Spagnolo P, Cullinan P, du Bois RM. Sarcoidosis. In: *Interstitial Lung Disease*, 5th edition, eds. Schwarz MI and King Jr TE. People's Medical Publishing House, 2011: pp. 433–497.

3 James JG, Neville E, Siltzbach LE. A worldwide review of sarcoidosis. *Ann N Y Acad Sci* 1976; 278: 321–334.

4 Moller DR. Potential etiologic agents in sarcoidosis: state of the art. *Proc Am Thor Soc* 2007; 4: 465–468.

5 Song Z, Marzili L, Greenlee BM et al. Mycobacterial catalase-peroxidase is a tissue antigen and target of the adaptive immune response in systemic sarcoidosis. *J Exp Med* 2005; 201: 755–767.

6 Newman LS, Rose CS, Terrin ML et al. A case control etiologic study of sarcoidosis: environmental and occupational risk factors. *Am J Respir Crit Care Med* 2004; 170: 1324–1330.

7 Gupta D, Agarwal R, Aggarwal AN et al. Molecular evidence for the role of mycobacteria in sarcoidosis: a meta-analysis. *Eur Resp J* 2007; 30: 508–516.

8 Sharma OP. Murray Kornfield, American College of Chest Physicians and Sarcoidosis: a historical footnote. 2004 Kornfield Memorial Founders Lecture. *Chest* 2005; 128: 1830–1835.

9 Criado E, Sanchez M, Ramirez J et al. Pulmonary sarcoidosis: typical and atypical manifestations at high-resolution CT with pathologic correlation. *Radiographics* 2010; 30: 1567–1586.

10 Scadding JG. Prognosis of intrathoracic sarcoidosis in England: a review of 136 cases after five years observation. *BMJ* 1961; 2: 1165–1172.

11 Wells AU, Hirani N, British Thoracic Society ILD Guideline Group. Interstitial lung disease guideline: the British Thoracic Society in collaboration with the Thoracic Society of Australia and New Zealand and the Irish Thoracic Society. *Thorax* 2008; 63: v1–v58.

12 Hostettler KE, Studler U, Tamm M et al. Long-term treatment with infliximab in patients with sarcoidosis. *Respiration* 2012; 83: 218–224.

INDEX